Y0-BWR-624

Antimicrobial Pharmacodynamics in Theory and Clinical Practice

INFECTIOUS DISEASE AND THERAPY

Series Editor

Burke A. Cunha

Winthrop-University Hospital
Mineola, and
State University of New York School of Medicine
Stony Brook, New York

1. Parasitic Infections in the Compromised Host, *edited by Peter D. Walzer and Robert M. Genta*
2. Nucleic Acid and Monoclonal Antibody Probes: Applications in Diagnostic Methodology, *edited by Bala Swaminathan and Gyan Prakash*
3. Opportunistic Infections in Patients with the Acquired Immunodeficiency Syndrome, *edited by Gifford Leoung and John Mills*
4. Acyclovir Therapy for Herpesvirus Infections, *edited by David A. Baker*
5. The New Generation of Quinolones, *edited by Clifford Siporin, Carl L. Heifetz, and John M. Domagala*
6. Methicillin-Resistant *Staphylococcus aureus*: Clinical Management and Laboratory Aspects, *edited by Mary T. Cafferkey*
7. Hepatitis B Vaccines in Clinical Practice, *edited by Ronald W. Ellis*
8. The New Macrolides, Azalides, and Streptogramins: Pharmacology and Clinical Applications, *edited by Harold C. Neu, Lowell S. Young, and Stephen H. Zinner*
9. Antimicrobial Therapy in the Elderly Patient, *edited by Thomas T. Yoshikawa and Dean C. Norman*
10. Viral Infections of the Gastrointestinal Tract: Second Edition, Revised and Expanded, *edited by Albert Z. Kapikian*
11. Development and Clinical Uses of Haemophilus b Conjugate Vaccines, *edited by Ronald W. Ellis and Dan M. Granoff*
12. *Pseudomonas aeruginosa* Infections and Treatment, *edited by Aldona L. Baltch and Raymond P. Smith*
13. Herpesvirus Infections, *edited by Ronald Glaser and James F. Jones*
14. Chronic Fatigue Syndrome, *edited by Stephen E. Straus*
15. Immunotherapy of Infections, *edited by K. Noel Masihi*
16. Diagnosis and Management of Bone Infections, *edited by Luis E. Jauregui*

17. Drug Transport in Antimicrobial and Anticancer Chemotherapy, *edited by Nafsika H. Georgopapadakou*
18. New Macrolides, Azalides, and Streptogramins in Clinical Practice, *edited by Harold C. Neu, Lowell S. Young, Stephen H. Zinner, and Jacques F. Acar*
19. Novel Therapeutic Strategies in the Treatment of Sepsis, *edited by David C. Morrison and John L. Ryan*
20. Catheter-Related Infections, *edited by Harald Seifert, Bernd Jansen, and Barry M. Farr*
21. Expanding Indications for the New Macrolides, Azalides, and Streptogramins, *edited by Stephen H. Zinner, Lowell S. Young, Jacques F. Acar, and Harold C. Neu*
22. Infectious Diseases in Critical Care Medicine, *edited by Burke A. Cunha*
23. New Considerations for Macrolides, Azalides, Streptogramins, and Ketolides, *edited by Stephen H. Zinner, Lowell S. Young, Jacques F. Acar, and Carmen Ortiz-Neu*
24. Tickborne Infectious Diseases: Diagnosis and Management, *edited by Burke A. Cunha*
25. Protease Inhibitors in AIDS Therapy, *edited by Richard C. Ogden and Charles W. Flexner*
26. Laboratory Diagnosis of Bacterial Infections, *edited by Nevio Cimolai*
27. Chemokine Receptors and AIDS, *edited by Thomas R. O'Brien*
28. Antimicrobial Pharmacodynamics in Theory and Clinical Practice, *edited by Charles H. Nightingale, Takeo Murakawa, and Paul G. Ambrose*

Additional Volumes in Production

Antimicrobial Pharmacodynamics in Theory and Clinical Practice

edited by

Charles H. Nightingale
Hartford Hospital
Hartford, Connecticut

Takeo Murakawa
Fujisawa Pharmaceutical Company, Ltd.
Osaka, Japan

Paul G. Ambrose
Cognigen Corporation
Buffalo, New York

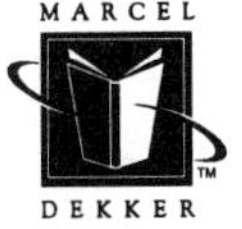

MARCEL DEKKER, INC. NEW YORK • BASEL

ISBN: 0-8247-0561-0

This book is printed on acid-free paper.

Headquarters
Marcel Dekker, Inc.
270 Madison Avenue, New York, NY 10016
tel: 212-696-9000; fax: 212-685-4540

Eastern Hemisphere Distribution
Marcel Dekker AG
Hutgasse 4, Postfach 812, CH-4001 Basel, Switzerland
tel: 41-61-261-8482; fax: 41-61-261-8896

World Wide Web
http://www.dekker.com

The publisher offers discounts on this book when ordered in bulk quantities. For more information, write to Special Sales/Professional Marketing at the headquarters address above.

Current printing (last digit):
10 9 8 7 6 5 4 3 2 1

PRINTED IN THE UNITED STATES OF AMERICA

Preface

To use antibiotics appropriately, the clinician needs to understand fundamental pharmacodynamic concepts. These concepts are essential, for they form the very basis for therapeutic strategies that maximize clinical benefit while minimizing toxicity to the patient. The objectives of this book are, first, to review the constellation of scientific and medical literature concerning antibiotics and pharmacodynamics. The relevance of this complex information is then synthesized into an easy-to-understand discussion of concept and theory. Finally, the reader is shown how to apply these theories and concepts, with specific examples, to the clinical practice of medicine and pharmacy. In other words, this book takes the reader from the test tube, through the animal and human volunteer laboratory, to the patient's bedside.

The book includes a thorough discussion of the pharmacodynamics of all major classes of the antimicrobial armamentarium. These include penicillins, cephalosporins, cephamycins, carbapenems, monobactams, aminoglycosides, quinolones, macrolides, antifungals, antivirals and others. Additionally, a pharmacodynamic discussion of new classes of antimicrobial agents that are upon the horizon, such as the ketolide antibiotics, is included.

This book is unique in that no other text of its kind currently exists. The information that this book provides integrates medical microbiology, clinical infectious diseases, and pharmacokinetics. This book pulls together in one text the essential elements of these disciplines and does so in a very understandable and practical manner.

The infectious disease physicians and pharmacists we selected as contributors are eminently qualified and are recognized experts in their field. Moreover, these authors were chosen on the basis of their ability to convey their perspective and expertise lucidly, which makes them ideal teachers. They all agreed that there was a need for such a book and were excited about joining in this venture.

This book will find an audience in a large array of healthcare disciplines, including college educators, medical, pharmacy, and microbiology students, infectious disease physicians and pharmacy specialists, medical house staff, clinical and staff pharmacists, clinical microbiologists, and other healthcare decision makers.

Charles H. Nightingale
Takeo Murakawa
Paul G. Ambrose

Contents

Contributors

George P. Allen, Pharm.D. Postdoctoral Fellow, Pharmacy Practice, Wayne State University, and Detroit Receiving Hospital and University Health Center Detroit, Michigan

Paul G. Ambrose, Pharm.D. Director, Infectious Disease Research, Cognigen Corporation, Buffalo, New York

Khanh Q. Bui, Pharm.D. Bristol-Myers Squibb Company, Chicago, Illinois

William A. Craig, M.D. Professor of Medicine and Therapeutics, Department of Infectious Diseases, University of Wisconsin, and William S. Middleton Memorial Veterans Hospital, Madison, Wisconsin

Burke A. Cunha, M.D. Chief, Infectious Disease Division, Winthrop-University Hospital, Mineola, and Professor of Medicine, State University of New York School of Medicine, Stony Brook, New York

George L. Drusano, M.D. Professor, Department of Medicine and Pharmacology, Clinical Research Institute, Albany Medical College, Albany, New York

Michael N. Dudley, Pharm.D. Vice President, Department of Pharmacology and Microbiology, Microcide Pharmaceuticals, Inc., Mountain View, California

Collin Freeman, Pharm.D. Clinical Science Specialist, Department of Scientific Affairs, Bayer Corporation, West Haven, Connecticut

David Griffith, B.S. Research Scientist, Department of Pharmacology, Microcide Pharmaceuticals, Inc., Mountain View, California

Ellie Hershberger, Pharm.D. Director, Infectious Disease Laboratory, Research Institute, William Beaumont Research Institute, Royal Oak, Michigan

Khalid H. Ibrahim, Pharm.D. Infectious Diseases Research Fellow, Department of Experimental and Clinical Pharmacology, University of Minnesota, Minneapolis, Minnesota

David T. Jones, Pharm.D., M.D. Department of Cardiology and Internal Medicine, University of California at Davis, Sacramento, California

Myo-Kyoung Kim, Pharm.D. Infectious Disease Fellow, Department of Pharmacy Research, Hartford Hospital, Hartford, Connecticut

Michael E. Klepser, Pharm.D. Associate Professor, College of Pharmacy, University of Iowa, Iowa City, Iowa

Melinda K. Lacy, Pharm.D. Assistant Professor, Department of Pharmacy Practice, School of Pharmacy, University of Kansas Medical Center, Kansas City, Kansas

Kenneth Lamp, Pharm.D. Medical Science Manager, Department of United States Medicines, Bristol-Myers Squibb, Plainsboro, New Jersey

Russell E. Lewis, Pharm.D. Assistant Professor, Department of Clinical Sciences and Administration, University of Houston College of Pharmacy, Houston, Texas

Philip D. Lister, Ph.D. Associate Professor, Department of Medical Microbiology and Immunology, Creighton University School of Medicine, Omaha, Nebraska

Holly M. Mattoes, Pharm.D. Scientific Communications Manager, DesignWrite Incorporated, Princeton, New Jersey

JoCarol J. McNabb, Pharm.D. Assistant Professor, College of Pharmacy, University of Nebraska Medical Center, Omaha, Nebraska

Eugene Moore, Pharm.D. Coordinator, Army Ambulatory Care Pharmacist Program, Department of Defense Pharmacoeconomic Center, Fort Sam Houston, Texas

Takeo Murakawa, Ph.D. Supervisor, International Development and Regulatory Affairs, Development Division, Fujisawa Pharmaceutical Company, Ltd., Osaka, and Lecturer (Part), Graduate School of Pharmaceutical Sciences, Kyoto University, Kyoto, and Graduate School of Pharmaceutical Sciences, Tokushima University, Tokushima, Japan

David P. Nicolau, Pharm.D. Division of Infectious Disease Pharmacy Research, Hartford Hospital, Hartford, Connecticut

Charles H. Nightingale, Ph.D. Vice-President for Research and Director of the Institute for International Healthcare Studies, Hartford Hospital, Hartford, Connecticut

Robert C. Owens, Jr., Pharm.D. Clinical Specialist, Infectious Diseases, Maine Medical Center, Portland, Maine, and University of Vermont College of Medicine, Burlington, Vermont

Peter J. Piliero, M.D. Assistant Professor, Department of Medicine, Albany Medical College, Albany, New York

Sandra L. Preston, Pharm.D. Assistant Professor of Medicine, Clinical Research Initiative, Albany Medical College, Albany, New York

Mark A. Richerson, Pharm.D., M.S. Commander, Medical Service Corps, United States Navy, and Department of Defense Pharmacoeconomic Center, Fort Sam Houston, Texas

Gigi H. Ross, Pharm.D. Infectious Diseases Scientific Liaison, Clinical Affairs, Ortho-McNeil Pharmaceutical, Raritan, New Jersey

John C. Rotschafer, Pharm.D., F.C.C.P. Professor, Department of Experimental and Clinical Pharmacology, College of Pharmacy, University of Minnesota, Minneapolis, Minnesota

René Russo, Pharm.D. Postdoctoral Fellow, College of Pharmacy, Rutgers University, Piscataway, New Jersey

Michael J. Rybak, Pharm.D., F.C.C.P., B.C.P.S. Professor of Pharmacy and Medicine and Director, Anti-Infective Research Laboratory, Department of Pharmacy Practice, Wayne State University, and Detroit Receiving Hospital and University Health Center, Detroit, Michigan

David H. Wright, Pharm.D. Manager, Professional Education and Scientific Affairs, Ortho-McNeil Pharmaceutical, Raritan, New Jersey

Annette Zoe-Powers, Pharm.D. Director, Department of Infectious Diseases, Bristol-Myers Squibb Company, Plainsboro, New Jersey

1

Pharmacodynamics of Antimicrobials: General Concepts and Applications

William A. Craig
University of Wisconsin and William S. Middleton Memorial Veterans Hospital, Madison, Wisconsin

1 INTRODUCTION

''Pharmacodynamics'' is the term used to reflect the relationship between measurements of drug exposure in serum, tissues, and body fluids and the pharmacological and toxicological effects of drugs. With antimicrobials pharmacodynamics is focused on the relationship between concentrations and the antimicrobial effect. Studies in the past have focused on pharmacokinetics and descriptions of the time course of antimicrobials in serum, tissues, and body fluids. Much less emphasis has been placed on the time course of antimicrobial activity. Studies over the past 20 years have demonstrated marked differences in the time course of antimicrobial activity among antibacterials and antifungals [15,20,84,88]. Furthermore, the pattern of antimicrobial activity over time is an important determinant of optimal dosage regimens [21]. This chapter focuses on general concepts and the application of pharmacodynamics to antimicrobial therapy.

2 MEASUREMENTS OF ANTIMICROBIAL ACTIVITY

2.1 Minimum Inhibitory and Minimum Bactericidal Concentrations

The minimum inhibitory and minimum bactericidal concentrations (MIC and MBC) have been the major parameters used to measure the in vitro activity of antimicrobials against various pathogens. Although the MIC and MBC are excellent predictors of the potency of an antimicrobial against the infecting organism, they provide essentially no information on the time course of antimicrobial activity. For example, the MBC provides minimal information on the rate of bactericidal and fungicidal activity and on whether killing can be increased by higher drug concentrations. In addition, the MIC provides no information on growth inhibitory effects that may persist after antimicrobial exposure. These persistent effects are due to three different phenomena: the postantibiotic effect (PAE), the postantibiotic sub-MIC effect (PAE-SME), and the postantibiotic leukocyte enhancement (PALE) [17,62,63]. The effects of increasing concentrations on the bactericidal and fungicidal activity of antimicrobials combined with the magnitude of persistent effects give a much better description of the time course of antimicrobial activity than that provided by the MIC and MBC.

2.2 Killing Activity

Antimicrobials exhibit two primary patterns of microbial killing. The first pattern is characterized by concentration-dependent killing over a wide range of concentrations. With this pattern, higher drug concentrations result in a greater rate and extent of microbial killing. This pattern is observed with the aminoglycosides, fluoroquinolones, ketolides, metronidazole, and amphotericin B [9,19,20,28]. The second pattern is characterized by minimal concentration-dependent killing. With this pattern, saturation of the killing rate occurs at low multiples of the MIC, usually around four to five times the MIC. Drug concentrations above these values do not kill microbes faster or more extensively. This pattern is also called time-dependent killing because the extent of microbial killing is primarily dependent on the duration of exposure. This pattern is observed with β-lactam antibiotics, macrolides, clindamycin, glycopeptides, tetracyclines, trimethoprim, linezolid, and flucytosine [4,8,15,20,29].

The different patterns of bacterial killing are illustrated in Fig. 1 by showing the effect of increasing drug concentrations on the in vitro antimicrobial activity of tobramycin, ciprofloxacin, and ticarcillin against a standard strain of *Pseudomonas aeruginosa* [20]. Increasing concentrations of tobramycin and ciprofloxacin produced more rapid and extensive bacterial killing, as exhibited by the steeper slopes of the killing curves. With ticarcillin, there was a change in slope as the concentration was increased from one to four times the MIC. However,

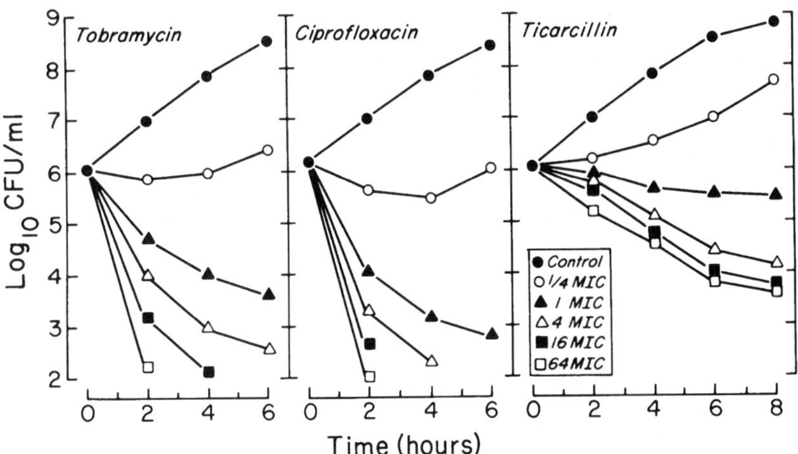

FIGURE 1 Time-kill curves of *Pseudomonas aeruginosa* ATCC 27853 with exposure to tobramycin, ciprofloxacin, and ticarcillin at concentrations from one-fourth to 64 times the MIC. (From Ref. 20.)

higher concentrations did not alter the slope. The slight reduction in bacterial numbers at the higher doses is due to an earlier onset of bacterial killing. From 2 h on, ticarcillin concentrations from 4 to 64 times the MIC produced the same rates of killing.

2.3 Persistent Effects

''Postantibiotic effect'' is the term used to describe the persistent suppression of bacterial growth following antimicrobial exposure [15,18,63]. If reflects the time it takes for an organism to recover from the effects of exposure to an antimicrobial and resume normal growth. This phenomenon was first observed in the 1940s in early studies with penicillin against staphylococci and streptococci [12,38]. Later studies starting in the 1970s extended this phenomenon to newer drugs and to gram-negative organisms. The postantibiotic effect is demonstrated in vitro by following bacterial growth kinetics after drug removal.

Moderate to prolonged in vitro postantibiotic effects are observed for all antibacterials with susceptible gram-positive bacteria such as staphylococci and streptococci [10]. Moderate to prolonged in vitro PAEs are also observed with gram-negative bacilli for drugs that are inhibitors of protein or nucleic acid synthesis. In contrast, short or no postantibiotic effects are observed for β-lactam antibiotics with gram-negative bacilli. The only exception has been for carbapenems, which exhibit moderate PAEs, primarily with strains of *Pseudomonas aeru-*

ginosa [16,47]. In vitro postantifungal effects (PAFEs) have been observed with various yeasts following exposure to amphotericin B and flucytosine but not to triazoles such as fluconazole [39,84].

The postantibiotic sub-MIC effect demonstrates the additional effect sub-MIC concentrations can have on the in vitro PAE. For example, exposure of streptococci in the PAE phase to macrolides at drug concentrations of one-tenth and three-tenths of the MIC increased the duration of the postantibiotic effect by about 50% and 100%, respectively [18,71]. The PAE phase can also make streptococci hypersensitive to the killing effects of penicillin [17]. The duration of the postantibiotic sub-MIC effects reported in the literature includes the duration of the PAE plus the enhanced duration due to sub-MIC concentrations. Morphological changes such as filaments can also be produced by sub-MIC concentrations [60].

Postantibiotic leukocyte enhancement describes the effects of leukocytes on bacteria during the postantibiotic phase. Studies have demonstrated that such bacteria are more susceptible to intracellular killing or phagocytosis by leukocytes [18,62]. This phenomenon can also prolong the duration of the in vitro postantibiotic effect. Antimicrobials that produce the longest postantibiotic effects tend to exhibit the most prolonged effects when exposed to leukocytes.

The postantibiotic effect has also been demonstrated in vivo in a variety of animal infection models [18,22]. The in vivo phenomenon is actually a combination of the in vitro PAE and sub-MIC effects from gradually falling drug concentrations. The largest number of studies have used the neutropenic mouse thigh infection model [88]. When performed in non-neutropenic mice, the in vivo PAE would also include any postantibiotic leukocyte enhancement effects.

There are several important differences between the in vivo and in vitro PAEs. In most cases, in vivo PAEs are longer than in vitro PAEs, most likely because of the additive effect of sub-MIC concentrations. Simulation of human pharmacokinetics can further enhance the duration of the in vivo PAE by a similar mechanism. Prolongation of sub-MIC concentrations of amikacin by simulating the human drug half-life (2 h) extended the duration of in vivo PAEs by 40–100% over values observed with a dose producing the same area under the concentration versus time curve (AUC) but eliminated with a murine half-life of 20 min [27]. In vivo PAEs with some drugs are further prolonged by the presence of leukocytes. In general, the presence of neutrophils tends to double the duration of the in vivo postantibiotic effect for aminoglycosides and fluoroquinolones with gram-negative bacilli [18,27]. However, leukocytes have no major effect on the minimal in vivo PAEs observed for β-lactams with gram-negative bacilli.

There are also some differences between the in vitro and in vivo PAEs that question the value of measuring the in vitro PAE. First, the duration of the in vitro PAE is not predictive of the duration of the in vivo PAE [40]. Second, prolonged PAEs for penicillin and cephalosporins with streptococci are observed in vitro but not in vivo [22,80,88]. Third, in vitro studies that suggest that the PAE of aminoglycosides decreases and disappears over a prolonged dosing interval or with repeated doses have not been confirmed in vivo [35,64]. Fourth, fluconazole exhibits a postantifungal effect in vivo but not in vitro [3,84].

3 PATTERNS OF ANTIMICROBIAL ACTIVITY

The pharmacodynamic characteristics described above suggest that the time course of antimicrobial activity can vary markedly for different antibacterial and antifungal agents. As shown in Table 1, these drugs exhibit three major patterns of antimicrobial activity. The first pattern in characterized by concentration-dependent killing and moderate to prolonged persistent effects. Higher concentrations would kill organisms more rapidly and more extensively than lower levels. The prolonged persistent effects would allow for infrequent administration of large doses. This pattern is observed with aminoglycosides, fluoroquinolones, daptomycin, ketolides, metronidazole, and amphotericin B. The goal of a dosing regimen for these drugs would be to maximize concentrations. The peak level and the AUC should be the pharmacokinetic parameters that would determine in vivo efficacy.

The second pattern is characterized by time-dependent killing and minimal to moderate persistent effects. High drug levels would not kill organisms better than lower concentrations. Furthermore, organism regrowth would start very soon after serum levels fell below the MIC. This pattern is observed with β-lactams, macrolides, clindamycin, oxazolidinones, and flucytosine. The goal of a dosing regimen for these drugs would be to optimize the duration of exposure. The duration of time that serum levels exceed some minimal value such as the MIC should be the major pharmacokinetic parameter determining the in vivo efficacy of these drugs.

The third pattern is also characterized by time-dependent killing, but the duration of the persistent effects is much prolonged. This can prevent any re-growth during the dosing interval. This pattern is observed with azithromycin, tetracyclines, quinupristin-dalfopristin, glycopeptides, and fluconazole. The goal of a dosing regimen is to optimize the amount of drug administered to ensure that killing occurs for part of the time and there is no regrowth during the dosing interval. The AUC should be the primary pharmacokinetic parameter that would determine in vivo efficacy.

4 PHARMACOKINETIC/PHARMACODYNAMIC PARAMETERS

By using the MIC as a measure of the potency of drug–organism interactions, the pharmacokinetic parameters determining efficacy can be converted to

Table 1 Three Patterns of Antimicrobial Activity

	Pattern 1	Pattern 2	Pattern 3
Pharmacodynamic characteristics	Concentration-dependent killing and moderate to prolonged persistent effects	Time-dependent killing and minimal to moderate persistent effects	Time-dependent killing and prolonged persistent effects
Antimicrobials included	Aminoglycosides, ketolides, fluoroquinolones, daptomycin, metronidazole, amphotericin B	β-Lactams, macrolides, clindamycin, oxazolidinones, flucytosine	Azithromycin, tetracyclines, glycopeptides, quinupristin-dalfopristin, fluconazole
Goal of dosing regimen	Maximize concentrations	Maximize duration of exposure	Optimize amount of drug
PK parameter(s) determining efficacy	Peak level and AUC	Time above some threshold amount (e.g., MIC)	AUC

pharmacokinetic/pharmacodynamic (PK/PD) parameters [21]. Serum (or plasma) concentrations are used for determining the pharmacokinetic indices. Because most infections occur in tissues and the common bacterial pathogens are extracellular organisms, interstitial fluid concentrations at the site of infection should be the primary determinants of efficacy. Serum levels are much better predictors of interstitial fluid levels than tissue homogenate concentrations. Because tissue homogenates mix the interstitial, intracellular, and vascular compartments together, they tend to underestimate or overestimate the interstitial fluid concentration depending on the ability of the drug to accumulate intracellularly [74].

Identification of the primary PK/PD parameter that determines efficacy is complicated by the high degree of interdependence among the various parameters. For example, a larger dose produces a higher peak/MIC ratio, a higher AUC/MIC ratio, and a longer duration of time above MIC. If the higher dose produces a better therapeutic effect than a lower dose, it is difficult to determine which PK/PD parameter is of major importance, because all three increased. However, comparing the effects of dosage regimens that include different dosing intervals can reduce much of the interdependence among PK/PD parameters. Such studies are often referred to as dose-fractionation studies [37,58]. For example, dividing several total doses into 1, 2, 4, 8, and 24 doses administered at 24, 12, 6, 3, and 1 h intervals, respectively, can allow one to identify which PK/PD parameter is most important for in vivo efficacy.

Several investigators have used this study design in animal infection models to correlate specific PK/PD parameters with efficacy for various antimicrobials against gram-positive cocci, gram-negative bacilli, and *Candida* species [3,4,9,28,29,57,61,87]. This is demonstrated graphically in Fig. 2 for ceftazidime against *Klebsiella pneumoniae* and in Fig. 3 for temafloxacin against *Streptococcus pneumoniae*. In these studies pairs of mice were treated with multiple dosage regimens that varied both the dose and the dosing interval. The number of colony-forming units (CFUs) remaining in the thigh after 24 h of therapy was plotted against the peak/MIC and 24 h AUC/MIC ratios and the percentage of time that serum levels exceeded the MIC that was calculated for each dosage regimen from pharmacokinetic indices. As shown in Fig. 2, there was a very poor relationship between CFUs/thigh and the peak/MIC and 24 h AUC/MIC ratios. On the other hand, an excellent correlation was observed between the number of bacteria in the thighs and the percentage of time that serum levels exceeded the MIC. However, the best correlation in Fig. 3 was observed with the 24 h AUC/MIC ratio followed by the peak/MIC ratio.

The specific PK/PD parameters correlating with efficacy in animal infection models for different antibacterials and antifungals are listed in Table 2. As expected, time above MIC has consistently been the only PK/PD parameter correlating with the therapeutic efficacy of β-lactam antibiotics. Time above MIC is

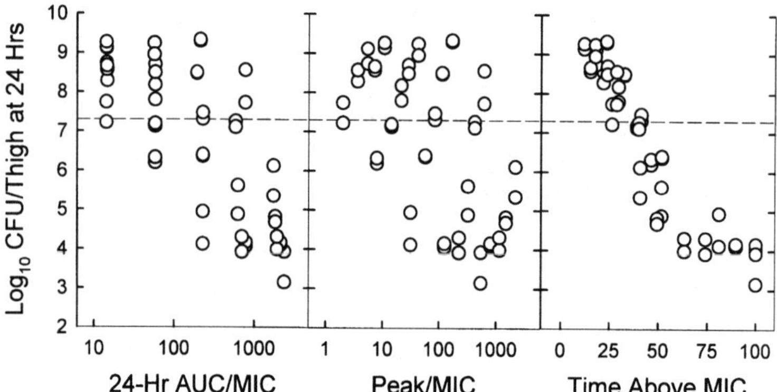

FIGURE 2 Relationship between three pharmacodynamic parameters (peak/MIC ratio, 24 h AUC/MIC ratio, and percentage of time that serum levels exceed the MIC) and the number of *K. pneumoniae* ATCC 53816 in the thighs of neutropenic mice after 24 h of therapy with ceftazidime. Each point represents data for one mouse. The dotted line reflects the number of bacteria at the beginning of therapy.

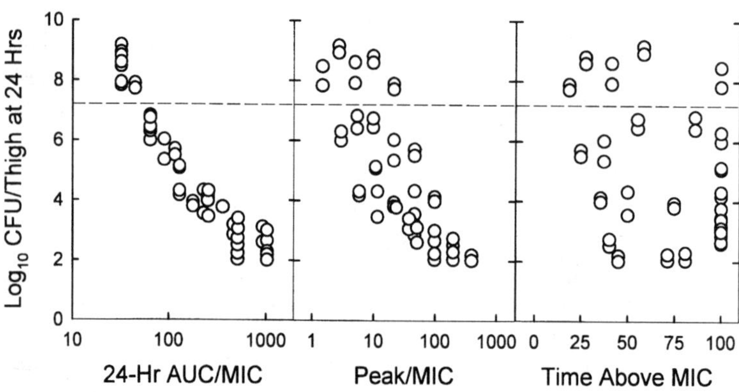

FIGURE 3 Relationship between three pharmacodynamic parameters (peak/MIC ratio, 24 h AUC/MIC ratio, and percentage of time that serum levels exceed the MIC) and the number of *S. pneumoniae* ATCC 10813 in the thighs of neutropenic mice after 24 h of therapy with temafloxacin. Each point represents data for one mouse. The dotted line reflects the number of bacteria at the beginning of therapy.

TABLE 2 PK/PD Parameters Determining Efficacy for Different Antimicrobials

PK/PD parameter	Antimicrobial
Time above MIC	Penicillins, cephalosporins, aztreonam, carbapenems, tribactams, macrolides, clindamycin, oxazolidinones, flucytosine
Peak/MIC ratio	Aminoglycosides, fluoroquinolones, daptomycin, vancomycin, teicoplanin, amphotericin B
AUC/MIC ratio	Aminoglycosides, fluoroquinolones, daptomycin, vancomycin, ketolides, quinupristin-dalfopristin, tetracyclines, fluconazole

also the parameter correlating with efficacy of the macrolides, clindamycin, oxazolidinones, and flucytosine.

The AUC/MIC and peak/MIC ratios have been the PK/PD parameters that correlate with efficacy for aminoglycosides and fluoroquinolones. Most studies have shown slightly better correlation with the AUC/MIC ratio than with the peak/MIC ratio. Peak/MIC ratios appear to be more important in infections where the emergence of resistant subpopulations is a significant risk and for drugs that act on the cell membrane, such as daptomycin and amphotericin B [9,37,76].

Although vancomycin, tetracyclines, azithromycin, and quinupristin-dalfopristin do not exhibit concentration-dependent killing, the AUC/MIC ratio has been the major PK/PD parameter correlating with therapeutic efficacy of these drugs in neutropenic animals [21,29]. A study in normal mice with vancomycin and teicoplanin against a strain of *S. pneumoniae* that used mortality as an endpoint demonstrated that the peak/MIC ratio was the most important parameter [55].

5 MAGNITUDE OF PK/PD PARAMETER REQUIRED FOR EFFICACY

Because PK/PD parameters can correct for differences in a drug's pharmacokinetics and intrinsic antimicrobial activity, one would expect that the magnitude of the PK/PD parameters required for efficacy would be similar in different animal species. Thus, results from studies in animal infection models could be predictive of the activity of drugs in humans. This would be especially helpful in designing dosage regimens for both old and new antibacterials in situations where it is difficult to obtain sufficient clinical data, such as with newly emerging resistant organisms. Studies in animals would also allow one to determine if the magnitude of the PK/PD parameter required for efficacy was similar for (1) different drugs within the same antimicrobial class, (2) different dosing regimens, (3) different pathogens, and (4) different sites of infection.

5.1 Animal Infection Models

The largest number of studies addressing the magnitude of the PK/PD parameters with various drugs, dosing regimens, pathogens, sites of infection, and animal species have been performed with β-lactams and fluoroquinolones. Time above MIC is the PK/PD parameter that correlates with the therapeutic efficacy of the various β-lactam antibiotics. Studies in animal infection models demonstrate that antibiotic concentrations do not need to exceed the MIC for 100% of the dosing interval to obtain a significant antibacterial effect [23,26,28,57,87]. In fact, an in vivo bacteriostatic effect is observed when serum levels exceed the MIC for about 30–40% of the dosing interval. Very similar percentages for time above MIC have been observed in murine thigh and lung infection models, for various dosing intervals from 1 to 24 h, and with several broad-spectrum cephalosporins against both gram-negative bacilli and gram-negative streptococci, provided unbound drug levels were used for highly protein bound cephalosporins such as ceftriaxone.

If one uses survival after several days of therapy as the endpoint for efficacy of β-lactams in animal infection models, then slightly higher percentages of time above MIC are necessary [2,30,70]. Figure 4 illustrates the relationship between time above MIC and mortality for animals infected with *S. pneumoniae* that were treated for several days with penicillins or cephalosporins. Several studies in-

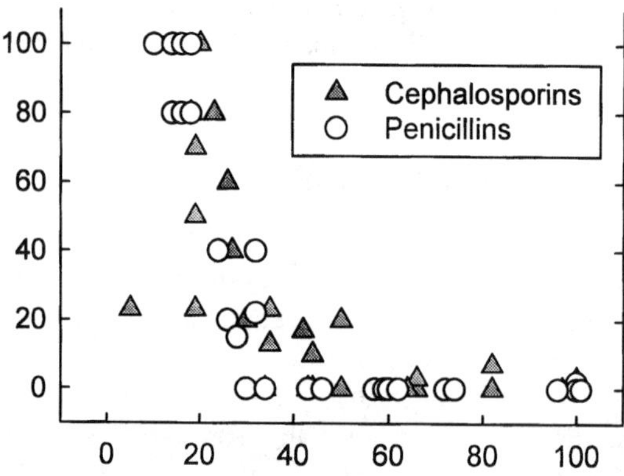

FIGURE 4 Relationship between the percentage of time serum levels of β-lactams exceed the MIC and survival in animal models infected with *S. pneumoniae*. (Data from Refs. 5, 30, and 70.)

cluded penicillin-intermediate and penicillin-resistant strains. The mortality was close to 100% if serum levels were above the MIC for 20% or less of the dosing interval. As soon as the percentage of time above MIC reached 40–50% or higher, survival was in the order of 90–100%.

The PK/PD parameter that best correlates with the efficacy of the fluoroquinolones is the 24 h AUC/MIC ratio [6,7,28]. The magnitude of this PK/PD parameter required to produce a bacteriostatic effect in animal infection models varied for most organisms from 25 to 50 [28,41]. These values are equivalent to averaging one to two times the MIC over a 24 h period [i.e., (1–2) × 24 = 24–48]. This magnitude was independent of the dosing interval, the site of infection, and the fluoroquinolone used, provided unbound drug concentrations were used for moderate to highly protein bound drugs such as gemifloxacin [7].

The relationship between the 24 h AUC/MIC values and outcome for fluoroquinolones as reported in the literature from studies that treated animals for at least 2 days, reported survival results at the end of therapy, and provided pharmacokinetic data is illustrated in Fig. 5 [28]. The infections in these studies included pneumonia, peritonitis, and sepsis produced by gram-negative bacilli and a few gram-positive cocci in immunosuppressed mice, rats, and guinea pigs. In general, 24 h AUC/MIC ratios less than 30 were associated with greater than 50% mortality, whereas AUC/MIC values of 100 or greater were associated with

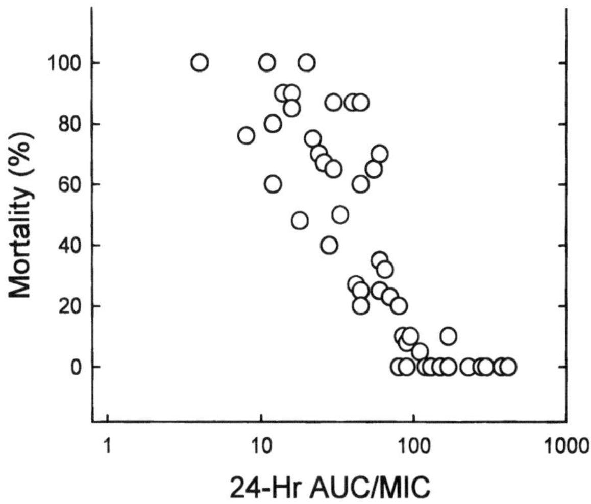

FIGURE 5 Relationship between 24 h AUC/MIC for fluoroquinolones and survival in immunosuppressed animals infected with gram-negative bacilli and a few gram-positive cocci. (From Ref. 28.)

almost no mortality. A value of 100 is equivalent to having serum concentrations average about four times the MIC over a 24 h period (i.e., 4 times 24 = 96).

Differences in the magnitude of the PK/PD parameter are observed with different classes of β-lactams, and with some organisms with both β-lactams and fluoroquniolones. For the same types of organisms, the percentages for time above MIC for a bacteriostatic effect were slightly lower for penicillins than for cephalosporins, and even lower for carbapenems [26]. These differences are due to the rate of killing, which is fastest with the carbapenems and slowest with the cephalosporins. In addition, the percentage for time above MIC required for efficacy with staphylococci was less than observed with gram-negative bacilli and streptococci [23]. This difference is due to the prolonged in vivo PAEs observed for β-lactams with staphylococci but not with gram-negative bacilli and streptococci. In non-neutropenic mice, the magnitude of the 24 h AUC/MIC for fluoroquinolones required for efficacy was about threefold lower for *S. pneumoniae* than for *Klebsiella pneumoniae* [7,28]. In vitro models have also demonstrated a lower AUC/MIC value for strains of *S. pneumoniae* [56,59].

5.2 Drug Combinations

Very little is known about determining the magnitude of PK/PD parameters when drugs are used in combination. Some investigators have suggested that one can add the magnitude of the 24 h AUC/MIC ratios for each of the drugs to estimate the pharmacodynamic activity of the combination [82]. However, a study in neutropenic mice infected with *Pseudomonas aeruginosa* demonstrated that the magnitudes of the PK/PD parameters required when a β-lactam, aminoglycoside, or fluoroquinolone is used alone are also important in predicting the efficacy of these drugs used in combination [66]. Thus, adding the 24 h AUC/MIC ratio of β-lactams to that of aminoglycosides or fluoroquinolones has a poor predictive value for their activity in combination. Instead, one must add the effect produced by the percentage of time above MIC for β-lactams to the effect resulting from the 24 h AUC/MIC ratio of aminoglycosides and fluoroquinolones to accurately predict the activity of these combinations. Adding the 24 h AUC/MIC ratios is appropriate for aminoglycoside-fluoroquinolone combinations, because that is the important PK/PD parameter for both drugs.

5.3 Human Infections

Bacteriological cure in patients with acute otitis media and acute maxillary sinusitis provides a sensitive model for determining the relationship between outcome and time above MIC for multiple β-lactam antibiotics. A variety of clinical trials have included pretherapy and repeat sinus puncture or tympanocentesis of middle ear fluid after 2–7 days of therapy to determine whether the initial organism isolated had been eradicted [25,32,33,48,54,77,79]. Figure 6 demonstrates the relationship between time above MIC and the bacteriological cure rate for many β-lactams against *S. pneumoniae* and *Haemophilus influenzae* in patients with these two infections. Several of the recent studies have included penicillin-intermediate and penicillin-resistant strains. In general, percentages for time above MIC greater than 40% were required to achieve an 85–100% bacteriological cure rate for both organisms including resistant pneumococci.

Commonly used parenteral doses of ceftriaxone, cefotaxime, penicillin G, and ampicillin provide free-drug concentrations above the MIC_{90} for penicillin-intermediate strains of *S. pneumoniae* for at least 40–50% of the dosing interval. A variety of clinical trials in severe pneumococcal pneumonia including bacteremic cases have demonstrated that these β-lactams are as effective against these organisms as against fully susceptible strains [43,50,72]. Thus, the magnitude of the PK/PD parameter determining efficacy for β-lactams against pneumococci is very similar in animal infection models and in human infections such as pneumonia, sinusitis, and otitis media.

As illustrated in Fig. 5, high survival in animal infection models treated with fluoroquinolones was observed with 24 h AUC/MIC values of 100 or higher. Very similar values were observed in two clinical trials. Forrest et al. [45] found

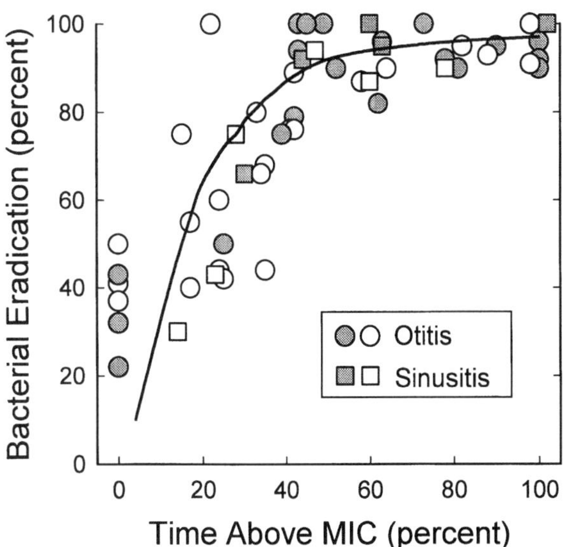

FIGURE 6 Relationship between time above MIC and bacteriological cure for various β-lactams against penicillin-susceptible (PSSP), penicillin-intermediate (PISP), and penicillin-resistant (PRSP) *S. pneumoniae* and *H. influenzae* in patients with acute otitis media and acute maxillary sinusitis. (Data from Refs. 25, 32, and 33.)

that a 24 h AUC/MIC value of 125 or higher was associated with satisfactory outcome in seriously ill patients treated with intravenous ciprofloxacin. Lower values resulted in clinical and microbiological cure rates of less than 50%. Another study in patients with a variety of bacterial infections treated with levofloxacin found that a peak/MIC ratio of 12 or higher and a 24 h AUC/MIC ratio of 100 or higher resulted in a statistically improved outcome [73]. These studies further demonstrate that the magnitude of the PK/PD parameter in animal infection models can be predictive of the magnitude of the parameter required for effective therapy in humans.

5.4 Prevention of Resistance

A peak/MIC ratio of 8–10 has been shown both in vitro and in vivo to prevent the emergence of resistant mutants during therapy with aminoglycosides and fluoroquinolones [13,31]. A 24 h AUC/MIC ratio greater than 100 has also been associated with a significantly reduced risk for the emergence of resistance during therapy [82]. The conclusion of this study was dependent almost entirely on the results with ciprofloxacin in patients with gram-negative bacillary infections, primarily those due to *P. aeruginosa*. A 24 h AUC/MIC ratio greater than 100 did not reduce the risk for the emergence of resistant organisms in patients treated with cephalosporins for infections due to gram-negative bacilli producing type 1 β-lactamase. Much more data are needed on the relationship between PK/PD parameters and the development of resistance.

6 APPLICATIONS OF PHARMACODYNAMICS

Knowledge of the pharmacodynamics of antimicrobials have proven useful for (1) establishing newer optimal dosing regimens for established drugs, (2) developing new antimicrobials or new formulations, (3) establishing susceptibility breakpoints, and (4) formulating guidelines for empirical therapy of infections.

6.1 New Dosage Regimens

Administration of β-lactams by continuous infusion enhances their ability to maintain serum levels above the MIC. Despite many potential advantages of continuous infusion, only a few clinical trials have documented the success of this type of dosage regimen [14,24]. Recent clinical trials have been designed to determine if continuous infusion will (1) allow for the use of daily dosages of drug lower than those required for intermittent administration or (2) improve efficacy against bacteria with reduced susceptibility. For example, equivalent outcomes have been observed with 3–4 g/day of ceftazidime by continuous infusion compared with 6 g/day administered intermittently [51,69]. Initial results with continuous infusion of large doses of ampicillin have demonstrated success for moderately ampicillin-resistant strains (ampicillin MIC = 32–64 mg/L) of vancomycin-resistant *Enterococcus faecium* [21].

The peak/MIC ratio appears to be the major PK/PD parameter determining the clinical efficacy of aminoglycosides. High rates of clinical success in severe gram-negative bacillary infections and rapid resolution of fever and leukocytosis in gram-negative bacillary nosocomial pneumonia require a peak/MIC ratio of 8–10 [53,65]. The once-daily dosage regimen for aminoglycosides was designed to enhance peak serum levels. In addition, once-daily dosing has the potential to decrease the nephro- and ototoxicity associated with these drugs [85]. Uptake of aminoglycosides into renal tubular cells and middle ear endolymph is more efficient with low sustained concentrations than with high intermittent levels [34,83,86].

Most meta-analyses of clinical trials have demonstrated a small but significant increase in clinical outcome with once-daily dosing and a trend toward decreased nephrotoxicity [1,10,11,44,46,49,67]. Studies have also demonstrated that the onset of nephrotoxicity occurs several days later when the drug is administered once daily than when multiple-daily dosage regimens are followed [52,75,81]. Nevertheless, once-daily dosing may not be ideal for all indications. Studies in experimental enterococcal endocarditis have shown a greater reduction in bacterial vegetation titers when the aminoglycoside is administered by multiple-dosing regimens than by once-daily administration [42,85].

6.2 New Antimicrobials and Formulations

Identification of the PK/PD parameter and its magnitude required for efficacy has proven useful for selecting the dosage regimen for phase III clinical trials of new antimicrobials. For example, the dosage regimen for linezolid (600 mg twice daily) was designed to produce serum levels above 8 mg/L for more than 50% of the dosing interval [8]. New extended release formulations of cefaclor and clarithromycin and the 14:1 amoxicillin-clavulanate formulation were all designed to enhance the duration of time serum levels exceed the MIC.

6.3 Susceptibility Breakpoint Determinations

The Subcommittee on Antimicrobial Susceptibility Testing of the National Committee for Clinical Laboratory Standards (NCCLS) recently incorporated pharmacodynamics as one of the factors to consider when establishing susceptibility breakpoints [68]. For example, pharmacodynamic breakpoints for β-lactam antibiotics would be defined as the highest MIC that serum concentrations following standard dosage would exceed for at least 40% of the dosing interval. Table 3 compares the old and new susceptibility breakpoints of several oral β-lactams for *S. pneumoniae* with the pharmacodynamic breakpoints predicted from serum concentrations in children and adults. The two values for cefaclor reflect the

TABLE 3 Pharmacodynamic and New and Old NCCLS Susceptibility Breakpoints for Oral β-Lactams with *Streptococcus pneumoniae*

Drug	Old NCCLS breakpoint (mg/L)	Pharmacodynamic ($T >$ MIC $> 40\%$) breakpoint (mg/L)	New NCCLS breakpoint (mg/L)
Amoxicillin	0.5	2	2
Cefaclor	—	0.5–1	1
Cefuroxime	0.5	1	1
Cefprozil	—	1–2	2
Cefpodoxime	—	0.5	0.5

difference in serum levels between standard doses and the extended-release formulation, and those for cefprozil reflect the difference in serum levels from children and adults. The NCCLS breakpoints are identical to the pharmacodynamic breakpoints.

6.4 Guidelines for Empirical Therapy

Because the magnitude of PK/PD parameters determined in animal infection models can be predictive of antimicrobial efficacy in human infections, it is easy to understand why pharmacodynamics is being used more and more in establishing guidelines for empirical therapy. Recently published guidelines for otitis media, acute bacterial rhinosinusitis, and community-acquired pneumonia have used the ability of antimicrobials to reach the magnitude of PK/PD parameters required for efficacy for both susceptible pathogens and those with decreased susceptibility to rank or select antimicrobials for empirical therapy of these respiratory infections [36,50,78].

7 SUMMARY

Studies over the past 20 years have demonstrated that antibacterials and antifungals can vary markedly in their time course of antimicrobial activity. Three different patterns of antimicrobial activity are observed. Specific PK/PD parameters, such as the peak/MIC and AUC/MIC ratios and the time above MIC, have also been shown to be major determinants of in vivo efficacy. The magnitude of the PK/PD parameters required for efficacy are relatively similar in animal infection models and human infections and are largely independent of the dosing interval, the site of infection, the drug used within each antimicrobial class, and the type of infecting pathogen. However, additional studies are needed to extend current observations to other antimicrobials and organisms and to correlate PK/PD parameters with therapeutic efficacy in a variety of animal infection models and human infections. Pharmacodynamics has many applications, including use for establishing optimal dosing regimens for old drugs, for developing new antimicrobials and formulations, for setting susceptibility breakpoints, and for providing guidelines for empirical therapy.

REFERENCES

1. Ali MZ, Goetz MB. A meta-analysis of the relative efficacy and toxicity of single daily dosing versus multiple daily dosing of aminoglycosides. Clin Infect Dis 1997; 24:796–809.
2. Andes D, Craig WA. In vivo activities of amoxicillin and amoxicillin-clavulanate against Streptococcus pneumonia: Application to breakpoint determinations. Antimicrob Agents Chemother 1998; 42:2375–2379.
3. Andes D, van Ogtrop M. Characterization and quantitation of the pharmacodynamics of fluconazole in a neutropenic murine disseminated candidiasis infection model. Antimicrob Agents Chemother 1999; 43:2116–2120.
4. Andes D, van Ogtrop ML. In vivo characterization of the pharmacodynamics of flucytosine in a neutropenic murine disseminated candidiasis model. Antimicrob Agents Chemother 2000; 44:938–942.
5. Andes DR, Craig WA. Pharmacokinetics and pharmacodynamics of antibiotics in meningitis. Infect Dis Clinics N Am 1999; 13:595–618.
6. Andes DR, Craig WA. Pharmacodynamics of fluoroquinolones in experimental models of endocarditis. Clin Infect Dis 1998; 27:47–50.
7. Andes D, Craig WA. Pharmacodynamics of gemifloxacin against quinolone-resistant strains of Streptococcus pneumoniae with known resistance mechanisms. Abstracts of the 39th Interscience Conference on Antimicrobial Agents and Chemotherapy. Am Soc Microbiol, Washington, DC, 1999.
8. Andes D, Van Ogtrop M, Craig WA. Pharmacodynamic activity of a new oxazolidinone in an animal infection model. Abstracts of the 38th Interscience Conference on Antimicrobial Agents and Chemotherapy. Am Soc Microbiol, Washington, DC, 1998.
9. Andes D. In-vivo pharmacodynamics of amphotericin B against Candida albicans. Abstracts of the 39th Interscience Conference on Antimicrobial Agents and Chemotherapy. Am Soc Microbiol, Washington, DC, 1999.
10. Bailey TC, Little JR, Littenberg B, Reichley RM, Dunagan WC. A meta-analysis of extended-interval dosing versus multiple daily dosing of aminoglycosides. Clin Infect Dis 1997; 24:786–795.
11. Barza M, Ioannidis JPA, Cappelleri JC, Lau J. Single or multiple daily doses of aminoglycosides: A meta-analysis. Br Med J 1996; 312:338–345.
12. Bigger JW. The bactericidal action of penicillin on Staphylococcus pyogenes. Irish J Med Sci 1994; 227:533–568.
13. Blaser J, Stone BB, Groner MC, et al. Comparative study with enoxacin and netilmicin in a pharmacodynamic model to determine importance of ratio of antibiotic peak concentration to MIC for bactericidal activity and emergence of resistance. Antimicrob Agents Chemother 1987; 31:1054–1060.

14. Bodey GP, Ketchel SJ, Rodriguez N. A randomized study of carbenicillin plus cefamandole or tobramycin in the treatment of febrile episodes in cancer patients. Am J Med 1979; 67:608–616.
15. Bundtzen RW, Gerber AU, Cohn DL, Craig WA. Postantibiotic suppression of bacterial growth. Rev Infect Dis 1981; 3:28–37.
16. Bustamante CL, Wharton RC, Wade JC. In vitro activity of ciprofloxacin in combination with ceftazidime, aztreonam, and azlocillin against multiresistant isolates of Pseudomonas aeruginosa. Antimicrob. Agents Chemother 1990; 34:1814–1815.
17. Cars O, Odenholt-Tornqvist I. The post-antibiotic sub-MIC effict in vitro and in vivo. J Antimicrob Chemother 1993; 31(suppl D):159–166.
18. Craig WA, Gudmundsson S. Postantibiotc effect. In: V Lorian, ed. Antibiotics in Laboratory Medicine. 4th ed. Williams and Wilkins, Baltimore, MD, 1996:296–329.
19. Craig WA, Andes D. Differences in the in vivo pharmacodynamics of telithromycin and azithromycin against Streptococcus pneumoniae. Abstracts of 40th Interscience Conference on Antimicrobial Agents and Chemotherapy. Am Soc Microbiol, Washington, DC, 2000.
20. Craig WA, Ebert SC. Killing and regrowth of bacteria in vitro: A review. Scand J Infect Dis 1991; suppl 74:63–70.
21. Craig WA. Pharmacokinetic/pharmacodynamics parameters: Rationale for antibacterial dosing of mice and men. Clin Infect Dis 1997; 26:1–12.
22. Craig WA. Postantibiotic effects in experimental infection models: Relationship to in vitro phenomena and to treatment of infections in man. J Antimicrob Chemother 1993; 31:149–158.
23. Craig WA. Interrelationship between pharmacokinetics and pharmacodynamics in determining dosage regimens for broad-spectrum cephalosporins. Diagn Microbiol Infect Dis 1995; 21:1–8.
24. Craig WA, Ebert SC. Continuous infusion of β-lactam antibiotics. Antimicrob Agents Chemother 1992; 36:2577–2583.
25. Craig WA, Andes D. Pharmacokinetics and pharmacodynamics of antibiotics in otitis media. Pediatr Infect Dis J 1996; 15:255–259.
26. Craig WA, Ebert S, Watanabe Y. Differences in time above MIC required for efficacy of beta-lactams in animal infection models. Abstracts of the 33rd Interscience Conference on Antimicrobial Agents and Chemotherapy. Am Soc Microbiol, Washington, DC, 1993.
27. Craig WA, Redington J, Ebert SC. Pharmacodynamics of amikacin in-vitro and in mouse thigh and lung infections. J Antimicrob Chemother 1991; 27(suppl C):29–40.
28. Craig WA, Dalhoff A. Pharmacodynamics of fluoroquinolones in experimental animals. In: J Kuhlman, A Dalhoff, HJ Zeiler, eds. Handbook of Experimental Pharmacology, Vol 127, Quinolone Antibacterials. pp 207–232.
29. Craig WA. Postantibiotic effects and the dosing of macrolides, azalides, and streptogramins. In: SH Zinner, LS Young, JF Acar, HC Neu, eds. Expanding Indications for the New Macrolides, Azalides and Streptogramins. Marcel Dekker, New York, 1997:27–38.
30. Craig WA. Antimicrobial resistance issues of the future. Diagn Microbiol Infect Dis 1996; 25:213–217.

31. Craig WA. Does the dose matter? Clin Infect Dis 2000; in press.
32. Dagan R, Abramason O, Leibovitz E, Greenberg D, Lang R, Goshen S, Yagupsky P, Leiberman A, Fliss DM. Bacteriologic response to oral cephalosporins: Are established susceptibility breakpoints appropriate in the case of acute otitis media? J Infect Dis 1997; 176:1253–1259.
33. Dagan R, Leibovitz E, Fliss DM, Leiberman A, Jacobs MR, Craig W, Yagupsky P. Bacteriologic efficacies of oral azithromycin and oral cefaclor in treatment of acute otitis media in infants and young children. Antimicrob Agents Chemother 2000; 44: 43–50.
34. De Broe ME, Verbist L, Verpooten GA. Influence of dosage schedule on renal cortical accumulation of amikacin and tobramycin in man. J Antimicrob Chemother 1991; 27(suppl C):41–47.
35. Den Hollander JG, Mouton JW, van Goor MP, et al. Alteration of postantibiotic effect during one dosing interval of tobramycin, simulated in an in vitro pharmacokinetic model. Antimicrob Agents Chemother 1996; 40:784–786.
36. Dowell SF, Butler JC, Giebink GS, Jacobs MR, Jernigan D, Musher DM, Rakowsky A, Schwartz B. Acute otitis media: Management and surveillance in an era of pneumococcal resistance—A report from the drug-resistant Streptococcus pneumoniae therapeutic working group. Pediatr Infect Dis J 1999; 18:1–9.
37. Drusano GL, Johnson DE, Rosen M. Pharmacodynamics of a fluoroquinolone antimicrobial agent in a neutropenic rat model of Pseudomonas sepsis. Antimicrob Agents Chemother 1993; 37:483–490.
38. Eagle H, Musselman AD. The slow recovery of bacteria from the toxic effects of penicillin. J Bacteriol 1949; 58:475–490.
39. Ernst EJ, Klepser ME, Pfaller MA. Postantifungal effects of echinocandin, azole, and polyene antifungal agents against Candida albicans and Cryptococcus neoformans. Antimicrob Agents Chemother 2000; 44:1108–1111.
40. Fantin B, Ebert S, Leggett J, et al. Factors affecting the duration of in-vivo postantibiotic effect for aminoglycosides against gram-negative bacilli. J Antimicrob Chemother 1990; 27:829–836.
41. Fantin B, Leggett J, Ebert S, Craig WA. Correlation between in vitro and in vivo activity of antimicrobial agents against gram-negative bacilli in a murine infection model. Antimicrob Agents Chemother 1991; 35:1413–1422.
42. Fantin B, Carbon C. Importance of the aminoglycoside dosing regimen in the penicillin-netilimicin combination for treatment of Enterococcus faecalis–induced experimental endocarditis. Antimicrob Agents Chemother 1990; 34:2387–2389.
43. Feikin DR, Schuchat A, Kolczak M, Barrett NL, Harrison LH, Lefkowitz L, McGreer A, Farley MM, Vugia DJ, Lexau C, Stefonek KR, Patterson JE, Jorgensen JH. Mortality from invasive pneumococcal pneumonia in the era of antibiotic resistance, 1995–1997. Am J Public Health 2000; 90:223–229.
44. Ferriols-Lisart R, Alos-Alminana M. 1996. Effectiveness and safety of once-daily aminoglycosides: A meta-analysis. Am J Health Syst Pharmacy 1996; 53:1141–1150.
45. Forrest A, Nix DE, Ballow CH, Goss TF, Birmingham MC, Schentag JJ. Pharmacodynamics of intravenous ciprofloxacin in seriously ill patients. Antimicrob Agents Chemother 1993; 37:1073–1081.

46. Galloe AM, Gaudal N, Christensen HR, Kampmann JP. Aminoglycosides: Single or multiple daily dosing? A meta analysis on efficacy and safety. Eur J Clin Pharmacol 1995; 48:39–43.
47. Gudmundsson S, Vogelman B, Craig WA. The in vivo postantibiotic effect of imipenem and other new antimicrobials. J Antimicrob Chemother 1986; 18(suppl E): 67–73.
48. Gwaltney JM, Savolainen S, Rivas P, Schenk P, Scheld WM, Sydnor A, Keyserling C, Leigh A, Tack KJ. Comparative effectiveness and safety of cefdinir and amoxicillin-clavulanate in treatment of acute community-acquired bacterial sinusitis. Antimicrob Agents Chemother 1997; 41:1517–1520.
49. Hatala R, Dinh T, Cook DJ. Once-daily aminoglycoside dosing in immunocompetent adults: A meta-analysis. Ann Intern Med 1996; 124:717–725.
50. Heffelfinger JD, Dowell SF, Jorgensen JH, et al. Management of community-acquired pneumonia in the era of pneumococcal resistance. Arch Intern Med 2000; 160:1399–1408.
51. Houlihan HH, Mercier RC, McKinnon PS, et al. Continuous infusion versus intermittent administration of ceftazidime in critically ill patients with gram-negative infection. Abstracts of the 37th Interscience Conference on Antimicrobial Agents and Chemotherapy. Am Soc Microbiol, Washington, DC, 1997.
52. Int Antimicrob Therap Coop Group of EORTC. Efficacy and toxicity of single daily doses of amikacin and ceftriaxone versus multiple daily doses of amikacin and ceftazidime for infection in patients with cancer and granulocytopenia. Ann Intern Med 1993; 119:584.
53. Kashuba AD, Nafziger AN, Drusano GL, Bertino JS. Optimizing aminoglycoside therapy for nosocomial pneumonia caused by gram-negative bacteria. Antimicrob Agents Chemother 1999; 43:623–629.
54. Klein JO. Microbiologic efficacy of antibacterial drugs for acute otitis media. Pediatr Infect Dis 1993; J 12:973–975.
55. Knudsen JD, Fuursted K, Raber S, Espersen F, Fridmodt-Moller N. Pharmacodynamics of glycopeptides in the mouse peritonitis model of Streptococcus pneumoniae and Staphylococcus aureus infection. Antimicrob Agents Chemother 2000; 44: 1247–1254.
56. Lacy MK, Lu W, Xu X, Tessier PR, Nicolau DP, Quintiliani R, Nightingale CH. Pharmacodynamic comparisons of levofloxacin, ciprofloxacin, and ampicillin against Streptococcus pneumoniae in an in vitro model of infection. Antimicrob Agents Chemother 1999; 43:672–677.
57. Leggett JE, Fantin B, Ebert S, Totsuka K, Vogelman B, Calame W, Mattie H, Craig WA. Comparative antibiotic dose-effect relations at several dosing intervals in murine pneumonitis and thigh-infection models. J Infect Dis 1989; 159:281–292.
58. Leggett JE, Ebert S, Fantin B, Craig WA. Comparative dose-effect relations at several dosing intervals for beta-lactam, aminoglycoside and quinolone antibiotics against gram-negative bacilli in murine thigh-infection and pneumonitis models. Scand J Infect Dis 1991 (suppl 74):179–184.
59. Lister PD, Sanders CC. Pharmacodynamics of levofloxacin and ciprofloxacin against Streptococcus pneumoniae. J Antimicrob Chemother 1999; 43:79–86.
60. Lorian V. Effect of low antibiotic concentrations on bacteria: Effects on ultrastruc-

ture, virulence, and susceptibility to immunodefenses. In: V Lorian, ed. Antibiotics in Laboratory Medicine. 4th ed. Williams and Wilkins, Baltimore, 1991:493–555.

61. Louie A, Drusano GL, Banerjee P, Liu QF, Liu W, Kaw P, Shayegani M, Taber H, Miller MH. Pharmacodynamics of fluconazole in a murine model of systemic candidiasis. Antimicrob Agents Chemother 1998; 42:1105–1109.
62. McDonald PJ, Wetherall BL, Pruul H. Postantibiotic leukocyte enhancement: Increased susceptibility of bacteria pretreated with antibiotics to activity of leukocytes. Rev Infect Dis 1981; 3:38–44.
63. McDonald PJ, Craig WA, Kunin CM. Persistent effect of antibiotics on Staphylococcus aureus after exposure for limited periods of time. J Infect Dis 1977; 135:217–223.
64. McGrath BJ, Marchbanks CR, Gilbert D, Dudley MN. In vitro postantibiotic effect following repeated exposure to imipenem, temofloxacin, and tobramycin. Antimicrob Agents Chemother 1993; 37:1723–1725.
65. Moore RD, Lietman PS, Smith CR. Clinical response to aminoglycoside therapy: Importance of the ratio of peak concentration to minimal inhibitory concentration. J Infect Dis 1987; 155:93–99.
66. Mouton JW, van Ogtrop ML, Andes D, Craig WA. Use of pharmacodynamic indices to predict efficacy of combination therapy in vivo. Antimicrob Agents Chemother 1999; 43:2473–2478.
67. Munckhof WJ, Grayson JL, Turnidge JD. A meta-analysis of studies on the safety and efficacy of aminoglycosides given either once daily or as divided doses. J Antimicrob Chemother 1996; 37:645–663.
68. National Committee for Clinical Laboratory Standards. Development of In-Vitro Susceptibility Testing Criteria and Quality Control Parameters; Approved Guideline. 2nd ed. Document M23–A2, January 2000.
69. Nenko AS, Cappelletty DM, Kruse JA, et al. Continuous infusion versus intermittent administration of ceftazidime in critically ill patients with suspected gram-negative infection. Abstracts of the 35th Interscience Conference on Antimicrobial Agents and Chemotherapy, Am Soc Microbiol, Washington, DC, 1995.
70. Nicolau DP, Onyeji CO, Zhong M, Tessier PR, Banevicius MA, Nightingale CH. Pharmacodynamic assessment of cefprozil against Streptococcus pneumoniae: Implications for breakpoint determinations. Antimicrob Agents Chemother 2000; 44: 1291–1295.
71. Odenholt-Tornqvist I, Lowdin E, Cars O. Postantibiotic sub-MIC effects of vancomycin, roxithromycin, sparfloxacin, and amikacin. Antimicrob Agents Chemother 1992; 36:1852–1858.
72. Pallares R, Linares J, Vadillo M, Cabellos C, Manresa R, Viladrich PF, Martin R, Gudiol F. Resistance to penicillin and cephalosporin and mortality from severe pneumococcal pneumonia in Barcelona, Spain. N Engl J Med 1995; 333:474–480.
73. Preston SL, Drusano GL, Berman AL, Fowler CL, Chow AT, Dornseif B, Reichi V, Natarajan J, Corrado M. Pharmacodynamics of levofloxacin: A new paradigm for early clinical trials. J Am Med Assoc 1998; 279:125–129.
74. Redington J, Ebert SC, Craig WA. Role of antimicrobial pharmacokinetics and pharmacodynamics in surgical prophylaxis. Rev Infect Dis 1991; 13(suppl 10):S790–S799.

75. Rybak MJ, Abate BJ, Kang SL, Ruffing MJ, Lerner SA, Drusano GL. Prospective evaluation of the effect of an aminoglycoside dosing regimen on rates of observed nephrotoxicity and ototoxicity. Antimicrob Agents Chemother 1999; 43:1549–1555.
76. Safdar N, Andes D, Craig WA. In-vivo pharmacodynamic characterization of daptomycin. Abstracts of 37th Infectious Diseases Society of America, Washington, DC, 1999.
77. Scheld WM, Sydnor A, Farr B, Gratz JC, Gwaltney JM. Comparison of cyclacillin and amoxicillin for therapy for acute maxillary sinusitis. Antimicrob Agents Chemother 1986; 30:350–353.
78. Sinus and Allergy Health Partnership. Antimicrobial treatment guidelines for acute bacterial rhinosinusitis. Otolaryngol Head Neck Surg 2000; 123(suppl 1):1–32.
79. Sydnor A, Gwaltney JM, Cocchetto DM, Scheld WM. Comparative evaluation of cefuroxime axetil and cefaclor for treatment of acute bacterial maxillary sinusitis. Arch Otolaryngol Head Neck Surg 1989; 115:1430–1433.
80. Tauber MG, Zak O, Scheld WM, Hengstler B, Sande MA. The postantibiotic effect in the treatment of experimental meningitis caused by Streptococcus pneumoniae in rabbits. J Infect Dis 1984; 149:575–583.
81. Ter Braak EW, De Vries PJ, Bouter KP, Van der Vegt SG, Dorrestein GC, Northier JW, Van Dijk A, Verkooyen RP, Verbrugh HA. Once-daily dosing regimen for aminoglycoside plus β-lactam combination therapy of serious bacterial infections: Comparative trial with netilmicin plus ceftriaxone. Am J Med 1990; 89:58–66.
82. Thomas JK, Forrest A, Bhavnani SM, Hyatt JM, Cheng A, Ballow CH, Schentag JJ. Pharmacodynamic evaluation of factors associated with the development of bacterial resistance in acutely ill patients during therapy. Antimicrob Agents Chemother 1998; 42:521–527.
83. Tran BH, Deffrennes D. Aminoglycoside ototoxicity: Influence of dosage regimen on drug uptake and correlation between membrane binding and some clinical features. Acta Otolaryngol (Stockholm) 1988; 105:511–515.
84. Turnidge JD, Gudmundsson S, Bogelman B, Craig WA. The postantibiotic effect of antifungal agents against common pathogenic yeast. J Antimicrob Chemother 1994; 34:83–92.
85. Urban A, Craig WA. Daily dosing of aminoglycosides. Curr Clin Top Infect Dis. 1997; 17:236–255.
86. Verpooten GA, Giuliano RA, Verbist L, Estermans G, De Broe ME. Once-daily dosing decreases renal accumulation of gentamicin and netilmicin. Clin Pharmacol Ther 1989; 45:22–27.
87. Vogelman B, Gudmundsson S, Leggett J, Turnidge J, Ebert S, Craig WA. Correlation of antimicrobial pharmacokinetic parameters with therapeutic efficacy in an animal model. J Infect Dis 1988; 158:831–847.
88. Vogelman B, Gudmundsson S, Turnidge J, Craig WA. The in vivo postantibiotic effect in a thigh infection in neutropenic mice. J Infect Dis 1988; 157:287–298.

2

Microbiology and Pharmacokinetics

Charles H. Nightingale
Hartford Hospital, Hartford, Connecticut

Takeo Murakawa
Fujisawa Pharmaceutical Company, Ltd., Osaka, Kyoto University, Kyoto, and Tokushima University, Tokushima, Japan

1 INTRODUCTION

Pharmacodynamics, as applied to antimicrobial agents, is simply the indexing of microbiological data to the drug's concentration in the body (pharmacokinetics). Antimicrobial agents are different from most therapeutic drugs in their mechanism of action. The major difference between the agents and other drugs involves the fact that the target of antimicrobial agents is not the human body but microorganisms that live in it. A strong understanding of microbiology and pharmacokinetics under dynamic in vivo conditions is needed to fully understand the topic of microbial pharmacodynamics. However, it is beyond the scope of this chapter to present such material in detailed survey form. Other chapters of this text will discuss specific drug classes and illustrate the important pharmacokinetic and microbiological properties of those drugs. We prefer to discuss the important aspects of microbiology and pharmacokinetics as they apply to antimicrobials and the treatment of infections. We refer the reader to other chapters of this textbook as well as to standard texts [1,2] and primary articles on microbiology and pharmacokinetics for a more basic explanation of these topics.

2 MICROBIOLOGY

2.1 Effect of Antimicrobial Agents on Microorganisms

To understand this topic one must first have a concept of what is meant by the term antimicrobial agent. In this chapter this term refers to a chemical entity (a substance of particular chemical structure) that has the ability to bind to some important site in a microorganism and cause microbial death. This important site is a place in the microorganism where the organism undergoes some biochemical reaction that is part of its life cycle. The binding substance (which we call an antimicrobial agent) blocks or interferes with the biochemical reaction and thus prevents the organism from completely fulfilling those acts necessary to support its life cycle. The results of this ''interference'' by a chemical (natural or synthetic) that we call an antimicrobial agent usually results in cell death if the agent is in high enough concentration for a long enough period of time. Assuming that this description is fundamentally correct, it follows, then, that three events must occur in order for the antimicrobial agent to eradicate the microorganism:

1. The antimicrobial agent must reach the action sites and bind to the binding sites in the microorganism. The binding site can be a penicillin-binding protein, a DNA gyrase, a topoisomerase, or a ribosome or any other point of attachment that interferes with the biochemical reactions in the microorganism. The actual site varies depending upon the chemical structure of the class of the agent and also varies somewhat within the same agent class. This ability to bind to an active site can be thought of as being roughly descriptive (although not completely) of what we would commonly call the microbiological activity of the antimicrobial agents.
2. The antimicrobial agent must occupy a sufficient number of active sites. The occupation of a sufficient number of sites is an interesting topic and is central to the definition of pharmacodynamics. The mechanism of action of the antimicrobial agent does not have to be fully elucidated for the purpose of this discussion. First it must be recognized that the number of active sites that must be occupied is largely unknown. Obviously, the number is greater than one, because we know, at least intuitively, that there are many active sites involving many molecules of active proteins such as enzymes or DNA, and we must describe them very qualitatively. One term that qualitatively describes the number of sites is ''sufficient.'' The drug must diffuse, usually (but not always) on the basis of the drug's concentration gradient, to the

metabolically active site of the microorganism. Because concentration is important, one might speculate upon the issue of identifying the important place where the drug concentration is favorable to its binding to active sites. Intuitively it is the drug concentration immediately surrounding the active site that ultimately controls this process. But that concentration is in the bacterial cell and is largely unknown.

3. The antimicrobial agent must reside on the active site for a period of time. Because antibiotics are not contact poisons but agents that interfere with a biochemical process essential for the bacterial life cycle, a definite time must evolve in order for the agent to elicit the desired response. The length of time at the active site is related to the strength of binding to that site.

When these three conditions exist, the antimicrobial agents will have the desired effect on the bacteria.

2.2 Parameters for Microbiological Activity of Antimicrobial Agents

The killing properties of antimicrobial agents are important for pharmacodynamic considerations. As described above, the killing properties of antimicrobial agents are dependent upon the antibiotic characteristics such as number of binding sites, and the binding or interfering properties at the active sites, i.e., the drug concentration and length of time required to lead to microbial death. It is difficult to completely characterize these properties. However, the overall results may be sufficient from a practical perspective—the killing concentration surrounding the bacterial cell should be a good surrogate for the actual drug concentration at the active site.

The following parameters of antimicrobial activity are of common or practical use:

1. The minimal inhibitory concentration (MIC) is the lowest drug concentration without visible growth for 16–20 h at 35°C in the medium.
2. The minimal bactericidal concentration (MBC) is the lowest concentration required to kill 99.9% of the bacterial cells of the inoculum after 16–20 h exposure to the drug at 35°C.

For pharmacodynamic considerations it is important to understand that (1) these parameters are determined under in vitro conditions and that (2) we cannot use only one cell of a microorganism for the tests—for example, a million cells are used as a unit.

Susceptibility of cells is not homogeneous, i.e., each cell of a million cell population has a different MIC or MBC, and the total bacterial population shows an MIC distribution that is different for each organism–drug combination.

2.3 Kinetic Killing Properties

The killing rate is an important parameter and will vary with the kind of microorganism and the strain of the organism as well as the type of antimicrobial agent. The killing properties of antimicrobial agents have two basic forms of relationships with drug concentration: concentration dependence and time-dependence. It should be noted that the issues of concentration-dependent and time-dependent bacterial killing are an abbreviated way of describing an antibiotic–bacterial interaction. This is shown in Fig. 1, which illustrates the usual in vitro experiments to determine whether a drug is static or cidal. If we grow bacteria in broth in the absence of antibiotic, the control curve results. If we add a small quantity of drug, the rate of growth still exceeds the rate of death and the organism continues to grow. Obviously that small amount of drug did not have much of an effect on the bacterial life cycle. If we add more drug, the rate of growth and death might be equal, and we say that the drug exhibits *static* properties. If we add even more drug, the rate of killing might exceed the rate of living and the drug is now termed a *cidal* agent. If we continue to add increasing amounts of drug, the rate of killing relative to the rate of living continues to increase, and if we look at just this concentration range we conclude that the drug exhibits *concentration-dependent killing*. If we add even more drug, we eventually reach a point where additional drug does not increase the rate of killing any further, and if we just look at its behavior in that concentration range we say that the drug exhibits *time-dependent killing* properties. In the example illustrated in Fig. 1, the same drug exhibited no effect, static behavior, cidal behavior, and concentration-dependent and time-dependent cidal behavior. In essence the same drug can have all of

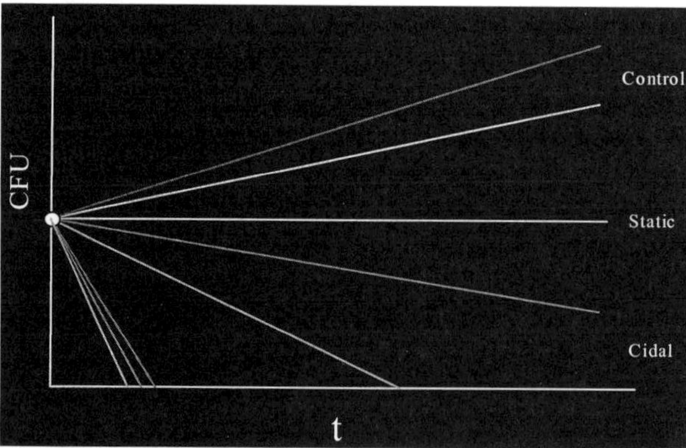

FIGURE 1 Relationship between net effect on bacterial growth and death, and time of exposure to antibiotic at various fixed concentrations.

these properties, depending on the drug's concentration in relation to its MIC. Therefore when we say that a drug is a concentration- or time-dependent killer, we seem to be speaking in incomplete sentences. A more complete description would be to add the phrase "under the concentrations achieved after clinical dosing." The importance of this phenomenon is that although investigators may study the properties of a drug and classify it as static or cidal, this is arbitrary, because the same experiment under different conditions would result in a different classification. This is why, for the tetracyclines, the official U.S. package insert has phrases that indicate that these agents are static but exhibit cidal properties against some bacteria.

It is important to also realize that the killing property of a drug is related to its rate of growth. If antibiotics interfere with certain biochemical reactions in the bacteria that are normally part of their life cycle, then the drug needs to be present, bound to the active site, at the time the biochemical reaction is to occur. As an example, penicillins or cephalosporins show bactericidal activity when cell growth is maximal but not for resting cells, because the drugs inhibit the synthesis of the bacterial cell wall and the bacteria must be actively making cell walls for the antibiotic to have its effect.

Sometimes the killing curve shows a reduction in the number of viable cells of an organism even at concentrations lower than the MIC ("subinhibitory concentrations"). This means that some cells in the population are more sensitive to the drug than the MIC reported for the entire population would indicate. In such a case, the MIC may change as a function of inoculum size.

A postantibiotic effect (PAE) is observed with cephalosporins against gram-negative bacteria: When the bacteria are exposed to antibiotics at several times the MIC for a certain period of time and then the antibiotic is removed, slow bacterial growth is observed for a certain period of time. Possible reasons for this phenomenon are that the drug continues to bind to the active sites of the bacteria or that the antibiotics remain in the cell even after the antibiotic has disappeared from outside the cell, or there may be some methodological problem associated with the removal of the drug from the test system.

The MIC, MBC, and killing kinetics properties such as concentration-dependent and time-dependent properties are commonly used as parameters for microbiological activity of antimicrobial agents and therefore are of major importance. However, it is important to understand that these definitions and most data are obtained in vitro, not at the actual sites of infection in the body. It is difficult or impossible to obtain the MIC in body fluids, and in addition the reported data have a large amount of variability associated with them due to the twofold dilutional techniques commonly used in the field of microbiology. This represents 100% variability in the reported MIC value. As a guide, the MIC values are very useful, but to consider them to be absolute, infallible numbers is misleading and confusing.

3 PHARMACOKINETICS

Parameters for the pharmacokinetic properties of antimicrobial agents are the same as for those of other therapeutic drugs. There is no particular issue in pharmacokinetic considerations with antimicrobial agents except that the target site is located in the infection site where microorganisms are living. The infection sites are distributed throughout the body, and an effective concentration of an antimicrobial agent is required to eradicate microorganisms in those infection sites where they are living.

3.1 Pharmacokinetic Parameters for Pharmacodynamic Consideration

We do not administer a drug directly into microorganisms, but into a human body. It must be driven to the place where the organism lives by the drug concentration in blood. Most organisms live in some interstitial fluid (IF) in the body, although some reside inside mammalian cells. Assuming we are considering organisms that live in IF, it is the drug concentration in this fluid that is important. Fortunately, drug transfer from the bloodstream into the IF is rather rapid, due to the leakiness of the capillary bed membrane, and blood (serum or plasma) concentrations control the IF drug concentration, which controls or influences the drug concentration around the bacterial active sites. In this way we ''back into'' the realization that drug concentrations in the serum (''serum'' will be used in this chapter to mean plasma, blood, or serum) are important for a sufficient number of active sites to be occupied by the drug. However, it is not true for every injection site. This forms the basis for modern pharmacodynamic theory, which allows one to index microbiological activity to the serum concentration of an antibiotic. The concentration of the drug in the serum is a major function of the drug's pharmacokinetics.

The pharmacokinetic parameters related to microbiological activity of an antibiotic are

Peak drug concentration: C_p
Half life: $T_{1/2}$
Area under the drug concentration curve: AUC
Time period during which drug concentrations exceed MIC or MBC

3.2 Difference of Pharmacokinetic Parameters in Serum and Tissues or Fluids

As mentioned above, pharmacokinetic parameters should be those based on the antibiotic concentration at the infection site. However, determination of the drug concentration at various infection sites is difficult in practice. A drug is distributed or penetrated into tissue or tissue fluids of infection sites via the bloodstream.

When the drug concentrations at the infection site and in the bloodstream are proportional, it is possible to use the serum or blood concentration to index to microbiological activity. If there is a big difference between the kinetic properties in the blood and those at the site of infection (tissues/fluids), then the drug concentration at the site of infection should be used to index to microbiological activity. Serum–tissue protein binding, drug distribution, penetration rate, and drug metabolism at these sites will be factors in effecting differences in blood and infection site drug kinetics.

4 CLINICAL ASPECTS

As mentioned before, there are major differences between antimicrobial agents and other therapeutic drugs, because the target of antimicrobial agents is not the human body but microorganisms that cause infectious diseases. The human body itself has host defense mechanisms to kill invasive microorganisms. Infectious diseases are caused by the bacteria creating, through the large number of them growing in the body, a condition that exceeds the body's host defense capability to recognize and eradicate the invasive microorganism. Therefore, eradication of microorganisms from the body or infection sites depends upon a combination of activities, partly provided by the body and partly provided by an antibacterial drug. If host defense activity is normal and the infecting organisms are not very pathogenic, clinical efficacy will result even when the activity of the antibiotic is modest. However, when the host defense mechanism is weak or impaired, as is the case with immunocompromised patients, the antimicrobial agents itself must kill and eradicate the infecting microorganisms. In such a situation, the dosing and activity of the antibiotic must be maximized.

5 PHARMACODYNAMICS

5.1 Pharmacodynamic Parameters

The drug concentration in the serum and the time that it remains there are related to the occupation of a sufficient number of binding sites in the bacteria and the length of time those sites are occupied. To produce a pharmacodynamic parameter it is only necessary to index a measure of microbiological activity such as the minimum inhibitory concentration (MIC) or minimum bactericidal concentration (MBC) to the area under the curve (AUC). In this chapter we will use the term MIC; however, the MBC or any other measure of microbiological activity could also be used. It is interesting that the mathematical product of drug concentration in the serum (C_p) multiplied by time is termed the drug's area under the serum concentration–time curve (AUC). A schematic representation of the AUC indexed to the MIC of bacteria is shown in Fig. 2. This pharmacodynamic parameter AUC/MIC is an important and fundamental parameter that relates microbiological activity to serum concentration. One simple way of thinking about the AUC/MIC ratio is that the AUC represents the concentration of drug and time of exposure that presents itself to the bacteria, over and above the minimum needed to do the job (MIC). The higher this ratio (AUC/MIC), the better is the chance of the antibiotic being successful. It should also be noted that in nature, antibiotics eradicate bacteria (fulfill the three requirements described earlier) by an interaction of microbiological activity and pharmacokinetics, not just one of the two. Decisions related to drug selection should therefore take both of these properties into consideration. Unfortunately, most clinicians, because of their training, will choose antibiotics on the basis of microbiological activity alone. We believe that this may result in poor decisions. The reason for this belief is that one can choose the most active antibiotic in the world (lowest MIC against the target organism), but if it does not go to where the bacteria reside, it will not kill anything. The reverse is also true. Good pharmacokinetics with very poor antimicrobial activity will also not result in a satisfactory outcome. Both need to be considered simultaneously; hence the importance of pharmacodynamics.

Under certain conditions, the AUC/MIC [(C_p × time)/MIC] ratio can be simplified. These simplifying assumptions are based upon whether the drug is classified as a concentration-dependent or time-dependent bacterial killer. This determination is made from in vitro experiments such as those for which data are shown in Fig. 3. For the aminoglycoside we can see that as the drug concentration increases, the rate of killing increases, and hence this drug is considered to be a concentration-dependent killer. If one makes the concentration high enough, the rate of killing is so fast that the contribution of drug exposure to the entire process is insignificant and can be ignored. The ratio AUC/MIC [(C_p × time)/MIC] sim-

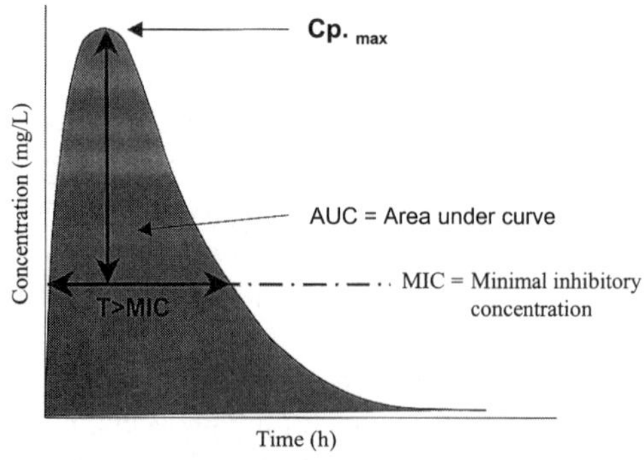

FIGURE 2 Pharmacodynamic relationship: AUC/MIC.

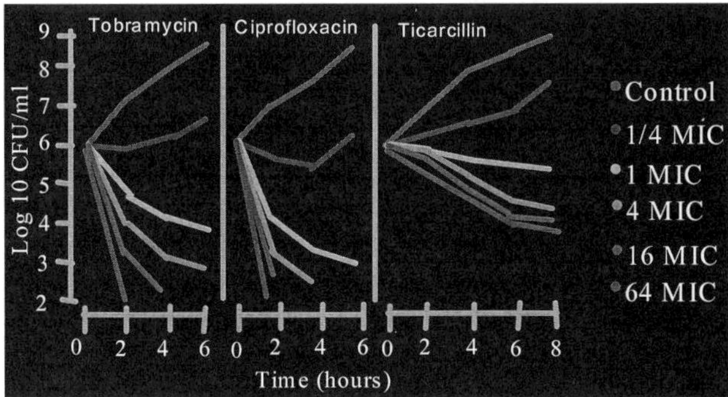

FIGURE 3 Concentration-dependent vs. independent bacterial killing. (From Ref. 21.)

plifies to C_p/MIC. For such a drug the question arises regarding how high the drug concentration must be in relation to the MIC in order to make this simplifying assumption. The answer is illustrated in Fig. 4, where it can be seen that when one reaches a C_p/MIC ratio of 10–12: 1, the simplifying assumption seems to hold. Several other investigators have demonstrated the same phenomenon [3,4]. Achieving a C_p/MIC ratio of 10 or greater forms the basis for high and infrequent dosing of aminoglycosides [5–7]. If such a ratio is achieved, bacterial killing is at a maximum. If it is not achieved, then the drug can still be quite effective; however, the simplifying assumption cannot be made, and the entire AUC must be applied to the ratio. A good dosing strategy for the clinical use of such drugs is to use the highest possible dose that achieves this ratio and does not cause toxicity.

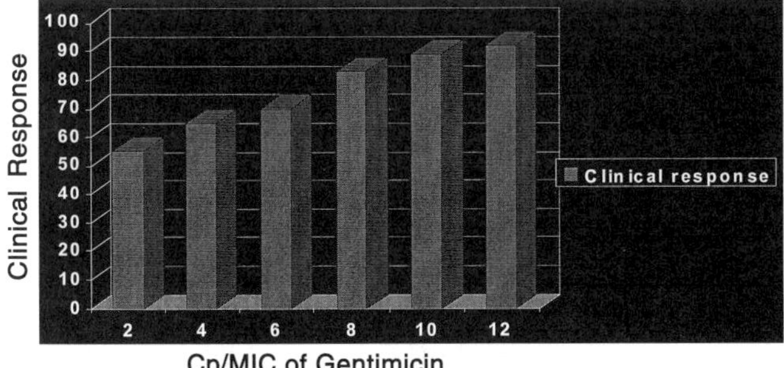

FIGURE 4 Clinical response vs. Cp/MIC. (from Ref. 7.)

Examination of Fig. 3 also reveals that other agents such as the β-lactams exhibit different bacterial killing attributes. It can be seen that once these drugs achieve concentrations of 2–4 times the MIC, further increases in concentration do not yield greater rates of bacterial killing. Bacterial killing is at a maximum under these conditions; the contribution of drug concentration to the entire killing process is minimal and can be ignored. The AUC/MIC ratio simplifies to drug exposure of the bacteria and is expressed pharmacodynamically as the time the serum concentrations remain above the MIC of the bacteria ($T >$ MIC). For drugs that display such behavior, the clinical dosing strategy is to maximize the $T >$ MIC. While the minimal $T >$ MIC varies with different drug–bug combinations, it appears from animal [8–11] and clinical [12] data that an acceptable working value of $T >$ MIC of about 50% of the dosing interval is associated with satisfactory outcomes. This number is appropriate for patients with intact or functioning immune systems. For immunocompromised patients, being 4–5 times the MIC is related to better outcomes and is roughly equivalent to being above the MIC for the entire dosing interval. [13]. The working number of 50% $T >$ MIC, or 100% $T >$ MIC for immunocompromised patients, is just a good approximation of what is necessary to achieve satisfactory clinical response. This will vary depending upon different conditions such as host factors and drug–bacteria interactions.

It is important to also realize that the pharmacodynamic classification of how a drug interacts with bacteria is directly related to the bacterial rate of growth. If antibiotics interfere with certain biochemical reactions in the bacteria that are normally part of their life cycle, then the drug needs to be present, bound to the active site, at the time the biochemical reaction would normally occur. Although this is intuitively obvious, what seems to be overlooked is that the pharmacodynamic parameter that correlates best with bacterial eradication will change with the growth properties of the bacteria. A good example of this is a recently published study by Lutsar et al. [14], who studied gatifloxacin pharmacodynamics in the cerebral spinal fluid (CSF) of rabbits. Because gatifloxacin is a quinolone, it is expected to be a concentration-dependent bactericidal agent. As such, one would expect that the pharmacodynamic parameters AUC/MIC or C_p/MIC might predominate. Whereas these investigators found that AUC_{csf}/MIC did correlate with outcomes, when the AUC_{csf} was held constant it was the $T >$ MIC that correlated with good outcome, not C_{pcsf}/MIC. This may at first seem counterintuitive, but it can be explained on the basis of the rate of growth of bacteria in CSF. If the rate of growth is relatively slow, the antibiotic will act only if it is present on the active site when that site is involved in the necessary biochemical reaction that is part of the bacteria's life cycle. When one considers this, it is not surprising that a relationship exists with $T >$ MIC rather than high and transitory peak concentrations.

Do bacteria grow more slowly in CSF? We believe they do, because rapidly growing bacteria in the CSF will probably kill the host before therapy can be initiated. We hypothesize that the CSF is a much poorer growth medium for bacteria than either broth or other sites in the body, and this slower growth allows therapy to be initiated but also changes the pharmacodynamic parameter that correlates with effective bacterial eradication.

5.2 Relationship Between Pharmacodynamics and Clinical Efficacy

The effective treatment of patients suffering from an infectious disease is a multifaceted process that depends upon many factors for a successful outcome. Generally speaking, there is an inverse relationship between the MIC of an organism and clinical efficacy, i.e., the lower the MIC the higher the cure rate. This is illustrated in Table 1. What can also be seen in this table is that the opposite—identifying the MIC that correlates to an effective clinical cure rate—is not so obvious, and many MIC values (e.g., <1, 1.0, 2.0, 3.0, 4.0) can be considered to result in an acceptable cure rate. Table 2 illustrates that eradication of bacteria can fail to occur even when the bacteria are susceptible to the antibiotic. Reports have been published, e.g., in the treatment of *S. pneumoniae* bacteremia, where the death rate is substantial in spite of aggressive and appropriate antimicrobial therapy. [15,16]. Obviously, the ability of the antibiotic to kill the organism is only one factor affecting patient outcome. Other factors such as the age of the patient, the vigor of the immune system, and psychological factors such as the will to live and the degree of confidence the patient has in the caregivers and the health system will affect outcomes. Although pharmacodynamic parameters are important and useful in guiding therapy, they are not the only issues that affect outcomes. The clinical practice of medicine still remains somewhat of an

TABLE 1 General Relationship Between MICs and Clinical Cures (Claforan)

MIC (μg/mL)	Clinical cures (%)
$\leq$1.0	94
8.0	90
16.0	77
32.0	84
$\geq$64.0	64

Source: Ref. 22.

TABLE 2 Success and Failure of Resistant and Sensitive Strains of *Haemophilus Influenza*

	Clinical correlation[a]		Number of strains with Indicated MIC							
Antibiotic	Antimicrobial outcome[b]	Number of Patients	<0.25	0.5	1	2	4	8	16	<32
Lorecarbef	C/1	186	4	7	52	74	28	8	7	6
	R/F	10			1	8		1		
Amox/ Clav	C/I	137	7	53	42	25	7	3		
	R/F	11		7	4					

[a] *Haemophilus influenza* AO MS, AMS, APECB, and pneumonia.
[b] C/I = cure or improve; R/F = relapse or failure.
Source: Ref. 23.

art rather than a pure science. Pharmacodynamic principles help move clinical medicine several steps toward the science side, but they are not the only issue of concern in clinical medicine.

Issues involving an antibiotic's properties such as protein binding, PAE, and volume of distribution are important properties of the drug; however, for licensed or marketed drugs further consideration of these properties is rarely needed. The rationale behind this statement is related to the process of drug licensing. Using the drug development process, the first step is to do preclinical studies followed by clinical studies. Phase I studies are designed to observe and detect gross human toxicity and to explore the drug dose and dosing issues. Once this is completed, a value judgment is made concerning a useful and safe clinical dose. The next step, phase II, is to carry out small-scale clinical trials, the main purpose of which is to confirm the efficacy of using the dose derived from preclinical and phase I studies. When it is confirmed that the drug is safe and effective with the chosen dosage and dosing regimen, the development proceeds to larger scale clinical trials, phase III. If the dose and dosing regimen are found to be acceptable, phase III trials eventually lead to licensing. The point of this is that the licensed drug has been found to be acceptable, useful, and nontoxic on the basis of all its properties. For an antibiotic these include its pharmacokinetics and pharmacodynamic properties, which involve considerations of volumes of distribution, half-life, PAE, protein binding, and tissue penetration. If the antibiotic were not acceptable, the dose would be changed until it met the criteria for licensing. In other words, the observed (empirical) result is due to the dose used based upon the agent's overall properties. The issues of protein binding, PAE, and other issues, although important, have already been taken into account and contribute to the net effect one observes. Further consideration of these issues with respect to clinical outcomes is rarely necessary. Considering a drug's protein binding as a separate and unrelated issue does not make an approved agent less or more effective in clinical use. It will change the pharmacodynamic parameters, e.g., AUC/MIC, and on a comparative basis will affect the rank order of drugs depending upon their protein binding.

5.3 The Application of Pharmacodynamic Parameters to Clinical Practice

All pharmacodynamic parameters are simply calculated numbers that have no inherent value by themselves. In order for these numbers to have value, one must correlate them to an outcome. Because most practitioners are interested in treating infected patients, the most accepted correlation is between the pharmacodynamic parameter and the clinical outcome. It is important to realize that if one correlates the pharmacodynamic parameter to an outcome that is different than clinical effectiveness, then the important or critical value of the pharmacodynamic parameter will change. For example, if one correlates the AUC/MIC to clinical cures, one critical number appears such that if one exceeds that parameter one can expect good clinical cures. If one correlates the parameter to maximal eradication of bacteria, another AUC/MIC number appears that will probably be higher than that calculated in the first example. If one desires to correlate the pharmacodynamic parameter to the suppression of the emergence of resistance, then a third critical pharmacodynamic number will appear.

Considering the pharmacodynamic parameter AUC/MIC and correlating it to clinical cures when the target organism is *S. pneumoniae* and the drug class is quinolones, we can make two important observations. Figure 5 represents a schematic, hypothetical graph of the relationship between clinical cure rates and AUC/MIC ratio. This schematic is based upon a variant of a dose–response curve. At some point (to the right of the vertical line) a maximum clinical response is observed. Most clinical studies in humans lie within this plateau, because the usual clinical trials are designed for success and not failure. Data to complete the curve (the data to the left of the vertical line) are generally obtained from animal studies or in vitro experiments. The breakpoint (the point where the curve plateaus) is a value judgment based upon the composite of all of these data [17–19]. Our value judgment is that an AUC/MIC ratio of >30–40 is related to successful clinical outcomes. If one examines Table 3, which is derived from successful clinical studies, one can see that there are a variety of AUC/MIC ratios for total drug that correlate with successful clinical outcomes. [20]. This is expected on the basis of Fig. 5 and argues that a single AUC/MIC ratio for a particular drug class against a particular organism does not exist. If one performs a similar analysis with the same or different drug classes against different organisms, a different range of ratios will be found to correlate to acceptable clinical outcomes. This argues that although pharmacodynamic parameters are useful in determining proper dosing, they should be used as a guide rather than as absolute

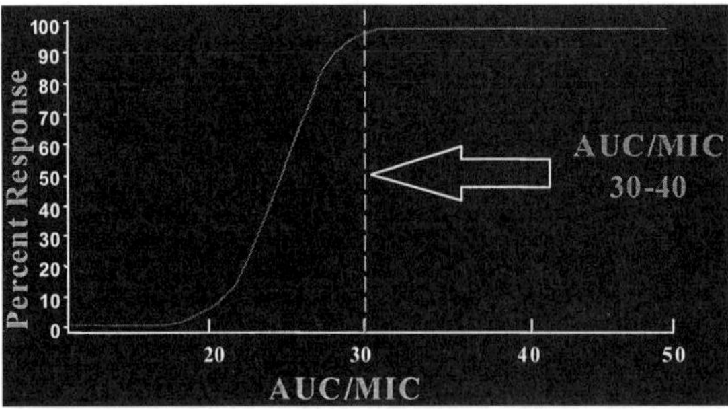

FIGURE 5 Dose–response curve for quinoloones vs. *S. pneumoniae*.

TABLE 3 Oral Quinolone Pharmacodynamics: *S. pneumoniae (Pharmacodynamic Order)*

Drug	Dose	MIC_{90}	AUC/MIC
Moxifloxacin	400 mg	0.25	142
Trovafloxacin	200 mg	0.25	138
Grepafloxacin	600 mg	0.25	90.8
Gatifloxacin	400 mg	0.5	67.8
Levofloxacin	500 mg	1	47.6
Sparfloxacin	200 mg	0.5	37.4

numbers. This concept is further strengthened by the realization that the AUC/MIC is a ratio with a numerator and a denominator. The numerator represents the AUC, but that is usually the AUC of the drug in normal, healthy volunteers. The clinical use of antibiotics is in patients, and it is the patient's AUC that should be used in the ratio. Unfortunately, this value is not readily available. The normal volunteer's AUC represents the worst-case situation, and this AUC is generally smaller than that of an actual patient. The denominator has even more error and variability associated with it. The MIC should be that of the drug and the bacteria in the host body, not in an artificial medium such as broth. Broth affords an ideal growth medium, whereas bodily fluids do not. The growth rates of organisms will be different in the body than in broth, and the interactions with the antimicrobial agents will be affected; i.e., the MIC will be different, as previously discussed. Unfortunately, it is difficult or impossible to obtain the MIC in bodily fluids; therefore we commonly use the incorrect MIC obtained in broth. A large degree of variability is associated with the usual technique of determining the MIC. Most MICs are measured using a twofold dilution technique, and one dilution to either side of the observed value is not considered to be an important or real difference. A reported MIC of 1.0 μg/mL can be 0.5, 1.0, or 2.0 μg/mL. That represents 100% variability in the reported MIC value. If the numerator is not accurate and the denominator is not accurate, then the entire ratio cannot be accurate. Reported AUC/MIC ratios are too variable to be considered absolute numbers and should be used only as guides to therapy. As a guide the MIC is very useful, but to consider it to be an absolute, infallible number is misleading and confusing.

REFERENCES

1. HP Kuemmerle, T Murakawa, CH Nightingale, eds. Pharmacokinetics of Antimicrobial Agents: Principles, Methods, Applications. Ecomed, 1993.

2. PR Murray, Editor in Chief, and EJ Baron, MA Pfaller, FC Tenover, and RH Yolken, eds. Manual of Clinical Microbiology. 6th ed. ASM Press, Washington, DC, 1995.
3. EJ Begg, BA Peddie, ST Chambers, DR Boswell. Comparison of gentamicin dosing regimens using an in-vitro model. J Antimicrob Chemother 1992;29:427–433.
4. BD Davis. Mechanism of the bactericidal action of the aminoglyocosides. Microbiol Rev 1987;51:341–350.
5. DP Nicolau, CD Freeman, PP Beleveau, CH Nightingale, JW Ross, R Quintiliani. Experience with a once-daily aminoglycoside program administered to 2,184 adult patients. Antimicrob Agents Chemother 1995;39:650–655.
6. MF Keating, GP Bodey, M. Valdivieso, V Rodriquez. A randomized comparative trial of three aminoglycosides—comparison of continuous infusions of gentamicin, amikacin, and sisomicin combined with carbenicillin in the treatment of neutropenic patients with malignancies. Medicine 1979;58:159–170.
7. RD Moore, PS Lietman, CR Smith. Clinical response to aminoglycoside therapy: Importance of the ratio of peak concentration to minimal inhibitory concentration. J Infect Dis 1987;155:93–99.
8. JE Leggett, S Ebert, B Fantin, WA Craig. Comparative dose-effect relations at several dosing intervals for beta-lactam, aminoglycoside and quinolone antibiotics against gram-negative bacilli in murine thigh-infection and pneumonitis models. Scand J Infect Dis 1991;74:179–184.
9. JE Leggett, B Fantin, S Ebert, K Totsuka, B Vogelman, W Calame, H Mattie, WA Craig. Comparative antibiotic dose-effect relations at several dosing intervals in murine pneumonitis and thigh-infection models. J Infect Dis 1989;159:281–292.
10. R Roosendaal, IAJM Bakker-Woudenberg, JC van den Berghe, MF Michel. Therapeutic efficacy of continuous versus intermittent administration of ceftazidime in an experimental Klebsiella pneumoniae pneumonia in rats. J Infect Dis 1985;156:373–378.
11. CO Onyeji, DP Nicolau, CH Nightingale, R Quintiliani. Optimal times above MICs of ceftibuten and cefaclor in experimental intra-abdominal infections. Antimicrob Agents Chemother 1994;38:1112–1117.
12. GP Bodey, SJ Ketchel, V Rodriguez. A randomized study of carbenicillin plus cefamandole or tobramycin in the treatment of febrile episodes in cancer patients. Am J Med 1979;67:608–616.
13. GP Bodey, SJ Ketchel, V Rodriguez. A randomised trial of carbenicillin plus cefamandole or tobramycin in the treatment of febrile episodes in cancer patients. Antimicrob Agents Chemother 1992;36:540–544.
14. I Lutsar, IR Friedland, L Wubbel, CC McCoig, HS Jafri, WN Ng, F Ghaffar, GH McCracken Jr. Pharmacodynamics of gatifloxacin in cerebrospinal fluid in experimental cephalosporin-resistant pneumococcal meningitis. Antimicrob Agents Chemother 1998;42:2650–2655.
15. EW Hook III, CA Horton, DR Schaberg. Failure of intensive care unit support to influence mortality from pneumococcal bacteremia. JAMA 1983;249:1055–1057.
16. WR Gransden, SJ Eykyn, I Phillips. Pneumococcal bacteremia: 325 episodes diagnosed at St. Thomas's Hospital. BMJ 1985;290:505–508.
17. PD Lister, CC Sanders. Pharmacodynamics of levofloxacin and ciprofloxacin against Streptococcus pneumoniae. J Antimicrob Chemother 1999;43:79–86.

18. Lacy M, Quintiliani R, et al. AAC 1999;43:672–677.
19. Lister P, Sanders C. AAC 1999;43:1118–1122.
20. P Ball, A Fernald, G Tillotson. Therapeutic advances of new fluoroquinolones. Exp Opin Invest Drugs 1998;7:761–783.
21. Craig WA et al. Scand J Infect Dis 1991;suppl 74.
22. Murry et al. Abstract, ICCAC meeting 1983.
23. Doern G, Pedi Infect Dis J 1995;14:420–423.

3

In Vitro Antibiotic Pharmacodynamic Models

Michael J. Rybak
Wayne State University Schools of Medicine and Pharmacy and
Detroit Receiving Hospital and University Health Center, Detroit, Michigan

George P. Allen
Wayne State University and Detroit Receiving Hospital and
University Health Center, Detroit, Michigan

Ellie Hershberger
William Beaumont Research Institute, Royal Oak, Michigan

1 INTRODUCTION

The traditional approach to in vitro assessment of antimicrobial action on organism viability has been through the use of typical susceptibility testing such as agar diffusion assay or broth dilution techniques. These tests give either a qualitative or quantitative assessment of antimicrobial activity at fixed concentrations of drug at a single point in time, usually 18–24 h. The killing curve approach allows for periodic or continuous monitoring of viable organisms after antibiotic exposure. This method significantly improves the ability to assess the interaction between antimicrobials and organisms. Factors such as the rate and extent of killing as a function of concentration can be determined. In addition, the impact of combination antibiotics can easily be evaluated. However, the major limitation of this method is the use of a fixed concentration of antibiotic throughout the experimental period. Therefore, it does not represent the clinical setting where antimicrobial concentrations continuously fluctuate as a function of delivery, penetration, metabolism and elimination.

These limitations prompted the development of antibiotic pharmacodynamic models that are capable of simulating antibiotic pharmacokinetics in the presence of viable bacteria. Controlled dilution of media containing the drug and organism inoculum is the basic function by which these dynamic models simulate antibiotic pharmacokinetics. One of the earliest attempts to use an in vitro antibiotic dynamic model system to simulate human infection was reported by Greenwood and O'Grady [1]. These investigators simulated bladder infection by using glass flasks in which the effect of antibiotics on bacteria in artificial media could be studied photometrically. Micturition was simulated by alterations in the volume and flow rate of medium so that the concentrations of organism and antibiotic in the model varied in a manner similar to in vivo infection. Although it was a very novel approach, there were a number of problems with this method, including the use of photometric analysis. The spectrophotometric method used in this experiment proved unreliable because it counted both viable and dead bacteria, and because of its dependence on light transmission through the artificial medium it was not useful for dense bacterial populations of 10^6–10^9 CFU/mL, which are often more relevant to human infection. Another inherent problem was that bacteria grew more rapidly in artificial media than was observed in urine. In subsequent models these limitations were corrected by plating and counting the number of viable bacteria over the course of the experiment and by using filtered sterilized urine as the growth medium. There remain some mechanical problems with this model, such as occasional adherence of organisms to the glass culture vessels during the washout phase and the inability to simulate cyclical variations in urine antibiotic concentrations due to renal clearance or micturition. However, these models have provided realistic simulations of the response of organism and antibiotics among patients in clinical trials [2]. In addition, the bladder model had a much higher correlation with a mouse infection protection test than did a variety of standard laboratory tests. Furthermore, conventional laboratory methods failed to predict antibiotic synergy observed in both the bladder model and mouse models [3,4].

Over the years there have been a variety of in vitro antibiotic dynamic models described in the literature that have attempted to characterize the pharmacokinetic profiles of various antibiotics while simulating an infection site. These models have ranged from simple simulations of bloodstream infections with one-compartment dynamic models to sequestered infections with more sophisticated multicompartmental approaches or hybrid systems incorporating infected tissue or cell lines. This chapter presents a description of these models and their inherent advantages and disadvantages for modeling infection and antimicrobial pharmacokinetics/pharmacodynamics.

2 ONE-COMPARTMENT MODEL

In the one-compartment model the antimicrobial agent is added to a central compartment that contains the appropriate culture medium and a known concentration of the organism. The medium inside the central compartment is then displaced via a peristaltic pump set at a fixed rate to simulate the clearance and half-life of the antibiotic (Fig. 1). This system represents a simple pharmacodynamic model that follows first order pharmacokinetics, resulting in an exponential decrease in the drug concentration. Desired pharmacokinetic drug parameters can be estimated using the equation

$$c = c_0 e^{-ket}$$

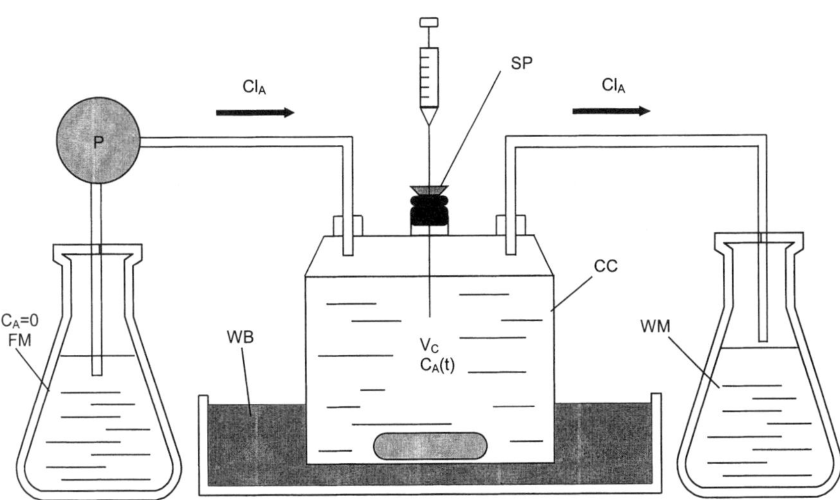

FIGURE 1 One-compartment model. The bacterial inoculum and antibiotic are introduced into the central compartment. C_A = concentration of antibiotic A, CC = central compartment, Cl_A = clearance of antibiotic A, FM = fresh medium, P = peristaltic pump, SP = sampling and injection port, V_C = volume of distribution of antibiotic A, SB = magnetic stir bar, WB = water bath (37.5°C), WM = waste medium.

where

c = antibiotic concentration
c_0 = concentration following drug administration
k_e = elimination rate constant
t = time

The elimination rate constant is defined by

$$k_e = \mathrm{Cl}/V_c \tag{1}$$

and

$$k_e = (\ln 2)/t_{1/2} \tag{2}$$

Therefore,

$$(\ln 2)/t_{1/2} = \mathrm{Cl}/V_c \tag{3}$$

Solving for Cl:

$$\mathrm{Cl} = (\ln 2)(V_c/t_{1/2}) \tag{4}$$

where

Cl = clearance
V_c = volume in the central compartment
$t_{1/2}$ = half-life of the drug

This system has the advantage of being able to simulate human kinetics by simply utilizing sterile flasks connected by tubing passed through a peristaltic pump. Because of their simplicity, one-compartment models have been used extensively throughout the years to evaluate pharmacodynamics of antimicrobial agents. Zabinski et al. [5] used a modified version of a one-compartment model previously described by Garisson and his colleagues to determine the effect of aerobic and anaerobic environments on the activities of different fluoroquinolones against staphylococci. The system used in this experiment consisted of a 1L glass vessel with inflow and outflow ports, silicone tubing, a peristaltic pump, a fresh media reservoir, and a stir hot plate (to maintain a normal body temperature of approximately 37°C). The entire system was then placed in a chamber containing an anaerobic gas mixture.

One of the disadvantages of this system is the clearance of bacteria from the central compartment along with the antibiotic. This clearance may vary significantly, depending on the half-life of the drug. For example, in an in vitro experiment using vancomycin (half-life 6 h) against *Staphylococcus aureus* (starting inoculum of 10^6 CFU/mL), an insignificant amount of organism will be lost because the doubling time of *S. aureus* is greater than the clearance of vancomycin. However, utilizing nafcillin (half-life 0.5 h) against the same isolate might overestimate the rate of kill, because its clearance rate is greater than the doubling time of *S. aureus*. Previously, membranes were used in these models to prevent the elimination of bacteria from the central compartment; however, accumulation of antibiotic on the surface of the membrane may result in the antibiotic being retained as well, thus confounding interpretation of antibiotic killing effects [6].

In an effort to circumvent the problem of bacterial dilution while preventing concomitant antibiotic retention, Navashin et al. [7] used a model that incorporated a modified membrane system that is washed continuously throughout the experiment. Their model is similar in construction to the models described above, consisting of a supply of fresh medium that is pumped into a chamber into which the bacterial inoculum is injected (Fig. 2). Medium is removed from this chamber by a second peristaltic pump; however, the medium is then eliminated through a filtration device that prevents the loss of bacteria. The filtration device includes

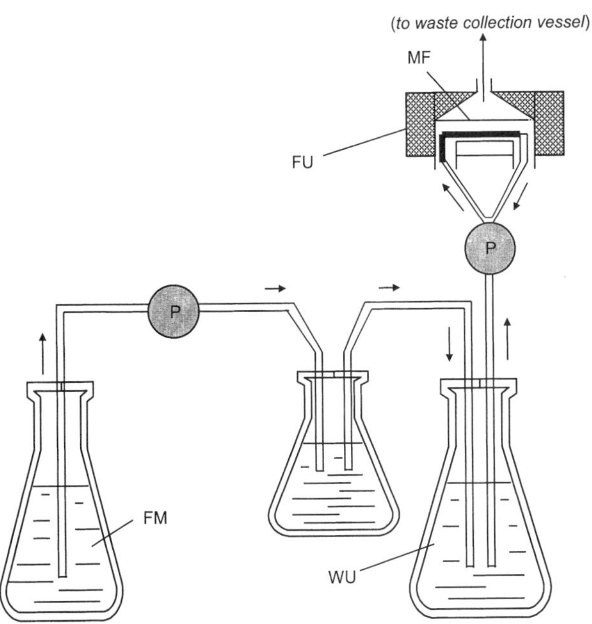

FIGURE 2 Two-compartment model with membrane-wash system. Medium is pumped from the working unit (a photometric cell) through a filtration unit designed to prevent bacterial loss. FM = fresh medium, FU = filtration unit, MF = membrane filter, P = peristaltic pump, WU = working unit of model. (Adapted from Ref. 7.)

a membrane with a pore size of 0.45 μm. To prevent blockage of this membrane with excreted antibiotic, outflow medium is continuously run over the surface of the membrane before being eliminated to a final reservoir.

In the absence of a membrane correction, the loss of bacteria becomes important when the action of an antibiotic on the bacteria is being evaluated. This is especially a problem when the activities of two drugs with considerably different half-lives are being compared. Haag et al. [8] developed differential equations to describe changes in the bacterial inoculum in the central compartment over time. Keil et al. [9] later examined these equations and developed an extension of them that can be used to compensate for the amount of bacteria being lost to the elimination rate.

The following are the equations developed by Haag and Keil, where $N(t)$ represents the number of colony-forming units per milliliter in the free medium (liquid compartment) at a given time, t; $N_B(t)$ represents the number of CFUs per milliliter in the model's biofilm layer (solid compartment) at the same time; $dN(t)/dt$ and $dN_B(t)/dt$ are the first derivatives of $N(t)$ and $N_B(t)$, respectively; k_w is the apparent bacterial growth rate constant; k_a is the rate constant for absorption of bacteria into the biofilm layer; and k_d is the rate constant for desorption of cells from the biofilm into the liquid medium [9,10]. The elimination rate constant is represented by k_e.

Assuming that k_w is the same in broth and biofilm, k_e, k_a, and k_d are constant over the course of the experiment; and $N(t)$ is far below the maximum bacterial density under nonflowing conditions, we have

$$\frac{dN(t)}{dt} = (k_w - k_e - k_a)N(t) + k_d N_B(t) \tag{5a}$$

$$\frac{dN_B(t)}{dt} = (k_w - k_d)N_B(t) + k_a N(t) \tag{5b}$$

When the bacterial culture is not diluted,

$$\frac{dN'(t)}{dt} = (k_w - k_a)N(t) + k_d N_B(t) \tag{6}$$

where $dN'(t)/dt$ describes the change in CFU/mL in an undiluted compartment over time.

The total time course of $N(t)$ is described by a second-order differential equation derived from Eqs. (5a) and (5b). Solving this equation (not shown) results in

$$N(t) = Ae^{m_1 t} + Be^{m_2 t} \tag{7}$$

and

$$A + B = N_0 \tag{8}$$

where N_0 is the initial number of CFU/mL in the model flask, $Ae^{m_1 t}$ describes the number of CFU/mL coming from the biofilm, $Be^{m_2 t}$ describes the number of CFU/mL coming from the liquid compartment, $m_1 > 0$, and $m_2 < 0$.

The factor $Be^{m_2 t}$ approaches 0 at high dilution rates and at $t = \infty$. Assuming that the development of a biofilm may be neglected ($k_e \gg k_a$ and k_d or $k_a = k_d = 0$, $A = 0$, and $B = N_0$), we arrive at

$$N'(t) = N(t)e^{k_e t} \tag{9}$$

In cases where the desorption of bacteria from the biofilm to the liquid medium far exceeds the loss of bacteria due to dilution, equation (9) becomes:

$$N'(t) = N(t)\ e^{(1/2)k_e t} \tag{10}$$

Comparison of Eqs. (9) and (10) shows that the effect of the presence of a biofilm layer on bacterial loss is compensated for by a factor f with a value between 0.5 and 1. The value of f approaches 0.5 as the influence of the biofilm is magnified. If k_e is constant throughout the course of the investigation, Eqs. (9) and (10) may be combined to give

$$N'(t) = N(t)e^{fk_e t} \tag{11}$$

If the antibiotic under study displays two different elimination rate constants for the α and β phases, the above equations must be altered. Assuming that there is no biofilm in the model flasks, manipulation of these equations results in

$$N'(t) = N(t)e^{\Sigma k_{ei}\Delta t_i} \tag{12}$$

where Δt_i and k_{ei} represent any number of time periods Δt, and their corresponding elimination rate constants k_e. If there is a biofilm present, we arrive at the equation

$$N'(t) = N(t)e^{(1/2)\Sigma(k_{ei}\Delta t_i)} \tag{13}$$

Combining Eqs. (12) and (13) gives

$$N'(t) = N(t)e^{f\Sigma(k_{ei}\Delta t_i)} \tag{14}$$

Again, the value of f is between 0.5 and 1. Equation (14) is valid only as long as bacteria are in the logarithmic phase of growth. For cultures approaching the stationary phase of growth the following equation is valid:

$$N'(t) = N_{\max} \frac{N(t)}{\{N(t) + [N_{\max} - N(t)]e^{-k_e t}\}} \tag{15}$$

Where there is an influence of biofilms and a variable k_e, the following equation should be used:

$$N'(t) = N_{\max} \frac{N(t)}{\{N(t) + [N_{\max} - N(t)]e^{-f\Sigma(k_{ei}\Delta t_i)}} \tag{16}$$

where the value of f is again between 0.5 and 1.

Keil and Wiedemann [9] evaluated the validity of these equations in a study of continuous infusions of meropenem with steady-state concentrations of 2.5–7.5 μg/mL against *Pseudomonas aeruginosa* and *Escherichia coli*. The resulting kill curves were compared to kill curves obtained from incubation of these bacteria in a static system with meropenem at constant concentrations of 2.5–7.5 μg/mL. Thus, the sole difference between experiments was the presence of dilution.

Equation (9) can be used to correct for bacterial loss when the duration of study does not exceed 8 h. However, results of Keil and Wiedemann's study revealed that Eq. (15) should be used when the duration of the experiment exceeds 12 h [9]. In addition, using a value of 1 for f results in kill curves representing the worst-case scenario, so that the antibacterial effect is not overestimated. Unfortunately, this study additionally showed that individual corrections must be performed for different bacterial species and model apparatuses.

Routine application of the above mathematical equations may prove to be cumbersome. The inclusion of growth control experiments, studying bacterial growth in the absence of antibiotic, can also help to address the severity of the problem of bacterial dilution. A typical growth curve is set to simulate the half-life of the antibiotic under study. To compensate for bacterial loss, the killing activity of the antibiotic can be compared to the growth control curve.

3 TWO-COMPARTMENT MODEL

The two-compartment model simulates biexponential pharmacokinetics following intravenous administration. Murakawa et al. [11] designed a model representing the central and peripheral compartments connected by tubing. This model consists of a central compartment that contains the antibiotic and organism. Medium constantly flows into this central compartment. Medium is then pumped from the central compartment to a peripheral compartment (free of antibiotic) and is subsequently pumped back into the central compartment via a second peristaltic pump. Finally, it is pumped out of the central compartment to a reservoir for bacterial counts. As with the one-compartment model, this system allows the organism to be pumped out of the central compartment; therefore, dilution of the organism according to the half-life of the antibiotic is a potential problem. An alternative design of the typical two-compartment model places the peripheral compartment within the central compartment (Fig. 3). The bacteria under study are placed into this inner chamber, and antibiotic is administered into the central compartment. The antibiotic may diffuse into the peripheral compartment, but bacteria are trapped within that compartment.

In an attempt to mimic drug concentration profiles in tissue versus serum, Zinner et al. [12] devised a model that uses a single capillary unit device as a system for studying antimicrobial effects (29). Later, Blaser et al. [13] chose a two-compartment capillary model that uses a series of artificial capillary units representing extravascular infection sites (Fig. 4). The Zinner and Blaser models can simulate human pharmacokinetics in interstitial fluid for one or two antibiotics. Each of the models uses an artificial capillary (dialysis) unit connected by silicone tubing to a peristaltic pump and a culture medium reservoir. A sampling port with a bidirectional stopcock is inserted into the tubing and allows injection

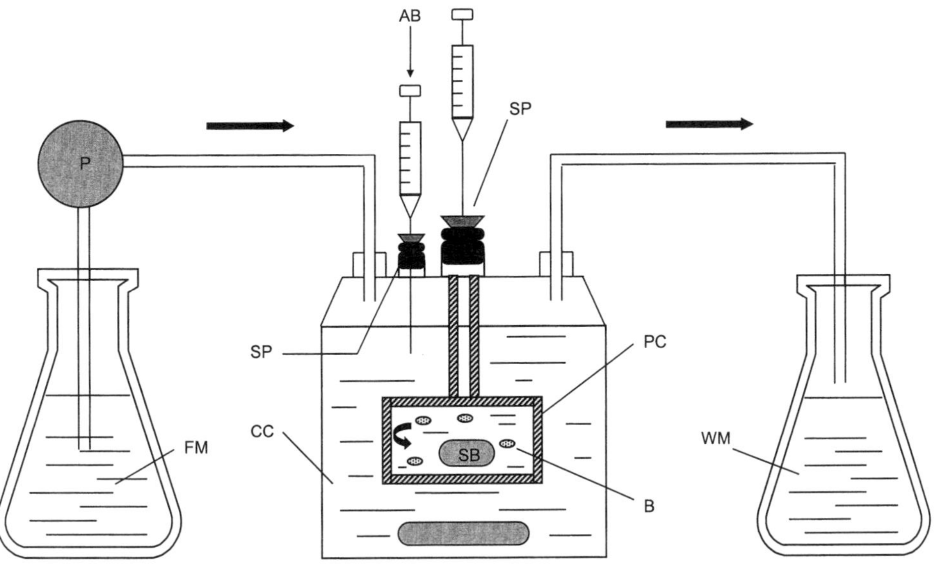

FIGURE 3 Two-compartment model. Bacteria are introduced into the peripheral compartment and are unable to pass into the central compartment (illustrated by heavy arrow). Antibiotic is injected into the central compartment. AB = antibiotic, B = bacteria, CC = central compartment, FM = fresh medium, PC = peripheral compartment, SB = magnetic stir bar, SP = sampling and injection port, WM = water medium. (Adapted from Ref. 22.)

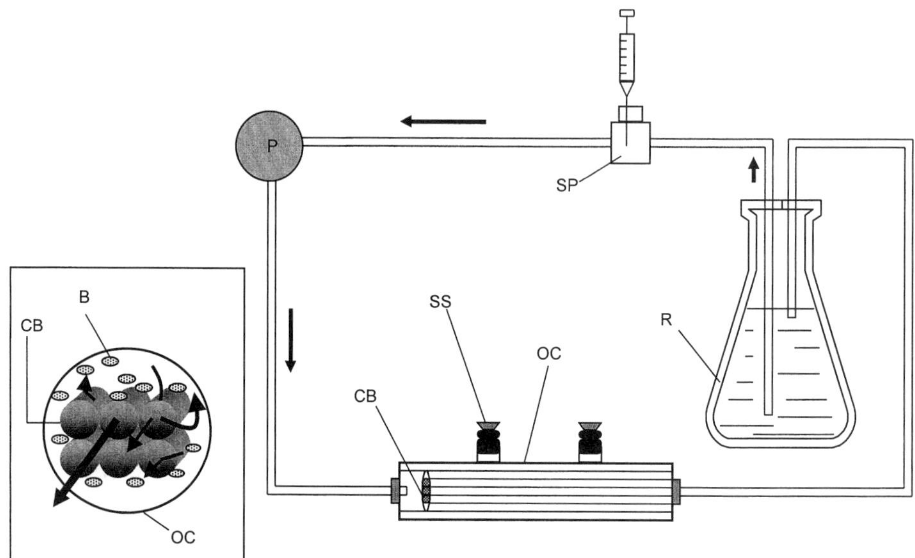

Figure 4 Two-compartment capillary model. The capillary device (dialyzer) is pictured at the bottom of the illustration. Inset shows a cross section of the capillary bundle. Medium flow through the bundle is represented by the heavy arrow. Bacteria are trapped in the outer compartment of the bundle, while antibiotic (light arrows) flow through the dialysis membranes. B = bacteria, CB = capillary bundle, OC = outer compartment, P = peristaltic pump, R = reservoir, SP = sampling and injection port, SS = sampling site (septum fittings). (Adapted from Ref. 12.)

of antibiotics either toward the capillary unit (bolus injection) or toward the medium reservoir (for continuous infusion dosing simulations).

Each capillary unit consists of two chambers: an outer chamber or culture tube and an inner chamber that comprises a bundle of 150 hollow polysulfone fibers. Each fiber (''capillary'') has an internal diameter of 200 μm and a wall thickness of 50–75 μm. In the study reported by Zinner and his colleagues, the capillaries used retained proteins of a size greater than 10,000 daltons. However, additional capillary units are available that retain proteins of sizes greater than 50,000 or 100,000 daltons. The entire capillary bundle is secured by silicone O-rings, which seal the outer chamber (extracapillary space) from the lumens of the capillary tubes.

An inoculum of bacteria is introduced into the outer chamber of the capillary system. Meanwhile, the antibiotic under study is injected into the silicone tubing and allowed to diffuse either directly to the capillary unit (to simulate intravenous bolus dosing) or indirectly through the medium reservoir (thus simulating a continuous infusion dosing strategy). Because bacteria do not diffuse out of the extracapillary space, this model simulates an infected tissue site. Depending on the molecular size of the antibiotic used and the permeability characteristics of the capillary tubing, antibiotic diffuses into the extracapillary space from the capillary tubing. Again, because the concentration of antibiotic obtained at the site where bacteria are present will be lower than that in the capillary tubing, this system allows simulation of the treatment of infections at tissue sites.

This model allows the study of a variety of pharmacokinetic and pharmacodynamic parameters, including the effects on bacterial killing of bolus dosing versus continuous infusions of antibiotics. In addition, the effects of single or combined agents can be assessed, and the model allows simulation of the fluctuations in concentrations that typically occur after dosing in humans. Furthermore, the model avoids the problem of bacterial dilution, as the volume of bacteria in the extracapillary space is not significantly changed during the experiment. However, controlled variation of antibiotic concentrations in the two chambers of this model may be difficult, given the variability inherent in relying on the diffusion of drugs through the walls of the capillary tubes.

Blaser et al. [13] compared the pharmacokinetics of netilmicin obtained in a two-compartment capillary model to those obtained in an experimental skin suction blister model in healthy volunteers. Netilmicin was administered according to two dosage schemes in the capillary model in order to achieve peak concentrations of 16 or 24 μg/mL. In the human blister model, netilmicin was given as an intramuscular injection of 2 mg/kg (lean body weight). The in vitro model demonstrated linear two-compartment pharmacokinetics. Peak concentrations obtained were higher than nominal for the central compartment and lower than nominal for the peripheral compartment. One hour after the end of a 60 min infusion, netilmicin concentrations were equivalent in the central and peripheral compartments. Overall, concentrations obtained in the in vitro model approximated those obtained in the human blister model (Fig. 5). Thus, this capillary model successfully simulates human pharmacokinetics.

4 COMBINATION THERAPY MODEL

In vitro models can also be used to simultaneously study the activity of two drugs with different half-lives in combination. Blaser [14] described the procedures for simulating combination therapy, using both one- and two-compartment models. In these models both drugs are placed in the central compartment and the clearance pump rate is set to simulate the half-life of the drug with the shorter half-life (Cl_A, drug A) (Fig. 6). A supplemental compartment is used to replace the

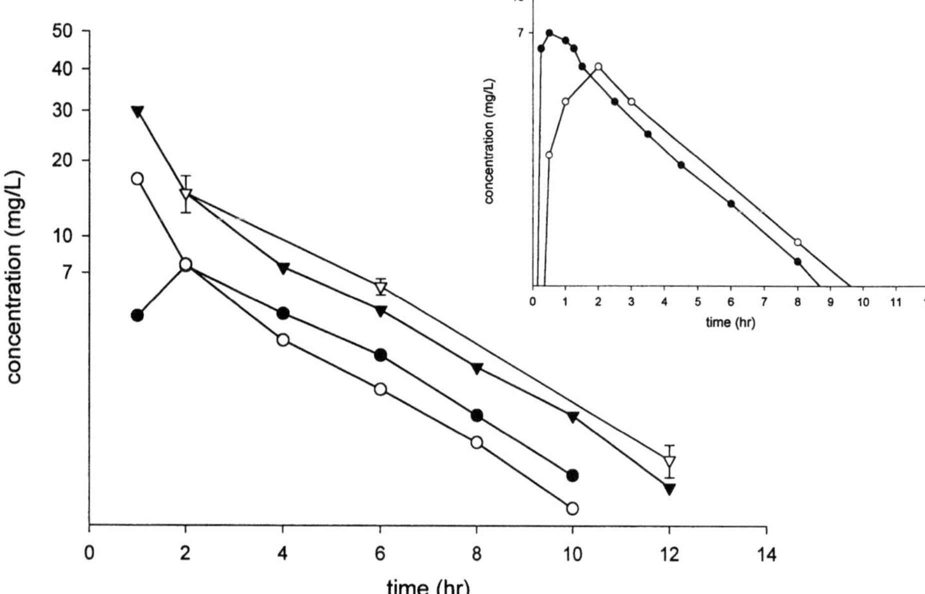

Figure 5 Comparison of in vitro and human models. Netilmicin concentrations in the central and peripheral compartments of an in vitro two-compartment capillary unit model are shown. The 2 sets of curves represent netilmicin concentrations after administration of infusions attaining peak concentrations of either 16 or 20 mg/L. The insert graph illustrates serum (●) and suction blister (○) netilmicin pharmacokinetics after administration in healthy human volunteers. Comparison of the main and insert graphs illustrates the similarity in pharmacokinetics between the in vitro and human models. (Adapted from Ref. 7.)

antibiotic with the longer half-life (drug B), which has been overeliminated. The pump rate for the supplemental compartment (Cl_S) is set to make up the difference between the clearance of the two drugs:

$$Cl_S = Cl_A - Cl_B$$

To maintain the same concentration of drug B in both compartments, the central and supplemental compartments should be dosed in a similar manner.

Meanwhile, drug-free medium is pumped into the central compartment so that the total amount of medium pumped into the system (M_{in}) equals the total volume of medium being pumped out of the system (M_{out}):

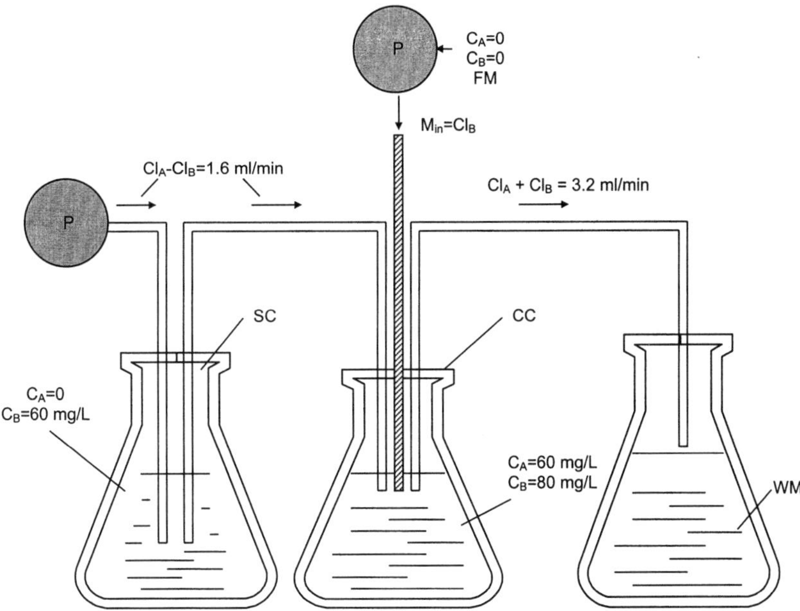

FIGURE 6 Combination therapy model. In this example, drug B is added from a supplemental chamber to the central reaction flask. C_A = concentration of drug A, C_B = concentration of drug B, CC = central compartment, Cl_A = clearance of drug A, Cl_B = clearance of drug B, FM = fresh medium, M_{in} = rate of inflow of fresh medium, P = peristaltic pump, SC = supplemental compartment, WM = waste medium. (Adapted from Ref. 14.)

$$M_{in} = Cl_A - Cl_S$$

Therefore; the pump rate for the drug free medium should be set as Cl_B.

The advantage of this system is that it can be used to determine synergistic, additive, or antagonistic effects of combinations of antibiotics simulating the actual pharmacokinetics of each agent. For example, Houlihan et al. [15] evaluated the activity of vancomycin alone and in combination with gentamicin against methicillin-resistant *Staphylococcus aureus*–infected fibrin–platelet clots in an infection model. Vancomycin was dosed at intervals of 6, 12, and 24 h, and gentamicin was given either as a single daily (every 24 h) dose or every 12 h. In plots of the bacterial inoculum versus time, synergism was defined as a >2 log increase in killing associated with a combination regimen in comparison to the most active single agent.

In preliminary fractional inhibitory concentration (FIC) testing, the combination of vancomycin and gentamicin displayed indifference. However, in the pharmacodynamic model, several combinations (e.g., vancomycin every 24 h + gentamicin every 24 h) demonstrated a synergistic effect. Thus, results from use of a static system (FIC testing) were not predictive of results obtained from a model where simulation of human pharmacokinetics is achieved. Blaser et al. [16] obtained similar results in a study of ceftazidime-netilmicin combinations against *Pseudomonas aeruginosa.* Using a two-compartment capillary model, synergism was noted for the combination against certain strains in the initial (4, 6, and 8 h) and final (24, 26, and 28 h) periods of evaluation. Synergism testing using the FIC method was predictive of the response seen in the in vitro model during the initial period only. This serves to reinforce the fact that results obtained from traditional susceptibility methodologies may not correlate with relationships seen with the use of pharmacodynamic models where in vivo pharmacokinetics are simulated.

5 BIOFILM-CATHETER MODEL

Nickel et al. [17] used a modified Robbins device to study the ability of tobramycin to penetrate a biofilm layer of *Pseudomonas aeruginosa.* The model consisted of a 41.5 cm long acrylic block with a 2 × 10 mm inner lumen and 25 evenly distributed sampling ports. The block was connected via tubing to a reservoir that was immersed in a 37°C water bath. Medium containing the bacterium under study was pumped from this reservoir (simulated bladder) through the modified Robbins device (simulated catheter) at a rate of 60 mL/h. The medium used consisted of artificial urine supplemented with nutrient broth. Discs cut from a commercially available catheter were suspended within the model and could be removed for analysis.

In the study performed by Nickel et al. a biofilm of *Pseudomonas aeruginosa* was formed by passing medium containing logarithmic-phase organisms through the model for 8 h. Formation of the biofilm was verified by examination of catheter surfaces using scanning electron microscopy (SEM) and epifluorescence microscopy. After the 8 h colonization period, medium was removed and transferred to flasks for subsequent exposure of these organisms to varying concentrations of tobramycin for a period of 8 or 12 h. Antibiotic-containing medium was then pumped through the model, and discs of catheter material were removed at 8 and 12 h intervals for determination of colony counts and microscopic examination. Thus, the killing of organisms in the sessile (biofilm) and planktonic states could be compared, as could the MICs and MBCs of these organisms. This model therefore allows study of the development of resistance among organisms in a biofilm and of the ability of antibiotics to penetrate the biofilm layer and exert an antimicrobial effect.

Walker et al. [18] developed an alternative form of the above model that consisted of a typical one-compartment vessel with plugged catheter segments (1.27 cm each) suspended within the chamber. Catheter material was inoculated with 5×10^6 CFU/mL of each organism, and counts of sessile and planktonic bacteria were performed using standard plate dilution and SEM. This model was used to test the antiadherence characteristics of various catheter coatings and impregnations.

Prosser et al. [19] developed a simplified adaptation of these models. In this model, 0.5 cm^2 discs composed of silicon latex catheter material were spotted with 80 μL of a bacterial suspension (confirmed to possess an optical density of 0.8 at 540 nm). Discs were then incubated for 1 h, washed with a buffer solution, and then transferred to broth-containing Petri dishes and incubated for an additional 20–22 h. The discs were then rewashed in buffer and placed in plain or antibiotic-containing broth, incubated for 4 h, washed, and resuspended in broth (with or without antibotic). This procedure was repeated at 8 and 24 h. At each time interval, surface film on all discs was scraped off into 5 mL of saline, and samples were plated for colony count determinations. Samples were also examined by light microscopy and SEM. One advantage of this model lies in the fact that planktonic bacteria are not contained within the model, so inactivation of antibiotic by these planktonic organisms does not occur. In addition, this model may be less cumbersome to operate than the modifed Robbins device.

6 INFECTED FIBRIN CLOT MODEL

One modification of a one-compartment model is the infected fibrin clot model developed by Rybak et al. [15,20], which uses fibrin clots to simulate a deep sequestered infection such as those associated with cardiac vegetations (Fig. 7). Fibrin clots made of human cryoprecipitate, organisms, and platelets (250,000–500,000 platelets per clot) are placed in 1.5 mL Eppendorf tubes. Bovine thrombin (5000 units) is then added to each tube, after insertion of a sterile monofilament line into the mixture. Each clot is then inserted into a sterile reaction vessel and removed at various time points for determination of bacterial counts. This model has been used to evaluate the activity of antimicrobial agents against organisms embedded in a simulated human tissue. With the incorporation of platelets and high inoculum of bacteria (10^9 CFU/g) the fibrin clots represent conditions of simulated endocardial vegetations (SEVs). The system does not consist of an airtight compartment; therefore, it requires two peristaltic pumps to pump the medium into and out of the central compartment. The SEVs have been shown to be viable in the models for up to 144 h.

Several studies have been performed to compare this model to an in vivo rabbit model of endocarditis. McGrath et al. [20] indirectly compared the results obtained from this model to those of a rabbit model of endocarditis done previously. They evaluated the effect of teicoplanin on colony-forming units (CFUs)

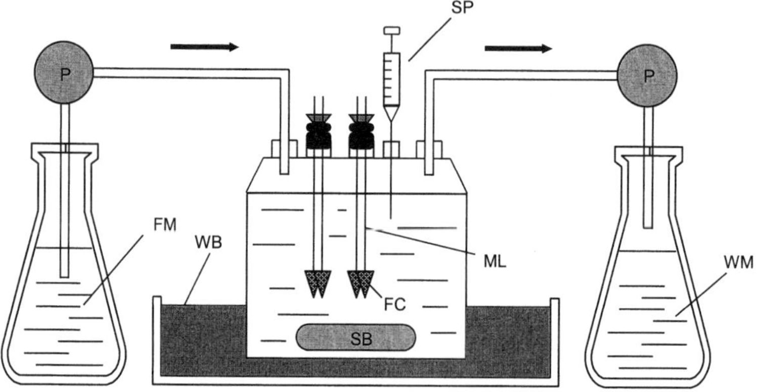

FIGURE 7 Fibrin clot model. Simulated fibrin clots or endocardial vegetations are suspended within the central compartment. The bacterial inoculum is introduced into this central compartment. FC = simulated fibrin clots, FM = fresh medium, ML = monofilament lines, P = peristaltic pump, SB = magnetic stir bar, SP = sampling and injection port, WB = water bath (37.5°C), WM = waste medium. (Adapted from Ref. 20.)

per gram of SEV in the model, using human pharmacokinetics, to the CFU/g of rabbit vegetations. This study demonstrated that the CFU/g of SEV were similar to those of the rabbit vegetations; however, the pharmacokinetics of teicoplanin varied between the two models, and samples were obtained at different time points for analysis.

A more recent study has retrospectively compared the simulated endocardial vegetation model to four different rabbit studies [10]. In this study authors compared the activities of four different fluoroquinolones—ciprofloxacin, clinafloxacin, sparfloxacin, and trovafloxacin—against various *Staphylococcus aureus* and enterococcal isolates, simulating pharmacokinetics obtained in the rabbit model. Models were conducted in the same fashion as the rabbits were treated, and SEVs were evaluated at the same time points as those at which the rabbit vegetations were assessed. The bacterial inocula in the SEVs were similar to those achieved in the rabbits' vegetations, prior to and following treatment, suggesting that this model may have a role in initial studies of antibiotics in the treatment of bacterial endocarditis (Fig. 8). To further define the model's role in the treatment of endocarditis, prospective studies comparing the in vitro model to rabbit models of endocarditis using various pathogens and antimicrobial agents are necessary.

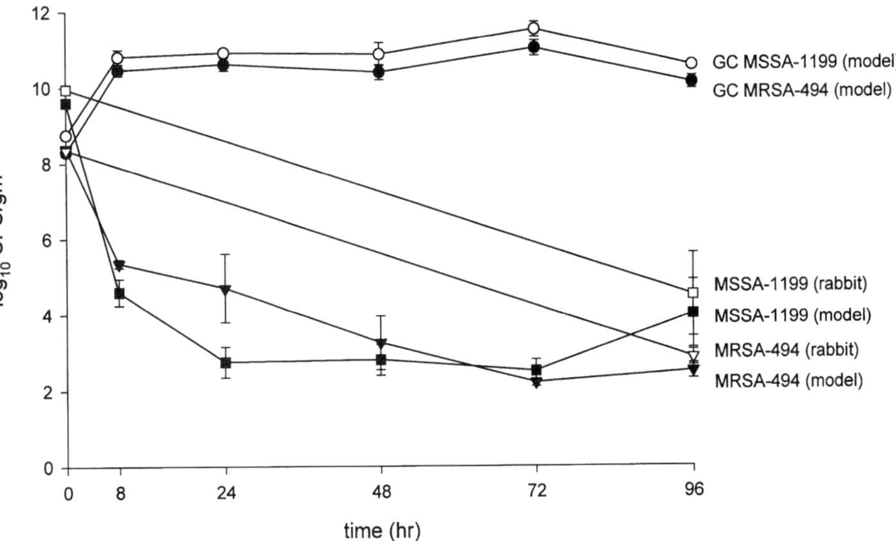

Figure 8 Comparison of in vitro and animal models. The activity of clinafloxacin against strains of methicillin-resistant (MRSA-494) and -susceptible (MSSA -1199) *Staphylococcus aureus* is illustrated in the graph. Bacterial killing observed with in vitro ("model") and animal ("rabbit") models of endocarditis are shown for each organism. Similarities between the animal and in vitro models in terms of the change in bacterial inoculum and final inoculum value (at 98 hours) may be seen. (Adapted from Ref. 16.)

7 IN VITRO MODEL OF INTRACELLULAR PATHOGENS

The previously mentioned models evaluate the activity of antibiotics against extracellular pathogens. However, many pathogens such as *Salmonella* spp., *Shigella* spp., *Campylobacter* spp., *Escherichia coli*, *Proteus mirabilis*, *Listeria monocytogenes*, *Haemophilus influenzae*, group B streptococci, and *Helicobacter pylori* can survive intracellularly, thereby escaping antimicrobial treatment. Certain antimicrobial agents such as azithromycin and clarithromycin possess intracellular activity, and an in vitro model can be a valuable tool in determining such activity. Several in vitro models, using different cell types, have been employed to determine intracellular activity of antimicrobial agents; however, continuous exposure to a fixed concentration of antibiotic does not reflect human pharmacokinetics.

Hultén et al. [21] have designed an in vitro model to study the intracellular activity of antimicrobial agents by simulating human pharmacokinetics (Fig. 9). In this model a human epithelial cell line is grown in the appropriate medium and seeded into cell culture inserts containing a 0.45 μm membrane. Inserts are exposed to a fixed concentration of the bacteria and incubated for several hours to allow the bacteria to penetrate into the cells. Extracellular bacteria are then removed, and inserts are placed in a metal rack that is fixed on a glass chamber connected to a pump simulating pharmacokinetics of the antibiotic. Inserts are removed, at various time points, and cells are processed and lysed prior to determination of bacterial inoculum. This model was used previously to determine the intracellular activity of amoxicillin, clarithromycin, and amoxicillin against *H. pylori*. This model was also used to evaluate the activity of different agents against *Mycobacterium tuberculosis* [21].

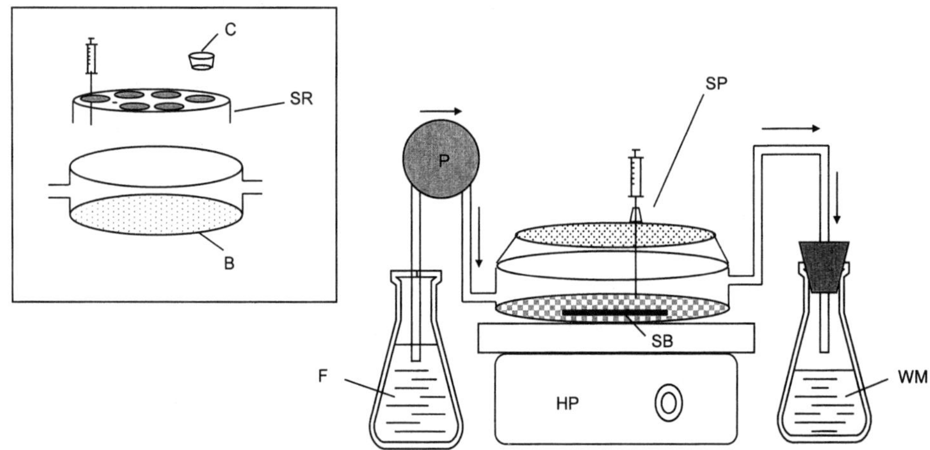

FIGURE 9 Intracellular pathogen model. Medium is pumped through the central compartment (glass chamber) at a rate to simulate antibiotic pharmacokinetics. Inset shows a cross section of the central compartment, with cell culture inserts suspended within a metal rack. B = bottom section of central compartment, CC = cell culture insert, FM = fresh medium, HP = hot plate (37.5°C), P = peristaltic pump, SB = magnetic stir bar, SP = sampling and injection port, SR = stainless steel rack, WM = waste medium. (Adapted from Ref. 21.)

8 LIMITATIONS OF IN VITRO MODELS

Although the in vitro models described in this chapter are widely used in the study of antimicrobial pharmacokinetics and pharmacodynamics, certain limitations to their use must be noted. The applicability of results obtained from in vitro models to the treatment of infections in vivo is limited by the factors described below.

8.1 Effects of the Immune System

The majority of in vitro models commonly used are devoid of immune system factors; that is, antimicrobial effects are studied in an environment that does not contain the host defense factors. The antimicrobial effect may thus be underestimated, because organisms are free from the inhibitory action of such immune system factors as leukocytosis, phagocytosis, and immunoglobulins.

Shah [22] employed a model that incorporated fresh human blood from healthy volunteers in an effort to replicate in vivo immune system effects. The model consisted of a glass chamber (similar to the one-compartment model previously described) with an inner cell suspended within. The inner cell, composed of plexiglass, was enclosed at each end with membrane filters designed to allow diffusion of antibiotics. Heparinized human blood was incorporated into the inner chamber, and the outer chamber contained a nutrient medium. The bacterial inoculum was injected into the inner chamber, and antibiotics were administered into the outer vessel.

Use of this model in a study of imipenem against *Escherichia coli*, *Klebsiella pneumoniae*, and *Pseudomonas aeruginosa* revealed that in the presence of blood alone, the bacterial count was reduced by 90–99%, but in all cases bacterial regrowth was noted. As expected, addition of antibiotic decreased the time to achieve 99% reduction of the bacterial inoculum, and the final bacterial count was decreased in comparison to that obtained in antibiotic-free models. Although the use of blood as a medium allowed incorporation of some aspects of the human immune system, the full range of host defense factors was not included in the model.

Incorporation of blood as a medium into in vitro models has not been widely employed, most likely due to the logistical concerns of working with human blood. However, it should be noted that the lack of an immune system in typical in vitro models is advantageous in some respects, in that the effect of antibiotic exposure alone on the development of bacterial resistance may be measured. Also, results from in vitro models lacking immune system effects may be satisfactorily applied to infection occurring in neutropenic hosts, although, again, not without some concerns over the clinical applicability of these results.

8.2 Altered Bacterial Growth Characteristics

Multiple investigations have confirmed that the behavior of bacteria in an in vitro environment is not equivalent to that in vivo. Microorganisms grown in vitro differ from those causing in vivo infection with respect to factors discussed in the following paragraphs.

8.2.1 Virulence

It has been noted in numerous experiments that bacterial virulence is progressively diminished with serial in vitro passage or cultivation [23]. The cause of this is unknown, but it may be due in part to adherence factors or derangements in biochemical pathways. The result of this loss of pathogenicity is potentially an overestimation of the effect of a given antimicrobial in an infection model. However, this reduction in virulence may be strain-specific, so the impact on clinical application of in vitro experimental results may be unclear.

8.2.2 Morphology

Bacteria adapt to life in a blood environment and undergo such morphological changes as encapsulation and mucus production [24]. Thus, bacteria in vivo possess an enhanced resistance to killing by serum factors. In vitro, these alterations in morphology are unstable, and organisms rapidly revert to a normal morphology. Thus, the effect of an antimicrobial in an infection model may be overestimated because the above-described morphological defense factors are absent.

8.2.3 Physiology

Microorganisms are known to rapidly develop adaptively to a variety of environments, possibly as a result of metabolic changes. In an in vitro environment, bacteria differ from those cultivated in vivo in terms of amino acid composition, the synthesis of toxic metabolites, and metabolic rate [24]. Overall, bacteria are more metabolically active in vivo than in vitro. However, replication generally occurs more rapidly in an in vitro environment, possibly due to the lack of immune system effects. For example, it has been shown that the typical growth rate of microorganisms in an in vivo animal model of infection may be on the order of 0.02–0.05 h^{-1}, wheras the growth rate in an in vitro batch culture may approach 2–3 h^{-1} [25]. Continuous culture of microorganisms, which allows precise control of growth rate, may allow maintenance of microorganisms in a state of growth more closely approximating that of organisms in the natural state [25].

In addition to changes in growth characteristics, differences in expression and/or structure of outer membrane proteins may occur such that microorganisms in vitro display reduced permeability. These effects are dependent on the composition of the nutrient medium used in model experiments. For example, the structure and composition of the outer membrane proteins of *Escherichia coli* may be altered by changes in growth medium and temperature as well as by the molecular size and osmolarity of sugars contained in the growth medium [24].

The overall effect of the above physiological changes on the applicability of results obtained from in vitro models is variable and may be difficult to determine. These alterations may be highly strain-specific, so general conclusions regarding methods to account for these changes are lacking.

8.2.4 Sensitivity to Serum Factors

As noted above, morphological changes of bacteria in vivo lead to a reduced susceptibility of those organisms to serum immune factors. For example, bacteria cultured in vitro display an enhanced susceptibility to phagocytosis [26]. Therefore, use of models incorporating, for example, human blood as a medium may fail to adequately account for immune effects, because the bacterial strain may be more susceptible to the effects of immune mediators than it would be in vivo.

8.3 Microorganism Viability

Certain organisms are difficult to work with in in vitro systems because of viability problems that are not apparent in vivo. For example, it is difficult to keep *Streptococcus pneumoniae* viable for periods longer than 12 h, because of the stationary-phase autolytic process that is common to this species. For this reason, in vitro killing curves obtained in test tubes do not usually exceed 6–12 h, so organism death can be correctly attributed to antibiotic effects rather than to autolytic processes.

In an in vitro infection model investigation, Cappelletty et al. [27] demonstrated that the viability of *S. pneumoniae* during growth control experiments is directly affected by the clearance of growth medium through the model. Simulations of antibiotics with longer half-lives were more likely to result in a slower rate of medium turnover, thus increasing the likelihood of autolysis induction. This serves to reinforce the idea that growth control experiments without antibiotic must always be performed to ensure that organism viability is optimal [27].

8.4 Effects of Protein Binding on Antimicrobial Action

Because plasma protein is usually not included in the nutrient broth medium, the effects of protein binding of antimicrobials may not be measured. For example, the antibacterial effect of drugs that are highly bound by plasma proteins may be overestimated in models where such protein binding is not replicated, because concentrations of the drug in the model will exceed those obtained in vivo. However, incorporation of protein, such as human albumin, may allow simulation of the free-drug concentrations that will be obtained after dosing in humans. For example, Garrison et al. [28] assessed the effects of physiological concentrations (3.8–4.2%) of human albumin on the activity of daptomycin and vancomycin against *Staphylococcus aureus*. Albumin was directly incorporated into the two-compartment in vitro model. It was found that the presence of albumin significantly diminished the bactericidal activity (as measured by kill rate and time to 99% kill) of both daptomycin (low- and high-dose regimens) and vancomycin. Rather than include protein in a model, if one knows the degree to which an antibiotic is bound to proteins one may simply dose in such a way as to simulate free concentrations that will be obtained in the presence of protein. This strategy is desirable because of the excessive cost associated with the use of albumin and other proteins in pharmacodynamic models.

8.5 Bacterial Adherence

In a study conducted by Haag et al., in vitro models with no dilution and/or elimination of growth medium (growth control) were compared to models where the addition and elimination of medium took place (addition and elimination were set to occur at the same rate). The investigators expected that, given a dilution rate higher than the bacterial growth rate, an artificial decrease in bacterial counts due to dilution of organisms would be observed. However, they instead noted that an *increase* in colony-forming units occurred after 1–2 h of simulation [8]. This phenomenon was ascribed to the presence of a subpopulation of bacteria that adhered to the inner surfaces of the model in a biofilm layer. It is thought that bacteria residing within the biofilm resist dilution but that a certain proportion of bacteria diffuse into the medium at a quantifiable rate.

As a result of this phenomenon, the effect of an antibiotic on cells in the liquid medium may be measured only in the early stages of an experiment. After this time, as the biofilm layer forms, the effect of the agent on the nondilutable adherent population is measured instead. Because organisms in this subpopulation typically display reduced antimicrobial susceptibility, the effect of the agent under study may be underestimated [8]. On the other hand, the effect of an agent on bacteria residing within sequestered sites of infection may be more reliably determined.

Attempts have been made to prevent bacterial adherence to model surfaces. For example, Gwynn et al. [29] found that siliconization of their model prevented the eventual increase in bacterial counts. It was postulated that the silicone's prevention of the formation of an adherent population was responsible for this effect. However, others have been unable to replicate these findings. Bacterial adherence may also depend on the geometry of vessels making up the model and on the material from which models are constructed.

8.6 Dilutionary Artifacts

Although in vitro models incorporating dilution (i.e., addition and elimination of medium at a rate to simulate the half-lives of antibiotics) more closely replicate the dosing of drugs in humans, dilution of the bacterial inoculum is a problem associated with these models. Such dilution (elimination) of microorganisms will result in an overestimation of the killing effect of an agent being studied. As described previously, investigators have employed a variety of strategies to overcome this effect, including construction of models that prevent elimination of bacteria, the use of static models in which dilution does not occur, and compensation for the effects of dilution by the use of mathematical correction [9].

8.7 Other Effects

In addition to the above limitations associated with in vitro modeling, problems may also arise during attempts to interpret results obtained from models incorporating either very highly or minimally bactericidal agents. With highly bactericidal antibiotics possessing an extended elimination half-life, complete eradication of bacteria to the limit of assay detection will rapidly occur. In this scenario, the extent of measurable effects of varying drug dosages will be minimized. In contrast, in models in which an agent with minimal bactericidal activity and a short elimination half-life is used, organism regrowth will rapidly overwhelm the model. The effect of regrowth is unknown, especially in light of the fact that organisms that regrow do not undergo changes in antimicrobial susceptibility. Again, the result of this phenomenon is that effects of the antimicrobial under study are difficult to measure.

9 SUMMARY

In vitro antibiotic pharmacodynamic models represent a significant advancement in the assessment of antimicrobial pharmacodynamics. The ability to simulate human pharmacokinetics while evaluating the effect of an antibiotic on viable bacteria is clearly superior to more traditional assessments such as basic susceptibility testing or kill-curve experiments performed in test tubes. These models are adaptable to a variety of conditions, allowing for evaluations of different organisms, environmental conditions, dosing schemes, combination therapies, or resistance mechanisms. Preliminary information suggests that results obtained from certain dynamic models correlate with those found in vivo. Although there are a number of limitations to the use and applicability of these models, they continue to evolve and are likely to add to our overall understanding of antimicrobial and microorganism interactions.

REFERENCES

1. D Greenwood, F O'Grady. Potent combinations of beta-lactam antibiotics using the beta-lactamase inhibition principle. Chemotherapy 1975;21:330–341.

2. JD Anderson, KR Johnson, MY Aird. Comparison of amoxicillin and ampicillin activities in a continuous culture model of the human urinary bladder. Antimicrob Agents Chemother 1980;17:554–557.
3. JD Anderson. Relevance of urinary bladder models to clinical problems and to antibiotic evaluation. J Antimicrob Chemother 1985;15(suppl A):111–115.
4. JD Anderson, F Eftekhar, R Cleeland, MJ Kramer, G Beskid. Comparative activity of mecillinam and ampicillin singly and in combination in the urinary bladder model and experimental mouse model. J Antimicrob Chemother 1981;8:121–131.
5. RA Zabinski, KJ Walker, AJ Larsson, JA Moody, GW Kaatz, JC Rotschafer. Effect of aerobic and anaerobic environments on antistaphylococcal activities of five fluoroquinolones. Antimicrob Agents Chemother 1995;39:507–512.
6. J Blaser, BB Stone, MC Groner, SH Zinner. Comparative study with enoxacin and netilmicin in a pharmacodynamic model to determine importance of ratio of peak antibiotic concentration to MIC for bactericidal activity and emergence of resistance. Antimicrob Agents Chemother 1987;31:1054–1060.
7. SM Navashin, IP Fomina, AA Firsov, VM Chernykh, SM Kuznetsova. A dynamic model for in-vitro evaluation of antimicrobial action by simulation of the pharmacokinetic profiles of antibiotics. J Antimicrob Chemother 1989;23:389–399.
8. R Haag, P Lexa, I Werkhäuser. Artifacts in dilution pharmacokinetic models caused by adherent bacteria. Antimicrob Agents Chemother 1986;29:765–768.
9. S Keil, B Wiedemann. Mathematical corrections for bacterial loss in pharmacodynamic in vitro dilution models. Antimicrob Agents Chemother 1995;39:1054–1058.
10. E Hershberger, EA Coyle, GW Kaatz, MJ Zervos, MJ Rybak. Comparison between a rabbit model of bacterial endocarditis and an in vitro infection model with simulated endocardial vegetations. Antimicrob Agents Chemother. 2000;44:1921–1924.
11. T Murakawa, H Sakamoto, T Hirse, M Nishida. New in vitro kinetic model for evaluating bactericidal efficacy of antibiotics. Antimicrob Agents Chemother 1980; 18:377–381.
12. SH Zinner, M Husson, J Klastersky. An artificial capillary in vitro kinetic model of antibiotic bactericidal activity. J Infect Dis 1981;144:583–587.
13. J Blaser, BB Stone, SH Zinner. Two compartment kinetic model with multiple artificial capillary units. J Antimicrob Chemother 1985;15(suppl A):131–137.
14. J Blaser. In-vitro model for simultaneous simulation of the serum kinetics of two drugs with different half-lives. J Antimicrob Chemother 1985;15(suppl A):125–130.
15. HH Houlihan, RC Mercier, MJ Rybak. Pharmacodynamics of vancomycin alone and in combination with gentamicin at various dosing intervals against methicillin-resistant *Staphylococcus aureus*-infected fibrin-platelet clots in an in vitro infection model. Antimicrob Agents Chemother 1997;41:2497–2501.
16. J Blaser, BB Stone, MC Groner, SH Zinner. Impact of netilmicin regimens on the activities of ceftazidime-netilmicin combinations against *Pseudomonas aeruginosa* in an in vitro pharmacokinetic model. Antimicrob Agents Chemother 1985;28:64–68.
17. JC Nickel, JB Wright, I Ruseska, TJ Marrie, C Whitfield, JW Costerton. Antibiotic resistance of *Pseudomonas aeruginosa* colonizing a urinary catheter in vitro. Eur J Clin Microbiol 1985;4:213–218.
18. KJ Walker, KJ Kelly, AJ Larsson, JC Rotschafer, DRP Guay, K Vance-Bryan. Adhe-

sion of *Staphylococcus epidermidis* (SE), *Staphylococcus aureus* (SA), and *Pseudomonas aeruginosa* (PA) to six vascular catheter materials (abstr). In: Program and Abstracts of the 33rd Interscience Conference on Antimicrobial Agents and Chemotherapy, New Orleans, LA, 1993.

19. BL Prosser, D Taylor, BA Dix, R Cleeland. Method of evaluating effects of antibiotics on bacterial biofilm. Antimicrob Agents Chemother 1987;31:1502–1506.
20. BJ McGrath, SL Kang, GW Kaatz, MJ Rybak. Bactericidal activities of teicoplanin, vancomycin, and gentamicin alone and in combination against *Staphylococcus aureus* in an in vitro pharmacodynamic model of endocarditis. Antimicrob Agents Chemother 1994;38:2034–2040.
21. K Hultén, R Rigo, I Gustafsson, L Engstrand. A new pharmacokinetic in vitro model for studies of antibiotic activity against intracellular microorganisms. Antimicrob Agents Chemother 1996;40:2727–2731.
22. PM Shah. Activity of imipenem in an in-vitro model simulating pharmacokinetic parameters in human blood. J Antimicrob Chemother 1985;15(suppl A):153–157.
23. DL Watson. Virulence of *Staphylococcus aureus* grown in vitro or in vivo. Microbiol Immunol 1979;23:543–547.
24. A Dalhoff. Differences between bacteria grown in vitro and in vivo. J Antimicrob Chemother 1985;15(suppl A):175–195.
25. P Gilbert. The theory and relevance of continuous culture. J Antimicrob Chemother 1985;15(suppl A):1–6.
26. A Dalhoff, G Stübner. Comparative analysis of the antimicrobial action of polymorphonuclear leucocytes in vitro, ex vivo and in vivo. J Antimicrob Chemother 1985; 15(suppl A):283–291.
27. DM Cappelletty, MJ Rybak. Bactericidal activities of cefprozil, penicillin, cefaclor, cefixime, and loracarbef against penicillin-susceptible and -resistant *Streptococcus pneumoniae* in an in vitro pharmacodynamic infection model. Antimicrob Agents Chemother 1996;40:1148–1152.
28. MW Garrison, K Vance-Bryan, TA Larson, JP Toscano, JC Rotschafer. Assessment of effects of protein binding on daptomycin and vancomycin killing of *Staphylococcus aureus* by using an in vitro pharmacodynamic model. Antimicrob Agents Chemother 1990;34:1925–1931.
29. MN Gwynn, LT Webb, GN Rolinson. Regrowth of *Pseudomonas aeruginosa* and other bacteria after the bactericidal action of carbenicillin and other β-lactam antibiotics. J Infect Dis 1981;144:263–269.

4

Animal Models of Infection for the Study of Antibiotic Pharmacodynamics

Michael N. Dudley
David Griffith
Microcide Pharmaceuticals, Inc., Mountain View, California

1 INTRODUCTION

Animal models of infection have had a prominent place in the evaluation of infection and its treatment. From early experiments demonstrating transmission of infectious agents to satisfy Koch's postulates to evaluation of chemotherapy in the antibiotic era, animal models have proven useful for understanding human diseases.

More recently, animal models for the study of infectious disease have been further refined to consider the importance of pharmacokinetic factors in the outcome of infection. This allows for the study of the relationship between drug exposure (pharmacokinetics) and anti-infective activity (pharmacodynamics). Consideration of these aspects has enhanced the information provided by animal models of infection and made the results more predictive of the performance of drug regimens in humans. This has largely been accomplished through a more thorough understanding of the importance of pharmacokinetics in the outcome of an infection, advances in quantitation of drug concentrations in biological matrices, and the development of metrics to quantify antibacterial effects in vivo.

This chapter will review approaches for design, analysis and application of these approaches in animal models for the study of optimization of anti-infective therapy and the discovery and development of new agents.

Use of animal models of infection to study the relationship between drug exposure in vivo and antibacterial effects dates back to the very early studies in penicillin. These early investigators noted that the duration of efficacy of penicillin in the treatment of streptococcal infections was dependent on the length of time for which serum concentrations exceeded the MIC [1–3]. How these early observations ultimately impacted on penicillin therapy in humans is difficult to ascertain; however, it is clear that pharmacodynamic studies in animal models have a crucial role in the preclinical evaluation of new anti-infectives, optimization of marketed agents, and the assessment of drug resistance.

2 RELEVANCE OF ANIMAL MODELS TO INFECTIONS IN HUMANS

It is largely assumed that efficacy of a drug in an animal model will correspond to that in humans. However, in many cases the induction and progression of infection in small animals does not correspond to that seen in the human setting. For example, humans rarely suffer from large, bolus challenges of bacteria by the intravenous route. A much more clinically relevant model for pathogenesis in humans involving translocation of bacteria from gastrointestinal membranes damaged by cytostatic agents has been developed [4]. Despite this major difference, the model of sepsis is a mainstay for early preclinical evaluation of anti-infectives in rodent models.

A few animal models have been widely accepted for prediction of effects in humans. The rabbit model of endocarditis (see below) has proven faithful in mimicking damage to valvular surfaces similar to that reported in human patients, and colonization of these vegetations by bacteria and growth corresponds closely to that observed in humans. For several years, prophylaxis regimens for endocarditis were based largely on experiments in this model.

3 ENDPOINTS IN ANIMAL MODELS OF INFECTION

Examples of major endpoints used in pharmacodynamic studies in animal models of infection are shown in Table 1. For lethal infections, the proportion of animals surviving at each dose/exposure level are determined to generate typical dose–response curves. With greater awareness of the potential for suffering in test animals during the later stages of overwhelming infection from a failing drug regimen, most investigators have substituted rapid progression to a moribund condition as a more humane alternative endpoint. Both endpoints require careful monitoring by the investigator and consistent application of these definitions to

Table 1 Summary of Advantages and Disadvantages of Various Endpoints in Animal Models of Infection

Endpoint	Advantages	Disadvantages
Death/moribund condition	Clear endpoint (death). Comparable endpoint in humans. Represents a difficult test of antibiotic/dosage regimen.	Animal stress and suffering. Short-term models require overwhelming inoculum that may trigger cytokine responses irrelevant to that seen in humans. Nonspecific effects of drugs (bacterial killing vs. other pharmacological effects). Cannot differentiate between cidal and static effects in vivo. Difficult to assess emergence of drug resistance during therapy. Outcomes can be very dependent on inoculum and other adjuvants and can obscure PK-PD analysis. Unanticipated changes in drug pharmacokinetics due to altered physiology during severe infection.
Quantitation of pathogens in body tissues and fluids	Can determine static/cidal activity of agent. Can assess emergence of drug resistance during treatment to test agents. Measure postantibiotic, subinhibitory effects and correlate with in vitro properties. May test strains that are avirulent in other models (e.g., sepsis). Assess relationship between drug concentrations in infected compartment with bacterial eradication (e.g., drug concentrations in CSF).	Relevance of tissue burden to clinical setting in humans often not established ("fuzzy test-tube"). Unrealistic introduction of pathogens into sterile body sites. Need to control for possible antibiotic carryover in processing specimens for quantitative culture.
Tissue damage and inflammation	Considers impact of both bacterial growth and resultant effects of antibiotics.	Relevance to human infection uncertain.

ensure reproducible results. Further, only the potency of the antimicrobial is estimated, because the maximum response is generally bounded (100% survival). However, given that death from infection often arises due to complex interplay between host factors, organ damage, etc., or even other factors that may be unrelated to antibacterial effects (e.g., a dropped cage), the investigator must be cautious in interpretating results.

In contrast, quantitation of bacteria in tissues at various time points allows for measurement of changes in bacterial numbers over time. The antibacterial effects often correlate with meaningful clinical outcomes in patients (e.g., relation between time to sterilization of CSF in meningitis and residual neurological effects in children). Quantification of bacterial counts in tissues or fluids detects more subtle changes in bacterial killing with dosage regimens. In addition, changes in susceptibility of the pathogens with treatment can be measured. The best approach is validation of the number of pathogens in tissues or fluids that correlates with survival in treated or untreated animals. Identification of an earlier endpoint that predicts survival in both treated and untreated animals meets the most rigorous definition for a true surrogate marker (i.e., a marker that predicts survival in treated and untreated groups).

3.1 Metrics for Quantifying Anti-Infective Effects In Vivo

Quantitation of antimicrobial effects in vivo usually measures the tissue or host burden of organism at specified intervals after the initiation of treatment. In view of the differences among drugs in in vitro pharmacodynamic properties (e.g., rate of bacterial killing and postantibiotic and subinhibitory effects) as well as pharmacokinetic properties, several approaches have been developed to measure the time course of antibacterial effects in vivo. These metrics tend to focus either on the overall extent of bacterial killing over time or on the rate of bacterial killing, either by measuring the time to reach a particular level of bacteria (e.g., time to 3 log decrease) or by calculation of a killing rate (e.g., reduction in log CFU/h). Table 2 summarizes several representative metrics used for describing the pharmacodynamic effects on bacteria in vivo.

4 PHARMACOKINETIC CONSIDERATIONS IN ANIMAL MODELS OF INFECTION

As described in earlier chapters, one objective of pharmacodynamic modeling is to relate the in vivo exposure of an anti-infective to the observed effects listed above. This requires careful study of antimicrobial pharmacokinetics in the test species.

Our approach is to measure the pharmacokinetic properties of readily available drugs in the infected animals. Although literature data are often available,

TABLE 2 Summary of Metrics Used to Describe Rate and Extent of Bacterial Killing Under In Vivo Conditions

Metric(s)	Typical units	Description	Comments	Refs.
Extent of bacterial killing				
Change in CFU	Log CFU per tissue weight, organ, or volume	Shows change in total bacterial numbers at sentinel time compared to starting inoculum or untreated control animals.	Most easily used to determine effects when destructive sampling is required.	Many
Area under the CFU vs. time curve; I_E	CFU · h/vol or wt of tissue	Quantifies the total burden of organisms over time by fitting function or by area estimation.	Comparisons assume similar starting inoculum (can correct by ratio of observation with starting inoculum to calculate survival fraction). Used to determine extent of anti-infective effect following single or multiple doses.	5–7
Static dose (exposure); EC-50, EC-90*	Log CFU per tissue weight, organ, or volume	Static: No change in CFU over the duration of the experiment compared to challenge inoculum. EC-50, EC-90: Corresponds to 50%, 90% of maximum effects.	Used for comparison of magnitude of PK-PD parameter for a given level of effect. Static dose observed to correlate with mortality in mice with some infections (e.g., pneumonia).	8
Rate and duration of bacterial killing				
Bactericidal rate	Log CFU/(mL · h)	Depicts the rate of bacterial killing over time by fitting slope to log CFU/mL vs. time curve.	Need complete depiction of curve to estimate accurate slope. Difficulty with simple models with data with biphasic killing pattern or bacterial regrowth.	9, 10

Table 2 Continued

Metric(s)	Typical units	Description	Comments	Refs.
Time to 99.9% decrease from starting inoculum	Hours	Describes the time necessary for a regimen to produce a specified level of reduction in CFU.	Choice of endpoint (99.9% reduction) often arbitrary.	11
Effective regrowth time (ERT)	Hours	Determines the time needed for a treatment regimen to resume growth and return to CFU counts at the start of treatment.	Adapted from in vitro PAE studies but may be applied to animal model results. Studies need to be prolonged to achieve a result. Evaluation of multiple dose regimens may not be possible.	12
Fully parameterized methods				
Estimates of growth, bacterial killing rates	Various parameters (e.g., kill rate, growth rate)	Models using polynomials or (more appropriately) parameterized for bacterial killing and regrowth phases.	Most adapted from in vitro curves but can be applied to results in animals. Many models unable to consider multiple doses. Limited application outside models of infection.	13–15

* EC-50, EC-90: 50% or 90% effective concentrated, respectively.

the results in a preclinical pharmacokinetic study (where the goal is to carefully measure pharmacokinetic properties) may differ from the values obtained in sick animals or with multiple doses. For novel compounds, the pharmacokinetics is not known, and studies in both infected and uninfected animals are needed to characterize the pharmacokinetic properties of the agent as well as to determine the actual exposure to drug in the experimental model. Nonlinear changes in exposure vs. dose (due to changes in drug clearance or bioavailability for extravascular administration) should be probed. When studying combinations of drugs, one must ensure that pharmacokinetic drug interactions do not occur; pharmacokinetic interactions could cause false interpretations of combination experiments (e.g., increased effects from antimicrobial synergism), where the effect was really due to elevated concentrations of an active component. We have also found that the formulation used for a second agent may also influence the pharmacokinetic properties of antibiotics (e.g., PEG plus levofloxacin in mice; unpublished observations).

4.1 Design Issues in Pharmacokinetic Studies for Animal Models

4.1.1 Sampling

Appropriate blood or tissue sampling strategies are key to getting robust estimates of pharmacokinetic parameters in animals. In mice, it is usually necessary to euthanize the animal using CO_2 or another AVMA-approved method to obtain adequate volumes of blood for drug assay. Cardiac puncture in a dead animal usually yields the greatest volume of blood. Harvest of tissues or other samples and immersion in a suitable matrix for sample processing (e.g., homogenization) can also be done to quantify tissue levels. In larger animal species (e.g., rats, rabbits), an indwelling intravenous or intra-arterial catheter allows collection of multiple samples over time. In these cases, placement of two cannulas in separate vessels should be undertaken to avoid possible carryover of drug-containing infusate into samples.

One can use *d*-optimality criteria to select sampling points [16]. However, we rarely use this, because the pharmacokinetics of drugs are rapid in small animals and the slight advantage of narrowing sampling times is easily lost. Further, for novel compounds there is no information upon which to base selection of sampling times. The maximal volume of blood to be collected over a pharmacokinetic study session should be estimated and approved upon consultation with a veterinarian and the Institutional Animal Care and Use Committee (IACUC).

After collection, samples can be centrifuged to separate cells from plasma or serum and aliquots of the sample transferred to screw-capped storage tubes. Pilot studies should consider possible loss of drug in polypropylene or other materials that may result in falsely low levels of drug. Administration of plasma expanders or volume replacement should be considered for prolonged studies in small animals. Patency of catheters can be maintained by gentle flushing of lines using heparin (10–100 U/mL) in 0.9% saline, but overzealous use can result in a systemic anticoagulant effect.

4.1.2 Drug Assay

Assay of serum and tissue concentrations of drug in the test animal species can be done using high performance liquid chromatographic (HPLC) or microbiological assays. The more widespread availability, precision, sensitivity, and rapidity of HPLC methods [particularly those using detection by tandem mass spectrometry (MS/MS)] has resulted in a shift toward the use of these methods, particularly in the early discovery or preclinical setting. Metabolites and their antimicrobial activity should be considered in the final pharmacokinetic–pharmacodynamic analyses. Preparation of standards in the appropriate biological matrix (e.g., serum; tissue homogenate) should be undertaken and the sensitivity, specificity, reproducibility, and ruggedness be validated to ensure reproducibility of results.

4.1.3 Modeling Pharmacokinetic Data

Serum or tissue concentration vs. time data can be analyzed using a variety of methods. Although noncompartmental (SHAM—slope, height, area, moment) methods are used by many investigators, we have found that a more informative analysis results when compartmental models are used. In addition, full parameterization allows for better simulations. Critical analysis of the selection of the appropriate pharmacokinetic model and generation of pharmacokinetic parameters and their confidence intervals is also helpful for performing simulations to calculate indices of pharmacokinetic parameters related to the MIC. Compartmental modeling is also particularly important for estimating pharmacokinetic parameters from studies that generate a single composite ''population'' curve of single data points gathered from destructive sampling (e.g., serum from mice). Many investigators have adopted WinNONLIN as the fitting program, but several other suitable programs include ADAPT II and MKMODEL. Even population modeling programs (e.g., NOMEM, NPEM) may be useful with some data sets.

After estimation of pharmacokinetic parameters, simulation of serum levels for various dosage regimens can be undertaken. Unbound drug concentrations should be simulated using protein binding values generated in the same species. It is particularly important to correlate effects with unbound drug exposure for studies where development of pharmacokinetic-pharmacodynamic relationships will be extended to other species, particularly humans. As will be discussed below, several studies have shown that the free concentration of drug in serum is linked to the efficacy of several anti-infectives. Differences in serum protein binding between preclinical species and humans could lead to errors in conclusions concerning target levels of total drug to obtain acceptable levels of efficacy. Examples include experience with cefonicid in the treatment of endocarditis due to *S. aureus* [17].

4.2 Animal vs. Human Pharmacokinetics

The pharmacokinetics of drugs are known to differ markedly between preclinical animal species (particularly small animals used in pharmacokinetic studies) and humans. These differences largely arise due to well-described allometric relationships that relate physiological variables measured within species to differences in body weight [18]. However, the differences in pharmacokinetic properties between animals and humans may arise due to differences in metabolism, biliary or renal transport, or a combination of these factors. For example, although meropenem is resistant to hydrolysis by human renal dehyropeptidases, it is highly susceptible to inactivation to a deydropeptidase produced in mouse tissues [19]. Table 3 depicts examples of differences in pharmacokinetic properties between humans and small animals for several classes of agents. These differences are often most marked for β-lactam agents.

In conducting pharmacokinetic-pharmacodynamic investigations in animal models with drugs used in humans, it is crucial that the differences between humans and animals be considered in the design and interpretation of experiments. This is particularly important for compounds whose activity in vivo is dependent upon the length of time concentrations exceed the MIC (e.g., β-lactams and *Pseudomonas aeruginosa*). When pharmacokinetic differences between humans and small animals are ignored, the results from animal models of infection can underestimate the efficacy of compounds in humans.

A vivid example of the importance of consideration of human vs. mouse pharmacokinetics was shown in studies with ceftazidime treatment of *Pseudomonas aeruginosa* infection in the neutropenic mouse thigh infection model by

TABLE 3 Comparison of Pharmacokinetic Parameters of Selected Antimicrobials in Small Animals and Humans

	Clearance [L/(h · kg)]			Elimination half-life (h)			
Drug	Human	Rat	Mouse	Human	Rat	Mouse	Ref.
Ceftizoxime	0.12	1.16	3.67	1.27	0.26	0.15	18, 20
Vancomycin	1.89	0.36	0.75	1.5	2.8	0.63	21, 22
Ofloxacin	0.15	0.45	N.A.	7.0	1.84	N.A.	23, 24
Azithromycin	1.29	3.85	3.33	65.9	6.8	0.72	25–27

N.A. = not available.

Gerber et al. in a neutropenic mouse model of infection (see Fig. 1) [28]. When human pharmacokinetics were simulated in the mice, the bacterial killing was much more sustained than that observed under normal mouse pharmacokinetic conditions.

Generally, two methods exist for simulation of human pharmacokinetic parameters in animals. In the simplest terms, they involve changing drug input or drug elimination.

4.2.1 Changing Drug Input

Several investigators have used multiple, frequent administration of drugs with rapid drug clearances and short serum elimination half-lives in mice or rats. This approach uses the principle of superposition of successive ''bolus'' doses given when concentrations are expected to have declined below target levels. The frequency of administration may be as short as every 30 min around the clock (Fig. 1).

The availability of computer-controlled pumps for delivery of intravenous fluids has enabled the use of these devices to use decreasing rates of drug delivery to simulate concentrations in humans [29]. Two approaches may be used: continuous infusion of diluent into the infusate, which is delivered as an infusion into the animal (much like what is done in in vitro pharmacodynamic models), or a continuously changing intravenous infusion rate of a fixed concentration of drug in infusate. The former approach has particular usefulness if one wishes to simulate human concentrations of two drugs in the animal. Both of these approaches have been used in larger animal species (rats, rabbits) in the evaluation of treatment of endocarditis, peritonitis, pneumonia, and meningitis.

The theoretical advantage associated with continuous infusion of antibiotics with certain in vitro pharmacodynamic properties has been studied in animal models of infection. Continuous infusion studies are considerably simpler than intermittent administration. One simply needs to divide the desired steady-state drug concentration by the drug clearance in the animal species to determine the infusion rate. Studies have evaluated delivery by this route for up to 5 days. Continuous infusion of drugs may also be obtained in mice using Alzet peritoneal or subcutaneous micro-osmotic pumps.

4.2.2 Changing Drug Elimination

An alternative (and perhaps more direct) way to mimic human drug pharmacokinetics in small animals is to slow drug elimination. For drugs largely excreted unchanged in urine, inducing renal impairment by administration of a nephrotoxin can result in slow excretion and allow for close simulation of human dosage regimens in mice. Several investigators have administered a single dose of uranyl nitrate (e.g., 10 mg/kg given 2–3 days prior to antibiotic treatment) to induce temporary renal dysfunction for studies of short-term duration (e.g., 24–30 h)

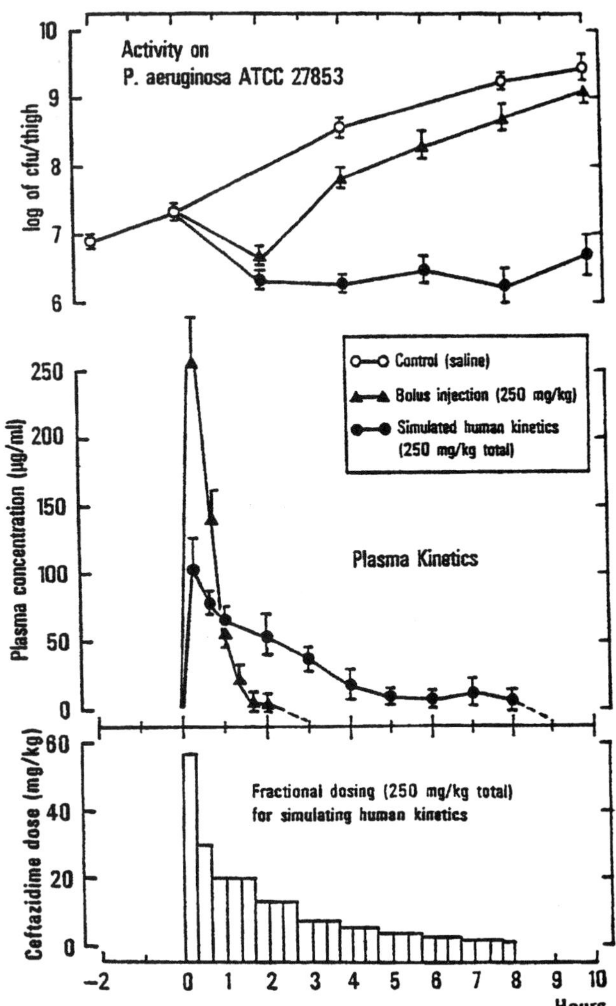

FIGURE 1 Comparison of the effects of a single dose of ceftazidime against a strain of *Pseudomonas aeruginosa* in the neutropenic mouse thigh infection model. When a single dose was given to a mouse, bacterial killing occurred only transiently, followed by regrowth. In contrast, when multiple frequent doses of drug were given to simulate the pharmacokinetic profile in humans, much more sustained bacterial killing was observed. (From Ref. 28.)

[8]. Although convenient, this substance is considered to have low-level radiation, and some states require special permits for its handling and disposal. Other substances have been reported to cause renal impairment in rodents (e.g., glycerol) [30]; however, we did not find that it significantly altered the pharmacokinetics of aztreonam in mice (Tembe, Chen, Griffith, and Dudley, unpublished observations).

Figure 2 compares the serum pharmacokinetic profile for amoxicillin in mice pretreated with a single dose of uranyl nitrate with concentrations in humans. When proper doses are administered, the serum concentration vs. time profile is comparable to that observed in humans. Simulation of human serum drug levels allowed for testing of the relationship between amoxicillin MIC and effects in a mouse model using drug exposures comparable to those observed in humans [8].

Other approaches for reducing drug clearance include administration of drugs that block renal tubular secretion. This requires that the agent of interest be excreted to a high degree by net renal tubular secretion in the animal species to be tested. Probenecid is one example; however, the magnitude of the effect may be variable and highly dose-dependent. In addition, probenecid may have effects on other nonrenal pathways for elimination, including phase II metabolism.

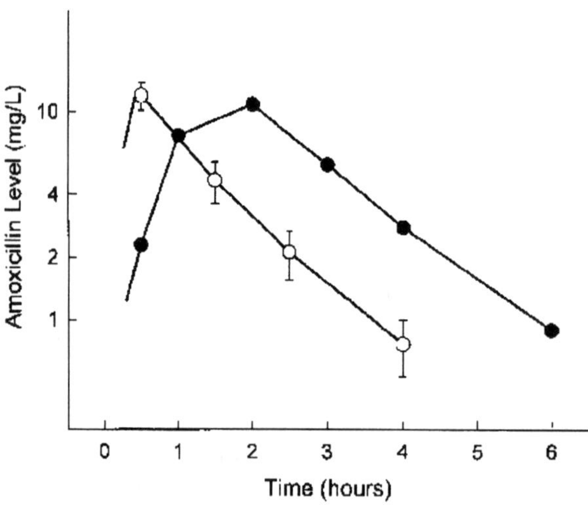

FIGURE 2 Comparison of serum amoxicillin concentrations found in renally impared mice with those in human volunteers. (From Ref. 8.)

5 PHARMACODYNAMIC MODELING USING MATHEMATICAL INDICES FOR RELATING PHARMACOKINETIC DATA WITH THE MIC

5.1 Pharmacokinetic-Pharmacodynamic Indices and Relationship to Dose, MIC, and Drug Half-Life

As described in earlier chapters, several indices for integrating pharmacokinetic data with the MIC have been applied for the study of anti-infective pharmacodynamics. Figure 3 depicts several indices that have been used to express these relationships. As shown in the figure, all of the parameters are highly correlated; e.g., an increase in dose results in an increase in all parameters. However, the magnitude of changes in each parameter with different doses, dosing intervals, drug clearance, and MIC will not increase proportionately with all the pharmacokinetic-pharmacodynamic (PK-PD) indices. This is especially important in the design and interpretation of studies of drugs with short half-lives in small animals where the percent of the dosing interval drug concentrations that exceed the MIC is the most important parameter for describing in vivo antimicrobial effects.

A brief consideration of the effects of dose on PK-PD parameters is helpful in recognizing the relative importance of each of these variables. For the ratios C_{max}/MIC or AUC/MIC, a change in dose results in proportional and linear (assuming linear pharmacokinetics) changes in AUC/MIC. Similarly, the MIC affects these parameters (inversely), but the proportion of change is linear.

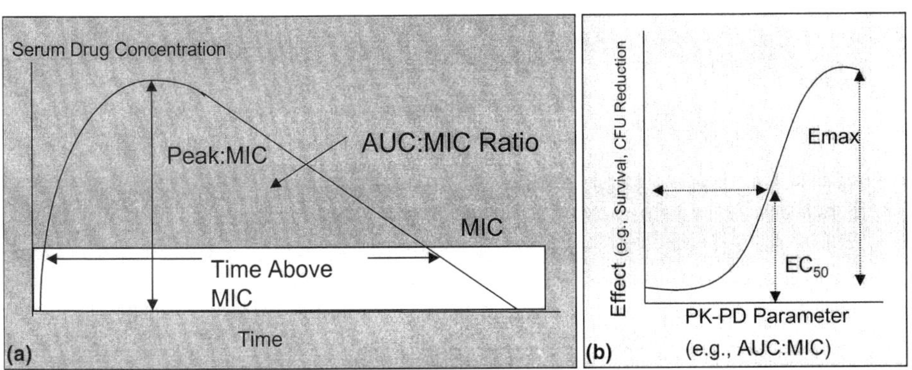

FIGURE 3 Examples of (a) pharmacokinetic parameters and the MIC and (b) pharmacodynamic relationship between a PK-PD parameter and effects in vivo.

The picture is considerably more complicated in calculation of the number of hours drug concentrations exceed the MIC. For a one compartment pharmacokinetic model and bolus drug input,

$$\text{Hours concn. exceeds MIC } (T > \text{MIC}) = \frac{\ln \text{dose}/V - \ln \text{MIC}}{\text{Cl}/V}$$

In contrast to the ratio metrics C_{max}/MIC and AUC/MIC, the magnitude of change in $T >$ MIC with dose or MIC is not directly proportional but changes as the natural logarithm of these values. Changes in drug clearance (half-life) produce the most marked change in this parameter.

The practical implications of this relationship for the design of studies and the evaluation of PK-PD data in animal models of infection for drugs where activity in vivo is dependent upon $T >$ MIC are profound. Figure 4 depicts changes in $T >$ MIC according to MIC or drug dose. When drug half-life is very fast (Cl/V is large), even high doses of drug will produce only minor changes in $T >$ MIC. Similarly, differences in in vitro potency (MIC) will have little effect on $T >$ MIC. Failure to incorporate these considerations into experiments results in erroneous conclusions concerning the effects of changes in MIC or drug dose and in vivo response for drugs where in vivo activity is linked to $T >$ MIC.

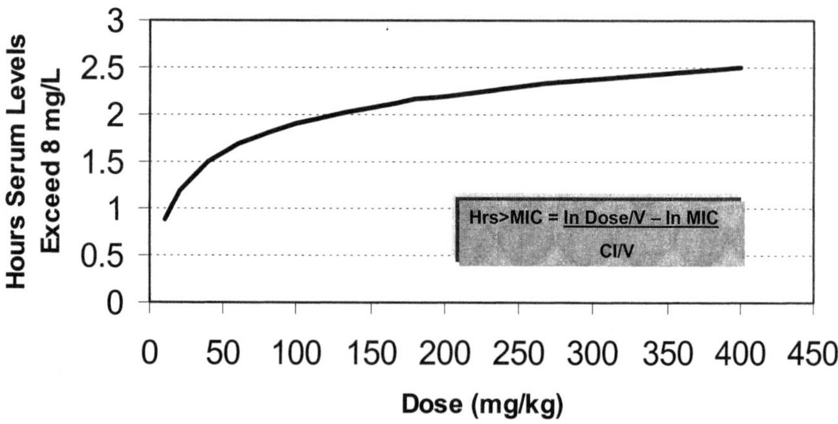

FIGURE 4 Relationship between MIC and $T >$ MIC and dose for vancomycin administered subcutaneously in mice.

5.2 Designing Experiments to Identify Relationships Between Pharmacokinetics, MIC, and In Vivo Effects

In planning experiments in which many regimens can be evaluated (e.g., short-term studies in mouse models), simulations of serum drug concentrations vs. time using pharmacokinetic parameters derived from infected animals should be performed. The parameters, MICs, and dosage regimens can easily be programmed into a spreadsheet to generate PK-PD data. One can assess a number of ''what if'' scenarios for several doses, dosage regimens, and MICs and generate two- or three-dimensional plots showing the correlation for each regimen. An example of uncorrelated PK-PD parameters for several vancomycin regimens in a mouse is shown in Fig. 5. One can finalize selection of dosage regimens that will minimize the covariance among different PK-PD parameters. In selecting regimens, it is also important to be mindful of the relationships of dose and MIC with the number of hours serum concentrations will exceed the MIC. In some cases it may be virtually impossible to design dosage regimens that produce a range of PK-PD parameters that correspond to those possible in humans. In these

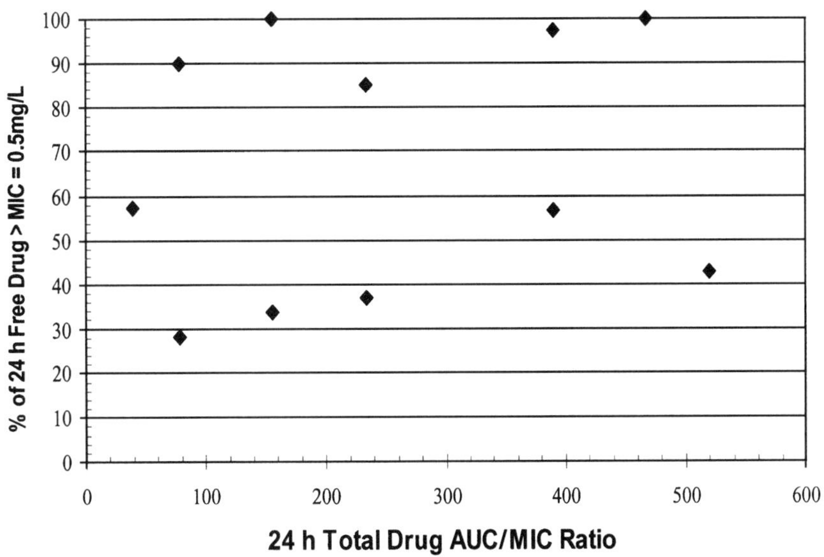

FIGURE 5 Lack of correlation between $T >$ MIC and AUC/MIC ratio for several regimens of vancomycin administered every 2–12 h in a mouse model of infection.

cases, the use of techniques to alter drug input or retard drug clearance may be required.

6 ANIMAL MODELS USED IN PK-PD STUDIES

6.1 Selection of Appropriate Models for Study of PK-PD Issues

For the study of pharmacokinetics and pharmacodynamics (PK-PD) in an animal model, one must take into consideration that the time course of antimicrobial activity will vary between different antimicrobial agents. For example, β-lactam antibacterials exhibit very little concentration-dependent killing and, in the case of staphylococci, long in vivo postantibiotic effects (PAEs). For these antibacterials, high drug levels will not kill bacteria more effectively or more rapidly than lower drug levels, because these agents should be bactericidal as long as the drug concentrations exceed the MIC. In contrast, fluoroquinolones and aminoglycosides show concentration-dependent killing. For these agents, the peak/MIC or AUC/MIC ratios should be the PK-PD parameters that most effectively describe their efficacy [1]. With these caveats in mind, the choice of an animal model to study PK-PD parameters will depend on the organism one wishes to study, the pharmacokinetics of the antimicrobial agent, and the type of infection one ultimately intends to treat in humans.

Of the animal models used to study PK-PD relationships, the most commonly used is the neutropenic mouse thigh model, fully described by Gerber and Craig in 1982 [20]. Other animal models used to study PK–PD relationships include animal models of pneumonia [21–23], kidney infections/pyelonephritis [24], peritonitis/septicemia [25, 26], meningitis [27, 31], osteomyelitis [32], and endocarditis [33–35]. In fact, almost any model can be used as long as drug exposure can be correlated with organism recovery or response.

6.2 Factors Influencing Endpoints

Factors that affect the results of all endpoints include the test strain and initial challenge inoculum, treatment-free interval (i.e., interval between bacterial inoculation and initiation of treatment), immunocompetence of test animal species, and administration of adjuvants. These all can contribute to outcome and the conclusion concerning the magnitude of the PK-PD parameter required for efficacy. Gerber et al. [36] showed that the efficacy of aminoglycosides and β-lactams was markedly affected by delaying treatment, requiring a higher dose. In fluoroquinolone treatment of pneumococcal infection in mice, the AUC/MIC ratio associated with the static effect is similar in immunocompetent or neutropenic mice. In contrast, AUC/MIC is considerably different between neutropenic and nonneutropenic mice in infections due to *Klebsiella pneumoniae* [37].

6.3 Animal Models

To study the pharmacodynamics of an antimicrobial agent, the pharmacokinetics of the agent in question should be determined in the animal species and under the same conditions that will be used in the infection model (e.g., neutropenic mice in the case of the neutropenic thigh model). The MICs of the organisms to be tested should be determined by an NCCLS reference method.

6.3.1 Thigh Infection Model

The thigh infection model has been used extensively to describe the pharmacodynamics of several classes of drugs, particularly fluoroquinolones, macrolides, β-lactams, and aminoglycosides. Most investigators have used Swiss albino mice for this model, although any mouse strain can be used. Although occasional studies are done in normal (nonneutropenic) animals, most of the experience with this model has been obtained in neutropenic mice [38]. Most investigators induce neutropenia by the administration of 150 mg/kg and 100 mg/kg of cyclophosphamide on days 0 and 3, respectively. This results in severe neutropenia by day 4, which is sustained over at least a 24–48 h period [38]. Inocula should be prepared in a suitable medium and allowed to grow into log phase. After dilution, 0.1 mL of bacterial suspension (10^5–10^6 CFU) is injected into each thigh while the animals are under light anesthesia (e.g., isoflurane, sodium pentobarbital, ether). For some experimental designs, a different organism may be injected in the contralateral thigh (e.g., when studying resistance mechanisms in isogenic strains), or mixtures of organisms can be used. The organisms are usually allowed to grow for 2 h prior to the start of treatment. Treatment is given in multiple dosing regimens over 24 h based on the pharmacokinetics of the drug and PK-PD parameters being tested. After 24 h of treatment, the animals are euthanized and their thighs are removed, homogenized in sterile saline, and serially diluted and cultured on a suitable medium to perform colony counts. In the event of agents with long half-lives (e.g., azithromycin), thigh homogenates can be assayed for the drug to exclude the possibility of drug carryover interfering with the results, or a substance to inactivate drug (e.g., β-lactamase) may be added. The CFU/thigh determined for each dosing regimen can be quantified, and relationships to drug exposure fit to a suitable pharmacodynamic model.

6.3.2 Pneumonia Models

The pneumonia model described below is a mouse model, however, there are a number of different models in rats [21, 39], hamsters [40], or rabbits [41]. Organisms used in pneumonia models include, but are not limited to, *S. pneumoniae*, *K. pneumoniae*, *P. aeruginosa*, *S. aureus*, *P. mirabilis*, *E. coli*, *L. pneumophila*, and *A. fumigatus*. Adjuvants are often used to increase virulence.

In the mouse model, most Swiss albino mice of either sex can be used.

Depending upon the organism, the mice may or may not need to be rendered neutropenic. Inocula should be prepared in a suitable medium and allowed to grow into log phase. After dilution, the animals are infected by intranasal instillation of 0.05 mL of bacterial suspension ($\sim 10^6$–10^7 CFU) while the animals are under anesthesia (isoflourane, sodium pentobarbital, ether, etc.). Treatment is given in multiple dosing regimens for up to 2 days starting 24 h after infection. After 24–48 h of treatment, the animals killed and their lungs are removed, homogenized, serially tenfold diluted, and then cultured on a suitable medium to perform colony counts. The CFU/lungs determined for each dosing regimen can then be fit to a suitable pharmacodynamic model. The advantages of this model are that the prolonged endpoint (24–48 h) allows for several cycles of bacterial growth.

Using this model, Woodnutt and Berry [21] found that the efficacy of amoxicillin-clavulanate (a combination of the two drugs) was best described by percentage time above the MIC, with the maximum bactericidal effect being achieved at a $T >$ MIC of 35–40%.

6.3.4 Pyelonephritis/Kidney Infection Models

Kidney infection models for study of antifungal activity have been described in both mice [24] and rats [42]. Organisms used in kidney infection models include, but are not limited to, *E. faecalis, E. coli, S. aureus, C. albicans,* and *A. fumigatus*.

For the mouse model, most Swiss albino, Balb/c, and DBA/2 mice can be used. Swiss albino mice can be rendered neutropenic to support growth of the organism. Inocula should be prepared in a suitable medium and allowed to grow into log phase. After dilution, the animals are infected by intravenous injection. Treatment is started 2 h after infection in the case of *C. albicans* but can be started as late as 24 h after infection in the case of *E. faecalis*. Treatment is given in multiple dosing regimens for 24 h or longer. After 24–120 h of treatment, the animals are killed and their kidneys are removed, homogenized, serially tenfold diluted, and then cultured on a suitable medium to perform colony counts. The CFU/kidneys determined for each dosing regimen can then be fit to a suitable pharmacodynamic model. The advantages of this model are endpoints that can range anywhere from 24 to 120 h, it generally uses an inoculum high enough to study resistance, and it allows for several growth and regrowth cycles. Using this model, it has been shown that the AUC/MIC best predicts the effects of fluconazole against strains with a wide range of susceptibilities to this drug [24,43, 44].

6.3.5 Peritonitis/Septicemia Models

The septicemia model described below is a mouse model [26,45]; however, there is a similar model in neutropenic rats [25]. Organisms used in peritonitis/sepsis models include, but are not limited to, *E. coli, S. aureus, S. epidermidis, P. aeruginosa, K. pneumoniae, S. pneumoniae, E. faecalis, S. marcescens, P. mirabilis,* group B *Streptococcus, C. albicans,* and *A. fumigatus.*

For this model, almost any mouse species can be used. Mice may or may not need to be rendered neutropenic. Inocula should be prepared in a suitable medium and allowed to grow into log phase. After dilution, the animals are infected by intraperitoneal injection of 0.1–0.5 mL of bacterial suspension (~1–10^9 CFU/ mouse). Treatment is given in multiple dosing regimens for up to 72 h. After treatment, animals still alive are considered long-term survivors. Deaths recorded throughout the experiment can be compared by Kaplan–Meier or probit analysis. Percent survival [(number alive/number treated) × 100] determined for each dosing regimen can then be fit to a suitable pharmacodynamic model.

Using this model, Knudsen et al. [45] found that the peak/MIC ratio and time above MIC were associated with survival for vancomycin and teicoplanin against *S. pneumoniae*. In a study using peritoneal washings and survival in mice for E_{max} modeling, der Hollander et al. [26] found that the peak/MIC ratio was associated with maximum bactericidal effects for azithromycin against *S. pneumoniae* and was achieved at a ratio of 4. In a similar model in rats, Drusano et al. [25] found that for lomefloxacin, a peak/MIC ratio that was 20:1 or 10:1 was associated with survival against *P. aeruginosa*. At peak/MIC ratios of <10:1, they found that the AUC/MIC ratio was associated with survival.

6.3.6 Meningitis Models

The meningitis model described below is a rabbit model [9,10]. There are also models in the rat, guinea pig, cat, dog, goat, and monkey, but studies in the higher species are discouraged. Organisms used in meningitis include *N. meningitidis, S. pneumoniae, H. influenzae, S. aureus, S. pyogenes, S. agalactiae, E. aerogenes, E. coli, K. pneumoniae, P. mirabilis, P. aeruginosa*, and *L. monocytogenes*.

For this model, male or female rabbits can be used. A dental acrylic helmet is attached to the skull of each rabbit by screws while it is under anesthesia. The helmet allows the animal to be secured to a stereotactic frame made for the puncture of the cisterna magna. Meningitis is induced by injection of a bacterial suspension directly into the cisterna magna. Treatment is started 18 h after infection and is given in multiple dosing regimens for up to 72 h. The CFU/mL CSF fluid or cure rates (sterile CSF cultures) determined for each dosing regimen can then be fit to a suitable pharmacodynamic model.

In this model, Tauber et al. [27] found that the peak CSF drug level/MBC ratio emerged as an important factor contributing to the efficacy of ampicillin against *S. pneumoniae*. In earlier studies these investigators also found that there was a linear correlation between β-lactam CSF peak concentrations and bactericidal activity in rabbits with *S. pneumoniae* meningitis [9]. Antibiotic concentrations in the CSF in the range of the MBC produced static effects, and concentrations of 10–30 times the MBC produced a maximal bactericidal effect.

In the same model of pneumococcal meningitis, Lutsar et al. [31] found that the bactericidal activity of gatifloxacin in the CSF was closely related to the AUC/MBC ratio but that maximal activity was achieved only when drug concentrations exceeded the MBC for the entire dosing interval. In another study of pneumococcal meningitis, Lutsar et al. [10] found that for ceftriaxone the time above MBC predicted the bacterial killing rate and that there was a linear correlation between time above MBC and bacterial killing rate during the first 24 h of therapy. Sterilization of the CSF was achieved only with $T >$ MBC of 95–100%. Ahmed et al. [46] found that concentrations of vancomycin needed to be at least four- to eightfold the MBC of *S. pneumoniae* in order to obtain adequate bacterial clearance. The suggestion was also that time above the MBC in the CSF was required for efficacy.

6.3.7 Osteomyelitis Models

The osteomyelitis model described below is both a rat model [32] and a rabbit model [47]. Organisms used in osteomyelitis models include *S. aureus* and *P. aeruginosa*. For this model, male or female rats or rabbits can be used. Animals are anesthetized, then the tibia is exposed, and a 1 mm hole is bored with a dental drill into the medullary cavity of the proximal tibia. Bones are infected by first injecting 5% sodium morrhuate followed by an injection of bacterial suspension. The hole is plugged with dental gypsum, and the wound is closed. Treatment is initiated 10 days after surgery and is given in multiple dosing regimens for up to 21 days for each compound.

In this model, O'Reilly et al. [32] chose single daily doses of 50 mg/kg for azithromycin, single daily doses of 20 mg/kg for rifampin, and three 90 mg/kg doses of clindamycin daily for treatment regimens against *S. aureus*. Despite having large bone peak/MIC and trough/MIC ratios, azithromycin failed to sterilize a single bone. Clindamycin sterilized 20% of the animals treated, and rifampin sterilized 53% of the animals treated. These results underscore the difficulties in predicting the efficacies of antibiotics in osteomyelitis based on in vitro studies and antibiotic levels in bone.

6.3.8 Endocarditis Models

The endocarditis model has been used extensively to evaluate antimicrobial regimens. Its advantages are that it produces an infection comparable to that observed in humans. The endocarditis model described below is a rabbit model [48]; however, there is also a rat model [49]. Organisms used in osteomyelitis models include, but are not limited to, *S. aureus*, *P. aeruginosa, S. epidermidis, E. aerogenes, E. faecalis, E. faecium, S. sanguis, S. mitis, C. albicans*, and *A. fumigatus*.

For this model, New Zealand rabbits are usually used. Rabbits are anesthetized; then a catheter is placed across the heart valve and left in place for the duration of the study. Animals are infected after 24 h by an intravenous injection of bacterial inoculum. Treatment begins 24 h after infection and is given as multiple dosing regimens for 3–10 days. Animals are killed; then heart valve vegetations are collected, homogenized, serially tenfold diluted, and then cultured on a suitable medium to perform colony counts. Terminal blood samples are taken to check for sepsis. The CFU/g vegetation determined for each dosing regimen can be fit to a suitable pharmacodynamic model.

In the rabbit model, Powell et al. [50] found that single daily doses or continuous infusion of tobramycin provided equally efficacious results, suggesting that the AUC/MIC ratio may be the variable that best describes the efficacy of this compound. In another rabbit model of endocarditis, Fantin et al. [51] found that RP 59500 was efficacious against *S. aureus* despite the fact that it was above the MIC for only 33% of the time. However, it was found that RP 59500 penetrated vegetations well with a vegetation/blood ratio of 4:1 and a prolonged in vitro postantibiotic effect.

In a rat model of endocarditis, Entenza et al. [49] found that despite having concentrations of the quinolone Y-688 that were the same as human concentrations, the compound failed to be efficacious against quinolone-resistant *S. aureus*. This failure may be due to insufficient vegetation penetration [52]. In separate in vitro time-kill studies with *S. aureus*, low concentrations of Y-688 selected for drug resistance. Poor drug penetration into vegetations could have provided ideal conditions for selection of resistance in vivo, and hence the failure of Y-688 in this model.

In an analysis of 19 publications on the treatment of experimentally induced endocarditis caused by *S. aureus*, S. *epidermidis*, viridians streptococci, *E. aerogenes*, and *P. aeruginosa* in rabbit or rat models, Andes and Craig [35] found that for fluoroquinolones, a 24 h AUC/MIC of ≥100, a peak/MIC of >8, and a time above the MIC of 100% were all associated with significant bactericidal activity after 3–6 days of therapy. However, they determined that the 24 h AUC/MIC ratio exhibited the best linear correlation. A conclusion was that the results found in endocarditis with quinolones were similar to those found in the neutropenic thigh model.

7 EXAMPLES OF USE OF ANIMAL MODELS TO STUDY PHARMACOKINETIC-PHARMACODYNAMIC ISSUES

7.1 In Vivo Postantibiotic Effects

Postantibiotic effects have been recognized since the very early studies of penicillin. Although in vitro studies can describe the persistent effects of a drug following its complete removal from a growing culture, they often have little relevance to the in vivo setting when drug concentrations fall more slowly over time. In contrast, demonstration of persistent antibiotic effects following a single dose can be helpful in determining the optimal dosage interval. Single dose experiments in animal models can be used to define the in vivo postantibiotic effect (in vivo PAE) [53,54]. In these experiments a single dose of drug is given and the serum concentration and tissue burden of the test organisms are measured over time. The in vivo PAE is calculated by the equation

$$\text{PAE} = T - C - M$$

where M is the time for which plasma levels exceeded the MIC, T is the time required for the bacterial counts of treated mice to increase by 1 $\log_{10}$ CFU/thigh above the count at time M; and C is the time necessary for the counts in control animals to increase by 1 $\log_{10}$ CFU/thigh. An example is shown in Fig. 6.

There are some important differences between the in vitro and in vivo PAEs. Most notably, the in vivo PAE tends to be longer than the in vitro PAE. A possible explanation for the differences between the in vitro and in vivo PAEs is the effect of subinhibitory drug concentrations on bacterial growth and re-

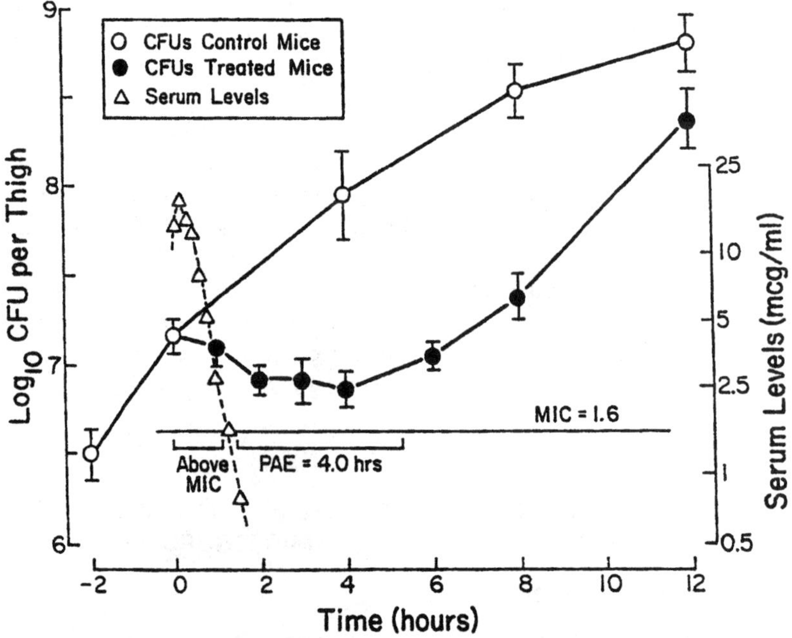

FIGURE 6 Example of an in vivo PAE for cefazolin. Growth curves of control (○) and antibiotic-exposed (●) *S. aureus* ATCC 25923 in mouse thighs after a single dose of cefazolin 12.5 mg/kg. Serum levels of cefazolin after a single dose at 12.5 mg/kg(Δ). (From Ref. 38.)

growth. Sub-MIC concentrations can increase the length of the PAE [55], as reflected in the in vitro measurement, PAE-SME. Measurements of the in vivo PAE from single-dose experiments can then be used to better define the duration of antimicrobial effects in vivo with declining concentrations.

7.2 Serum Protein Binding

Unfortunately, the effect of serum protein binding on antimicrobial activity still attracts considerable controversy and confusion among many clinicians and researchers. The proportional reduction of antimicrobial activity in the presence of serum or binding proteins has been thoroughly demonstrated for several anti-infectives in susceptibility testing.

Although of high interest, there are too few examples of well-controlled experiments that demonstrate the importance of serum protein binding on efficacy in vivo. The difficulty in showing the importance of protein binding in animal models largely lies in the fact that the class of anti-infectives with the greatest variability in serum protein binding are the β-lactam antibiotics. Since the in vivo efficacy of these agents is dependent upon $T >$ MIC and they have relatively short half-lives in small animals, large differences in serum protein binding are required to produce significant differences in free-drug $T >$ MIC. Merriken et al. [56] demonstrated the importance of serum protein binding on the efficacy of several structurally related analogs of penicillin in a mouse model of sepsis due to *Staphylococcus aureus*. All of the agents had similar in vitro potency against the test organism (MIC between 0.25 and 0.5 mg/L) and pharmacokinetic properties, but the percent bound to serum proteins ranged between 36% and 98%. Although the differences in pharmacokinetic properties of total drug were small (2.5-fold range), there was a 70-fold difference among agents in dose required for survival in 50% of animals (ED_{50} ranged from 0.7 to 49.7). In a neutropenic mouse thigh model, we also compared the efficacy of three cephalosporin analogs with varying MICs to 2 strains of methicillin-resistant *Staphylococcus aureus*, pharmacokinetics, and protein binding. As shown in Fig. 7, bacterial killing was best described by the number of hours that free-drug concentrations exceeded the MIC.

7.3 Drug Resistance

The increasing problem of resistance to anti-infective drugs has required critical analysis of the significance of novel resistance mechanisms. The study of drug pharmacodynamics in animal models of infection either using isogenic strains with or without a resistance factor or using relevant clinical isolates can assess the importance of resistance under in vivo conditions. This information can be important in establishing resistance breakpoints for in vitro MIC testing (see below) as well as for formulating optimal dosage regimens to prevent or overcome established resistance. Generally, if resistance in vivo is less than that observed in vitro, this will be reflected by the disruption of expected relationships between drug exposure (e.g., AUC) and MIC.

The clinical relevance of resistance to extended spectrum cephalosporins by novel plasmid-mediated β-lactamases was studied by Craig and colleagues in the neutropenic mouse thigh model against several isogenic strains producing extended-spectrum β-lactamases. Mice were pretreated with uranyl nitrate to simulate human exposures to the drug. The results showed that although MICs were elevated at a high inoculum, in vivo results were best correlated with MICs obtained at the lower inoculum (W. Craig, personal communication).

Reduced susceptibility to vancomycin in enterococci, and more recently *Staphylococcus aureus*, is of increasing clinical concern because of the absence of alternative therapies. In experiments in the neutropenic mouse thigh model with *S. aureus* strains that were vancomycin-susceptible or intermediate (VISA), the efficacy was best described by the C_{max}/MIC or AUC/MIC ratio. When results for the vancomycin susceptible strains were compared with those for VISA, only slightly higher vancomycin exposures (C_{max} or AUC) were required for the same level of efficacy despite the higher MICs. Although further studies are required, this suggests that these strains have a reduced level of susceptibility in vivo to vancomycin that is less than that predicted by the in vitro MIC [57]. Optimization of vancomycin dosage regimens could be a successful strategy for the clinical management of strains with reduced susceptibility to vancomycin.

Drug efflux is increasingly recognized as an important mechanism of resistance in bacteria and fungi. However, little is known concerning the efficiency of these pumps to produce resistance under in vivo conditions. Using isogenic strains of *Pseudomonas aeruginosa* with varying levels of expression of the multicomponent mexAB-oprM efflux pump, a reduced response to levofloxacin and ciprofloxacin in the neutropenic mouse thigh model and mouse sepsis model was observed; the reduction in efficacy due to efflux was proportional to the change in AUC/MIC [58]. In contrast, Andes and Craig [59] reported that AUC/MIC ratios associated with response in the neutropenic mouse thigh model for NOR-A efflux-related resistance to fluoroquinolones in *Streptococcus pneumoniae* were lower than that in susceptible strains or strains with reduced susceptibility due to non-efflux (e.g., gyrA) mechanisms. These data suggest that efflux mechanisms of resistance may be significant in some bacteria but not in others.

Resistance to fluconazole due to target modifications and/or efflux has also been shown to be significant in vivo using pharmacodynamic modeling. Sorensen et al. studied several strains of *C. albicans* with over a 2000-fold range in MIC in a mouse model of disseminated candidiasis. The reduction in counts in kidneys at 24 h following fluconazole was found to be described by the AUC/MIC ratio for all doses and strains tested [44], suggesting that elevated fluconzole MICs due to target or efflux-based mechanisms correspond to similar levels of reduced activity in vivo.

7.4 Establishing Susceptibility Breakpoints

Given the usefulness of pharmacokinetic-pharmacodynamic relationships for predicting efficacy in vivo, animal models using these analyses have been used for establishing breakpoints for in vitro susceptibility testing. The Antimicrobial Susceptibility Testing Subcommittee of the National Committee for Clinical Laboratory Standards (NCCLS) has used such analyses for consideration of breakpoints for certain classes of drugs where clinical data are scant as well as for new agents. A combined approach where data from human clinical trials involving treatment with organisms with varying MICs along with animal model PK-PD data provides a rational basis for establishing susceptibility breakpoints.

Pharmacokinetic-pharmacodynamic data derived in animal models of infection are used to establish susceptibility/resistance breakpoints for MIC testing in several ways. Studies in a relevant model of infection can be used to characterize the parameter that best describes efficacy in the model. The ''target'' PK-PD parameter (e.g., 24 h AUC/MIC ratio) for producing a bacteristatic drug, 50% or even 90% of the maximum response can be derived from the experiments. Based on the pharmacokinetic properties in humans at safe doses, PK-PD parameters for various dosage regimens can be calculated for various MIC values. The

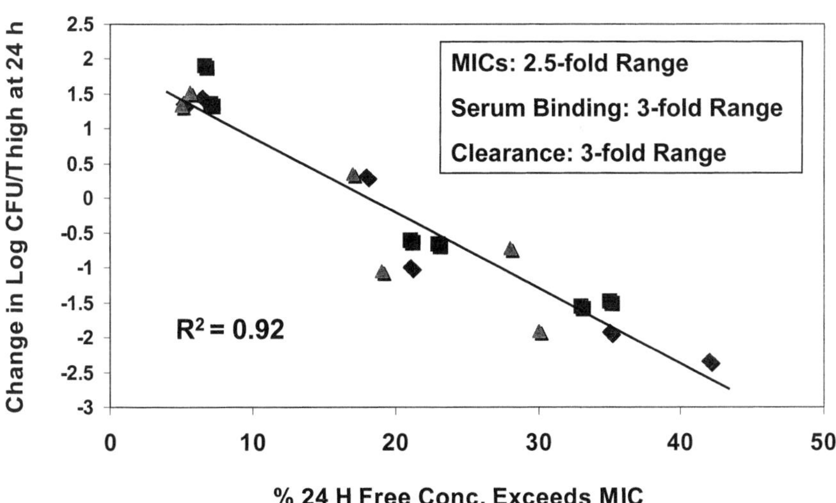

FIGURE 7 Relationship between exposure in vivo to free drug concentrations and bacterial killing in a neutropenic mouse thigh infected model due to 2 strains of methicillin-resistant *Staphylococcus aureus*, and three cephalosporin analogs (■, ▲, ◆ for each compound) with varying MICs and serum protein binding.

highest MIC value that still achieves the target PK-PD parameter for the drug would correspond to a suitable MIC breakpoint for susceptibility testing. For example, a drug whose efficacy in an animal model of infection is maximal when the 24 h free-drug AUC/MIC ratio exceeds 30 and safe regimens in humans produce a 24 h AUC of 60 mg · h/L, then a susceptibility breakpoint of 2 mg/L could be recommended. Of note is that although the exact serum concentration vs. time curve, dosing frequency, and protein binding may differ between humans and small animals, these differences are considered in reducing the exposure relative to the MIC by using pharmacokinetic measures (e.g., free-drug AUC, C_{max}).

The rigor of the selected breakpoint can be further evaluated using simulation. The availability of population pharmacokinetic parameters and their variability in target patient groups can be used to determine the probability of individual patients attaining a PK-PD target parameter using a selected breakpoint. The simulation can be even further developed by incorporating the distribution of MICs in organisms of interest and serum concentration data for individual pa-

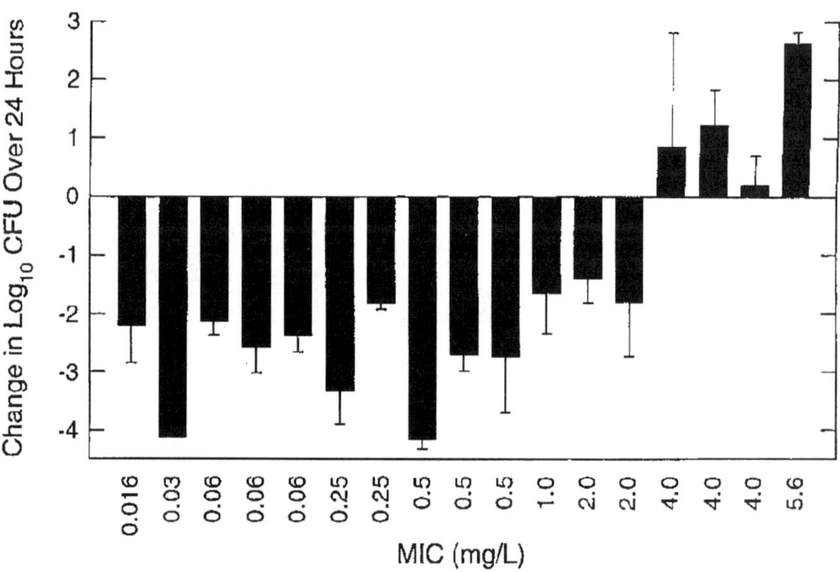

FIGURE 8 Effect of simulated human dosage regimens of amoxicillin on recovery of bacteria from the thighs of neutropenic mice according to amoxicillin MIC. Mice were pretreated with uranyl nitrate to enable simulation of amoxicillin levels corresponding to that observed in humans with usual doses as shown in Fig. 2. Organisms with an MIC ≤2 mg/L all showed a reduction in CFU/thigh, thus supporting a susceptibility breakpoint of this value. (From Ref. 8.)

tients for the population means and variances [60]. This corresponds to the equivalent of a simulated clinical trial.

An alternative approach employs direct simulation of human pharmacokinetics in the animal and testing of strains with varying MICs to the test agent. One would expect to see a graded response according to MIC and ultimately a ''no effect'' at a threshold MIC value. This approach is shown in Fig. 8. Human dosage regimens of amoxicillin were simulated in neutropenic mice, whose thighs were then infected with several strains of *S. pneumoniae* with varying levels of susceptibility to the drug. For strains with MICs exceeding 2 mg/L, little or no effect was seen on bacterial counts recovered from mice at 24 h, thus supporting a susceptibility breakpoint of 2 mg/L or less.

8 CONCLUSIONS

Animal models of infection are a pivotal tool in the study of PK-PD properties of anti-infectives. Consideration of PK-PD issues in the design and interpretation of experiments in animals have strengthened the usefulness of these models for the study of human infection. Animal experimentation has been greatly improved because of recognition of the importance of these issues. In addition, many of the recognized limitations of animal models for application to treatment of human infections have been overcome by recognition of the importance of pharmacokinetics in the outcome of infection. These principles are routinely applied in the study of new drugs in all phases of drug discovery and development as well as in the optimization of dosage in the pre- and postmarketing evaluation of agents.

ACKNOWLEDGMENTS

We acknowledge the excellent assistance of scientists and animal care personnel in Discovery and Preclinical Pharmacology at Microcide Pharmaceuticals, who contributed to generating data for some of the examples provided.

REFERENCES

1. H Eagle, R Fleishman, M Levy. ''Continuous'' vs. ''discontinuous'' therapy with penicillin. N Engl J Med 1953; 248:481–488.
2. H Eagle, R Fleishman, M Levy. On the duration of penicillin action in relation to its concentration in the serum. J Lab Clin Med 1953; 40:122–132.
3. H Eagle, R Fleishman, A Musselman. Effect of schedule of administration on the therapeutic efficacy of penicillin. Am J Med 1950; 9:280–299.
4. H Collins, A Cross, A Dobek, S Opal, J McClain, J Sadoff. Oral ciprofloxacin and a monoclonal antibody to lipopolysaccharide protect leukopenic rats from lethal infection with *Pseudomonas aeruginosa*. J Infect Dis 1989; 159:1073–1082.

5. J Tisdale, M Pasko, J Mylotte. Antipseudomonal activity of simulated infusion of gentamycin alone or with piperacillin assessed by serum bactericidal rate and area under the killing curve. Antimicrob Agents Chemother 1989; 1989:9.
6. A Firsov, S Vostrov, A Shevchenko, G Cornaglia. Parameters of bacterial killing and regrowth kinetics and antimicrobial effect examined in terms of area under the concentration-time curve relationships: Action of ciprofloxacin against Escherichia coli in an in vitro model. Antimicrob Agents Chemother 1997; 1997:6.
7. M Dudley, D Gilbert, T Longest, S Zinner. Dose ranging of the pharmacodynamics of cefoperazone plus sulbactam in an in vitro model of infection: Comparison using a new parameter—area under the survival fraction versus time curve. Pharmacotherapy 1989; 9:189.
8. D Andes, W Craig. In vivo activities of amoxicillin and amoxicillin-clavulanate against *Streptococcus pneumoniae*: Application to breakpoint determinations. Antimicrob Agents Chemother 1998; 42:2375–2379.
9. M Tauber, C Doroshow, C Hackbarth, M Rusnak, T Drake, M Sande. Antibacterial activity of β-lactam antibiotics in experimental meningitis due to *Streptococcus pneumoniae*. J Infect Dis 1984; 149:568–574.
10. I Lutsar, A Ahmed, I Friedland, M Trujillo, L Wubbel, K Olsen, GH McCracken Jr. Pharmacodynamics and bactericidal activity of ceftriaxone therapy in experimental cephalosporin-resistant pneumococcal-meningitis. Antimicrob Agents Chemother 1997; 41:2414–2417.
11. K Madaras-Kelly, A Larsson, J Rotschafer. A pharmacodynamic evaluation of ciprofloxacin and ofloxacin against two strains of *Pseudomonas aeruginosa*. J Antimicrob Agents Chemother 1996; 37:703–710.
12. H Hanberger. Pharmacodynamic effects of antibiotics. Studies on bacterial morphology, initial killing, postantibiotic effect and effective regrowth time. Scand J Infect Dis Suppl 1992; 81:1–52.
13. H Mattie. A predictive parameter of antibacterial efficacy in vivo, based on efficacy in vitro and pharmacokinetics. Scand J Infect Dis Suppl 1990; 74:133–136.
14. J Zhi, C Nightingale, R Quintiliani. A pharmacodynamic model for the activity of antibiotics against microorganisms under measurable conditions. J Pharm Sci 1986; 75:1063–1067.
15. M Dudley, S Zinner. Simultaneous mathematical modeling of the pharmacokinetic and pharmacodynamic properties of cefoperazone. 89th Meeting of the American Society of Clinical Pharmacology and Therapeutics, San Diego, CA, 1988.
16. D D'Argenio, A Schumitsky. ADAPT II: A program for simulation, identification, and optimal experimental design: User manual. Biomedical Simulations Resource, Univ Southern California, Los Angeles, 1992.
17. M Dudley, W Shyu, C Nightingale, R Quintiliani. Effects of saturable protein binding on the pharmacokinetics of unbound cefonicid. Antimicrob Agents Chemother 1986; 30:565–569.
18. J Mordenti. Pharmacokinetic scale-up: Accurate prediction of human pharmacokinetic profiles from animal data. J Pharm Sci 1985; 74:1097–1099.
19. M Tsuji, Y Ishii, A Ohno, S Miyazaki, K Yamaguchi. In vitro and in vivo antibacterial activities of S-4661, a new carbapenem. Antimicrob Agents Chemother 1998; 42:94–99.

20. A Gerber, W Craig. Aminoglycoside-selected subpopulations of *Pseudomonas aeruginosa*: Characterization and virulence in normal and leukopenic mice. J Lab Clin Med 1982; 100:671–681.
21. G Woodnutt, V Berry. Two pharmacodynamic models for assessing the efficacy of amoxicillin-clavulanate against experimental respiratory tract infections caused by strains of *Streptococcus pneumoniae*. Antimicrob Agents Chemother 1999; 43: 29–34.
22. R Roosendaal, I Bakker-Woudenber, J v d Bergh, M Michel. Therapeutic efficacy of continuous versus intermittent administration of ceftazidime in an experimental *Klebsiella pneumoniae* pneumonia in rats. J Infect Dis 1985; 152:373–378
23. E Azoulay-Dupuis, E Vallee, J Bedos, M Muffat-Joly, J Pocidalo. Prophylactic and therapeutic efficacies of azithromycin in a mouse model of pneumococcal pneumonia. Antimicrob Agents Chemother 1991; 35:1024–1028.
24. D Andes, M v Ogtrop. Characterization and quantitation of the pharmacodynamics of fluconazole in a neutropenic murine disseminated candidiasis infection model. Antimicrob Agents Chemother 1999; 43:2116–2120.
25. G Drusano, D Johnson, M Rosen, M Standiford. Pharmacodynamics of a fluoroquinolone antimicrobial agent in a neutropenic rat model of Pseudomonas sepsis. Antimicrob Agents Chemother 1993; 37:483–490.
26. J der Hollander, J Knudsen, J Mouton, K Fuurstad, N Frimodt-Moller, H Verbrugh, F Espersen. Comparison of pharmacodynamics of azithromycin and erythromycin in vitro and in vivo. Antimicrob Agents Chemother 1998; 42:377–382.
27. M Tauber, S Kunz, O Zak, M Sande. Influence of antibiotic dose, dosing interval and duration of therapy on outcome in experimental pneumococcal meningitis in rabbits. Antimicrob Agents Chemother 1989; 33:418–423.
28. A Gerber, H Brugger, C Feller, T Stritzko, B Stalder. Antibiotic therapy of infections due to *Pseudomonas aeruginosa* in normal and granulocytopenic mice: Comparison of murine and human pharmacokinetics. J Infect Dis 1986; 153:90–97.
29. L Mizen. Methods for obtaining human-like pharmacokinetic patterns in experimental animals. In: O Zak, M Sande, eds. Handbook of Animal Models of Infection. Academic Press, New York, 1999, pp 93–103.
30. J Lin, T Lin. Renal handling of drugs in renal failure. I: Differential effects of uranyl nitrate- and glycerol-induced acute renal failure on renal excretion of TEAB and PAH in rats. J Pharmacol Exp Ther 1988; 246:896–901.
31. I Lutsar, I Friedland, L Wubbel, C McCoig, J Jafri, W Ng, F Ghaffar, GH McCracken Jr. Pharmacodynamics of gatifloxacin in cerebrospinal fluid in experimental cephalosporin-resistant Pneumococcal meningitis. Antimicrob Agents Chemother 1998; 42: 2650–2655.
32. T O'Reilly, S Kunz, E Sande, O Zak, M Sande, M Tauber. Relationship between antibiotic concentration in bone and efficacy of treatment of staphylococcal osteomyelitis in rats: Azithromycin compared with clindamycin and rifampin. Antimicrob Agents Chemother 1992; 36:2693–2697.
33. F Genko, T Mannion, C Nightingale, J Schentag. Integration of pharmacokinetics and pharmacodynamics of methicillin in curative treatment of experimental endocarditis. J Antimicrob Chemother 1984; 14:619–631.
34. T Carpenter, C Hackbarth, H Chembers, M Sande. Efficacy of ciprofloxacin for

experimental endocarditis caused by methicillin-susceptible or -resistant strains of *Staphylococcus aureus*. Antimicrob Agents Chemother 1986; 30:382–384.
35. D Andes, W Craig. Pharmacodynamics of fluoroquinolones in experimental models of endocarditis. Clin Infect Dis 1998; 27:47–50.
36. A Gerber, W Craig, H-P Brugger, C Feller, A Vastola, J Brandel. Impact of dosing intervals on activity of gentamicin and ticarcillin against *Pseudomonas aeruginosa* in granulocytopenic mice. J Infect Dis 1983; 145:296–329.
37. D Andes, M V Ogtrop, W Craig. Impact of neutrophils on the in-vivo activity of fluoroquinolones. 37th Annual Meeting of the Infectious Disease Society of America, Infect Dis Soc Am, Philadelphia, PA, 1999.
38. W Craig, S Gudmundsson. The postantibiotic effect. In: V Lorian, ed. Antibiotics in Laboratory Medicine, Williams and Wilkins, Baltimore, MD, 1996, pp 296–329.
39. G Smith, K Abbott. Development of experimental respiratory infections in neutropenic rats with either penicillin-resistant *Streptococcus pneumoniae* or β-lactamase-producing *Haemophilus influenzae*. Antimicrob Agents Chemother 1994; 38:608–610.
40. S Arai, Y Gohara, A Akashi, K Kuwano, N Nishimoto, T Yano, K Oizumi, K Takeda, T Yamaguchi. Effects of new quinolones on *Mycoplasma pneumoniae*-infected hamsters. Antimicrob Agents Chemother 1993; 37:287–292.
41. L Piroth, L Martin, A Coulon, C Lequeu, M Duong, M Buisson, H Portier, P Chavanet. Development of an experimental model of penicillin-resistant *Streptococcus pneumoniae* pneumonia and amoxicillin treatment by reproducing human pharmacokinetics. Antimicrob Agents Chemother 1999; 43:2484–2492.
42. T Rogers, J Galgiani. Activity of fluconazole (UK 49,858) and ketoconazole against *Candida albicans* in vitro and in vivo. Antimicrob Agents Chemother 1986; 30: 418–422.
43. A Louie, G Drusano, P Banerjee, Q-F Liu, W Liu, P Kaw, M Shayegani, H Taber, H Miller. Pharmacodynamics of fluconazole in a murine model of systemic candidiasis. Antimicrob Agents Chemother 1998; 42:1105–1109.
44. K Sorensen, E Corcoran, S Chen, D Clark, V Tembe, O Lomovskaya, M Dudley. Pharmacodynamic assessment of efflux- and target-based resistance to fluconazole (FLU) on efficacy against *C. albicans* in a mouse kidney infection model. 39th Interscience Conference on Antimicrobial Agents and Chemotherapy, San Francisco, CA, 1999.
45. J Knudsen, K Fuursted, F Esperson, N Frimodt-Moller. Activities of vancomycin and teicoplanin against penicillin-resistant pneumococci in vitro and in vivo and correlations to pharmacokinetic parameters in the mouse peritonitis model. Antimicrob Agents Chemother 1997; 41:1910–1915.
46. A Ahmed, H Jafri, I Lutsar, C McCoig, M Trujillo, L Wubbel, S Shelton, GH McCracken Jr. Pharmacodynamics of vancomycin for the treatment of experimental penicillin- and cephalosporin-resistant pneumococcal meningitis. Antimicrob Agents Chemother 1999; 43:876–881.
47. M Smeltzer, J Thomas, S Hickmon, R Skinner, C Nelson, D Griffith, TR Parr Jr, R Evans. Characterization of a rabbit model of staphylococcal osteomyelitis. J Orthop Res 1997; 15:414–421.

48. M Sande, M Johnson. Antimicrobial therapy of experimental endocarditis caused by *Staphylococcus aureus*. J Infect Dis 1975; 131:367–375.
49. J Entenza, O Marchetti, M Glauser, P Moreillon. Y-688, a new quinolone active against quinolone-resistent Staphylococcus aureus: Lack of in vivo efficacy in experimental endocarditis. Antimicrob Agents Chemother 1998; 42:1889–1894.
50. S Powell, W Thompson, M Luthe, R Stern, D Grossniklaus, D Bloxham, D Groden, M Jacobs, A Discenna, H Cash, J Klinger. Once-daily vs. continuous aminoglycoside dosing: Efficacy and toxicity in animal and clinical studies of gentamicin, netilmicin, and tobramicin. J Infect Dis 1983; 147:918–932.
51. B Fantin, R Leclercq, M Ottaviani, J Valois, B Maziere, J Duval, J Pocidalo, C Carbon. In vivo activities and penetration of the two components of the streptogramin RP 59500 in cardiac vegetations of experimental endocarditis. Antimicrob Agents Chemother 1994; 38:432–437.
52. A Cremieux, B Maziere, J Vallois, M Ottaviani, A Azancot, H Raffoul, A Bouvet, J Pocidalo, C Carbon. Evaluation of antibiotic diffusion into cardiac vegetations by quantitative autoradiography. J Infect Dis 1989; 159:938–944.
53. W Craig. Post-antibiotic effects in experimental infection models: Relationship to in-vitro phenomena and to treatment of infections in man. J Antimicrob Chemother 1993; 31:149–158.
54. B Vogelman, S Gudmundsson, J Turnidge, J Leggett, W Craig. In vivo postantibiotic effect in a thigh infection in neutropenic mice. J Infect Dis 1988; 157:287–298.
55. O Cars, I Odenholt-Tornqvist. The post-antibiotic sub-MIC effect in vitro and in vivo. J Antimicrob Chemother 1993; 31:159–166.
56. D Merrikin, J Briant, G Rolinson. Effect of protein binding on antibiotic activity in vivo. J Antimicrob Chemother 1983; 11:233–238.
57. M Dudley, D Griffith, E Corcoran, C Liu, K Sorensen, V Tembe, S Chamberland, D Cotter, S Chen. Pharmacokinetic-pharmacodynamic (PK-PD) indices for vancomycin (V) treatment of susceptible (VSSA) and intermediate (VISA) *S. aureus* in the neutropenic mouse thigh model. 39th Interscience Conference on Antimicrobial Agents and Chemotherapy, San Francisco, CA, 1999.
58. D Griffith, O Lomovskaya, L Harford, A Lee, MN Dudley, V Lee. Effect of efflux pumps (EPs) on the activity of fluoroquinolones against *Pseudomonas aeruginosa* in murine models of infection. 37th Interscience Conference on Antimicrobial Agents and Chemotherapy, Toronto, Canada, 1997.
59. D Andes, W Craig. Pharmacodynamics of gemifloxacin (GEM) against quinolone-resistant strains of *S. pneumoniae* (SP) with known resistance mechanisms. 39th Interscience Conference on Antimicrobial Agents and Chemotherapy, San Francisco, CA, 1999.
60. M Dudley, PG Ambrose. Pharmacodynamics in the study of drug resistance and establishing in vitro susceptibility breakpoints: ready for prime time. Curr Opin Microbiol 2000; 3:515–521.

5

β-Lactam Pharmacodynamics

JoCarol J. McNabb
University of Nebraska Medical Center, Omaha, Nebraska

Khanh Q. Bui
Bristol-Myers Squibb Company, Chicago, Illinois

1 INTRODUCTION

1.1 Historical Overview

Penicillin G, the original β-lactam antibiotic, was discovered by Fleming in 1928 and used for the first time in 1941 to treat a staphylococcal infection in a British policeman. By the end of World War II, penicillin was commercially available in the United States [1]. Although initially given as a continuous infusion, due to the abundance of penicillin and the difficulties with the intravenous drip delivery system, long-acting repository forms of penicillin G became popular with clinicians. The pharmacodynamic concepts that apply to β-lactams were actually pioneered in the late 1940s by Harry Eagle, an immunologist at the National Institutes of Health. Calling upon both in vitro and in vivo animal studies, Eagle was the first investigator to propose the concept of time-dependent bactericidal killing for β-lactams. Eagle demonstrated in vivo that a penicillin-free interval prolongs the duration of treatment necessary for cure and that less total daily drug given in frequent, multiple doses is more effective than larger, infrequent doses. Eagle also demonstrated in vivo with nonneutropenic mice and rabbits that the duration of the penicillin concentration above the MIC of a specific pathogen correlates to drug efficacy. In Eagle's experiments, a serum concentration 2–5 times the MIC of the bacteria correlated with penicillin's bactericidal activity [2]. The concept of dividing antibacterials into groups based on the pattern of bactericidal activity was not formally proposed by investigators until the late 1970s. As early as 1953, however, Eagle clearly discussed not only the time-dependent bactericidal activity of penicillin but also the concentration dependence of streptomycin, the first aminoglycoside [3].

In like manner, Eagle also elucidated the effect of antibiotic concentration on the rate at which a pathogen is killed both in vitro and in vivo. Marked differences in the effective concentration of penicillin and the maximal rate of kill exist between organisms, depending on the generation time and the MIC of the organism. For gram-positive bacteria, however, 3–10 times the MIC of the pathogen kills at a maximal rate that does not continue to increase as the concentration of penicillin increases [4–7]. Excessively high concentrations of penicillin do not increase its bactericidal effect. In fact, in relation to *S. pneumoniae*, Eagle observed a paradoxical decrease in the rate of killing in vitro at very high concentrations of penicillin [8]. Although two case reports of streptococcal endocarditis cured by reducing the dose of penicillin appear in the literature, the clinical significance of this paradoxical phenomenon, now termed the ''Eagle effect,'' has never been studied in a clinical trial [9–10].

As experience with penicillin increased, clinicians soon realized that in practice the concentration did not have to be continuously maintained above the MIC of a given pathogen to effect a cure in humans [11]. Several investigators, most notably Bigger and Parker, demonstrated in vitro that once gram-positive bacteria were exposed to a lethal dose of penicillin, a period of delayed organism regrowth ensued during which surviving organisms did not immediately begin to multiply [12–14]. Schmidt and Eagle were the first investigators to report this phenomenon in animal studies of *S. pneumoniae* infection [15–17]. Eagle proposed an elegant hypothesis explaining what is now known as the post antibiotic effect. Calling this phenomenon the ''slow recovery of bacteria from the toxic effects of penicillin,'' he proposed that bacteria that are damaged but not killed by exposure to penicillin remain susceptible to host defenses for several hours after the penicillin is removed [18,19]. Eagle's in vitro and in vivo experiments are the foundation for β-lactam pharmacodynamics. His experiments, however, were not designed to answer one of the most crucial pharmacodynamic questions: What is the optimal time above the MIC for the β-lactams? Although not specifically proven by his own experiments, Eagle consistently asserted throughout his work that the best dosing strategy for penicillin is to maintain antibiotic concentrations above the pathogen's MIC for the entire dosing interval. This concept guided the dosing of β-lactams for the next 50 years.

1.2 Pharmacokinetics Versus Pharmacodynamics

The differentiation between pharmacokinetics and pharmacodynamics has been discussed earlier in this book. To review these concepts, the reader is encouraged to refer back to Chapter 2. Because of the large number of β-lactam antibiotics available, a complete review of each product will not be undertaken. Where possible, generalizations will be made to simplify the discussion as it pertains to this class. β-Lactams are best represented by a two-compartment model in which they undergo rapid distribution followed by an elimination or terminal phase. The pharmacokinetic parameters of the β-lactams show many similarities in relation to the steady-state volume of distribution. In a review of eight β-lactams (including members of the semisynthetic penicillin, cephalosporin, and carbapenem group), Drusano [20] showed that the volume of distribution following the post-distributive phase for these agents is much less than 1 L/kg (range 0.15–0.24 L/kg), indicating that they remain in the extracellular water as opposed to moving into mammalian cells. β-Lactams can be found in most body sites and secretions, making them an option for many infections.

Although the volumes of distribution are similar for the compounds in this class, other pharmacokinetic parameters such as clearance, route of elimination and half-life show more variability. The clearance can vary by threefold, from 7 to 24 L/h [20]. Because the volume of distribution falls within a narrow range, this change in clearance is the primary determinant of half-life variation for this class. The terminal half-life for penicillin and its analogs tends to be shorter (0.8–1.2 h) than those of the cephalosporins (1.4–8 h) [20–23]. This is the rationale for different dosing regimens, as some require administration every 4 h, whereas others produce reliable outcomes with more extended dosing intervals of every 12 or 24 h.

The renal route of elimination is the primary pathway for the clearance of β-lactams. The notable exceptions for this would be ceftriaxone, cefoperazone and nafcillin, which undergo extensive nonrenal elimination as well [22].

2 FACTORS AFFECTING PHARMACODYNAMICS

2.1 Postantibiotic Effect

The postantibiotic effect (PAE) is the suppression of bacterial growth that persists when drug is removed after a short exposure of a microorganism to an antimicrobial. All antimicrobials appear to have a PAE to gram positive bacteria in vitro. The mechanism of the PAE is not well understood. It may relate to nonlethal damage of the bacteria or limited persistence of the drug at a cellular site of action. Factors that have been shown to influence the PAE include the type of organism, the dose and concentration of antibiotic, the duration of exposure, and the size of the bacterial inoculum.

In vitro, one determines the PAE by observing bacterial growth kinetics after antibiotic is removed. The PAE retards the growth of antibiotic-exposed culture in relation to a control and is usually defined as the difference between the time for each culture (exposed and control) to increase in concentration by 1 $\log_{10}$ (tenfold) after removal of the drug [24]. There is no standard protocol for measurement of the PAE in vitro, however. Some investigators measure the PAE indirectly by viable colony counts. Others use direct methods, including bioluminescense or optical density [25]. The methodology will affect the results. A PAE obtained from a bioluminescense assay is typically longer than the PAE determined by viable counts [26]. This knowledge is important in evaluating results from different studies. The magnitude of the PAE depends upon drug exposure time and antibiotic concentration, up to some maximal response [27, 28]. By viable counts, the PAE of penicillins and cephalosporins to gram-positive bacteria is consistently 1–3 h [29]. Imipenem and meropenem are the only β-lactams that demonstrate a PAE to gram-negative bacteria, primarily *P. aeruginosa* [30–32]. The PAE of these carbapenems to *P. aeruginosa* appears to be strain-dependent and varies up to 2 h in length depending on the particular strain [33].

In general, the PAE observed in vivo is of greater duration than the PAE observed in vitro for the same bacteria. Several theories have been proposed to explain this phenomenon. The sub-MIC effect is one possible explanation. Investigators evaluating the effects of residual drug on bacterial growth have shown that, in vitro, a post antibiotic sub-MIC effect will prolong the duration of the PAE. For example, the PAE of benzylpenicillin is 2.4 h to *S. pyogenes*. When exposed to sub-MIC concentrations of penicillin (0.3 × MIC), the PAE increases to 22 h. Continued exposure to antibiotics at sub-MIC concentrations is actually closer to the reality of declining in vivo drug levels than the in vitro models where antibiotic is completely removed from the system when PAE is tested [34]. Another possible explanation for the longer in vivo PAE is the postantibiotic leukocyte enhancement (PALE) effect. As long as there is otherwise a PAE, leukocytes have been shown in vitro to enhance the killing of antibiotic-damaged bacteria and prolong the PAE [35].

The neutropenic mouse thigh model and the neutropenic mouse pneumonia model are the two most widely accepted animal models used by investigators to study the PAE in vivo. By eliminating the effects of white blood cells, one can determine the PAE attributable solely to the antibiotic. In a neutropenic mouse thigh model of infection, all β-lactams induce a PAE of 1.2–4.5 h to *S. aureus,* no PAE to gram-negative bacteria, and no PAE to *S. pneumoniae* [36]. These results are consistent with in vitro results with the exception of penicillin in relation to *S. pneumoniae* [37]. Even though penicillin does exert an in vitro PAE to *S. pneumoniae*, investigators have not been able to reproduce the effect in vivo. Using the mouse thigh model to evaluate the effect of combination antibiotics, investigators have also shown that when both drugs (an aminoglycoside plus a β-lactam to treat *S. aureus)* induce a PAE alone, then the combination prolongs the PAE beyond the longer of the individual PAEs [38].

The most important clinical application of the PAE as a pharmacodynamic parameter is in defining optimal dosing schedules for β-lactams. The PAE is crucial in determining the optimal time above the MIC for any given drug–pathogen combination. The existence of a PAE implies that the time above the MIC can be less than 100% of the dosing interval and, in fact, the PAE is the theoretical rationale for the intermittent dosing of β-lactams.

2.2 Protein Binding

The effect of protein binding continues to be a topic of debate even as more is learned about the pharmacodynamics of β-lactams. It is recognized that protein binding is a rapid process that produces a reversible interaction between antibiotic and protein, principally albumin [39]. A constant equilibrium exist between the total (T) drug concentration and free/unbound (F) and protein bound (DB) fractions: $T \leftrightarrow F + DB$. It is accepted that only the free drug is able to diffuse from the bloodstream to the site of infection and subsequently into the bacteria. This concept is important for the time-dependent antibiotics that rely on maintaining unbound serum concentrations in excess of the MIC for a prolonged period of time. For highly protein bound drugs, failures may be predicted as free-drug concentrations drop below the MIC.

In vivo models with mice and rabbits have demonstrated that the degree of β-lactam protein binding correlates with the penetration into implanted tissue cages. When table tennis balls were implanted into rabbits, it was found that the penetration of cephalothin (65% protein bound) was 27% versus 12% that of cefazolin (86% protein bound) [40]. This was further substantiated with work in a mouse peritonitis infection model with *S. aureus* showing that the degree of protein binding was inversely proportional to the dose of antibiotic required to produce a protective dose [41]. Merrikin et al. [41] used a set of β-lactams that had the same intrinsic activity to the test strain while maintaining the pharmacokinetics relatively constant to derive their data. They also noted that the more highly protein bound drugs had a longer half-life but that this did not correlate with the protective dose because the MICs of all agents were identical.

Studies evaluating the effect of protein binding and clinical outcome in humans are difficult to perform. Instead, the skin blister fluid model has been used in healthy subjects to estimate the relationship between serum protein binding and tissue penetration. This is interpreted as a movement of drug from the intravascular to the extravascular space that is necessary during the treatment of an active infection. When flucloxacillin (95% protein-bound) was compared to amoxicillin

(17% protein-bound), penetration into blister fluid was markedly less for the highly protein bound antibiotic [42]. This suggests that amoxicillin is a better agent for treatment, but many other factors (intrinsic antimicrobial activity, solubility) must be considered when making a determination for the appropriateness of use. The authors also pointed out that the effect of protein binding on penetration becomes more pronounced only when the proportion of bound drug is high. Because most β-lactams exhibit less than 70% protein binding, their penetration will be minimally affected [42].

The in vitro and in vivo reduction in cephalosporin activity is less predictable when cephalosporins are tested against gram-negative organisms. Leggett and Craig [43] found that the ceftriaxone, cefoperazone, moxalactam, and ceftizoxime MICs for *E. coli* and *K. pneumoniae* in human serum ultrafiltrate were less than predicted by simply examining the protein binding alone. The same effect was not observed with *S. aureus* or *P. aeruginosa.* A disproportionate rise in the MIC was observed when the antibiotics were placed into 25%, 50%, and 95% serum. The hypothesis for this observation was that the serum contained products that enhanced the killing of gram-negative bacilli. In essence, a protein found in the serum effectively lowered the MIC when these cephalosporins were exposed to Enterobacteriaceae. This finding may explain why ceftriaxone (95% protein bound) provides activity at or slightly below its MIC, even though failure would be predicted.

Clinical data in humans to show that protein binding can alter the outcome of an infection were presented in a case report by Chambers et al. [44]. These workers reported three therapeutic failures with cefonicid used once daily for the treatment of *S. aureus* endocarditis. This is a highly bound (95%) cephalosporin, and it was suggested that free drug concentrations were not sustained for a long enough period of time. The measured total drug concentrations (free and bound) exceeded 150 μg/mL, but the serum bactericidal titer (SBT) was $<1:8$. Successful outcomes are predicted when the SBTs are $\geq 1:8$. Another consequence of the high protein binding was the MIC difference of cefonicid in broth versus serum. When the organisms were originally tested in broth, the geometric mean for all patients was 4.6 μg/mL, whereas use of 50% serum as the diluent resulted in a six fold increase (27.9 μg/mL). As noted previously, protein binding, particularly in situations with highly bound cephalosporins against gram-positive bacteria, will result in an increase of the MIC. This latter observation is often overlooked when susceptibility tests are performed. From these data, it appears that this regimen allowed free-drug concentrations to remain above the MIC for only a very short period of time. The role of protein binding may affect the pharmacodynamics of specific antibiotic–bacterium combinations, especially in situations where the free drug concentrations do not exceed the time above the MIC for β-lactams.

3 RESEARCH STUDIES

3.1 In Vitro Studies

The in vitro evidence supporting the role of β-lactams as concentration-independent (time-dependent) agents was reported by Craig and Andes [45], who used a standard time-kill method with ticarcillin, ciprofloxacin, and tobramycin. Following the addition of antibiotic to the experimental strain of *Pseudomonas aeruginosa*, they found that only ticarcillin failed to produce a faster rate of bacterial killing after concentrations of 4 × MIC were achieved. The rate and extent of bacterial killing between 4 × MIC as compared to 16 × MIC and 64 × MIC were similar, leading them to suggest that exceeding the MIC by more than fourfold is not necessary.

3.2 In Vivo Animal Studies

The in vivo data with animals correlate with observations from in vitro experiments. An undertaking to describe and highlight all of the previous work in this area will not be attempted here. Instead, studies describing important results that contribute to the understanding of β-lactam pharmacodynamics will be used. To minimize the confusion related to host factors, most of the experimental data were derived using a neutropenic infection model. Eliminating the activity of white blood cells from these models has a distinct advantage over using normal animals: only antibiotic–organism interactions are studied, without any additional interference from neutrophils.

Using a mouse model, Gerber et al. [46] correlated bacterial regrowth to the time above the MIC ($T >$ MIC). When ticarcillin was administered as either a single bolus or a fractionated dose (more closely simulating human pharmacokinetics, resulting in similar AUCs), neutropenic animals were found to have reduced bacterial growth, with more frequent dosing extending the $T >$ MIC. The extremely large peak/MIC ratio produced from a bolus dose (20:1) did not reduce the bacteria count more than the fractionated doses (5:1). This same study evaluated the effect of these two dosing schemes in normal mice. Unlike previous results, the bacterial regrowth with the bolus dose was not demonstrated, suggesting that the effect of the combination with antibiotic and white blood cells was significant in suppressing *P. aeruginosa*. No attempt was made to determine the optimal $T >$ MIC required to produce a good outcome, but an examination of these data show that concentrations during bolus dosing were above the MIC for only 25% of the dosing interval.

The required $T >$ MIC for obtaining the best outcome may vary for individual antibiotic–pathogen combinations. A univariate analysis of ticarcillin, cefazolin and penicillin all demonstrated that the $T >$ MIC was the most important parameter in determining outcome as opposed to the AUC or peak concentrations [47]. To produce a bactericidal effect, *E. coli* required a longer exposure to cefazolin (>60% versus 20%) compared to *S. aureus*. This large difference is the result of a significant PAE of cefazolin for *S. aureus*. This evidence supports earlier work with cephalosporins and *S. pneumoniae* that found a relationship between $T >$ MIC and the effective dose required for protection of 50% of the animals [48].

Studies comparing normal and neutropenic animals can show the pharmacodynamic influence of host defenses. As described previously, the work of Gerber et al. [46] demonstrated that normal mice could suppress bacterial growth regardless of the optimal dosing scheme. Roosendaal et al. [49] also discovered a striking difference between normal and leukopenic rats. For normal rats, the intermittent (every 6 h) and continuous administration of ceftazidime required equivalent doses (0.35 and 0.36 mg/kg, respectively) to reach the protective dose for 50% (PD_{50}) of the animals. For leukopenic rats, the continuous infusion required 3.75 mg/kg to produce the PD_{50}, whereas 30 mg/kg of ceftazidime was needed with the intermittent dosing. This study highlights two important differences between normal and neutropenic animals: (1) Host defenses can overcome the deficiencies when the pharmacodynamics are not maximized and (2) neutropenic hosts require larger doses than normal hosts to eradicate organisms.

3.3 Clinical Studies

Human studies to determine the optimal pharmacodynamics of β-lactams have focused on infections in acute otitis media (AOM) or continuous infusion (CI) settings. AOM is an attractive model because of the relative ease of fluid collection that can be used for determining antibiotic concentation or MIC over time. A more in-depth discussion of AOM is presented in Section 7. Clinical data with continuous infusion provide important information because the pharmacodynamics are maximized with a prolonged time above the MIC. The following section presents a summary of relevant continuous infusion studies.

4 CONTINUOUS INFUSION

The goal of antibiotic therapy is to achieve the best possible clinical outcomes while consuming the least amount of hospital resources. Health care systems are under intense pressure to increase quality of care and at the same time reduce costs. Pressure to reduce the cost of antimicrobial therapy is especially intense because these drugs may account for up to 50% of a hospital pharmacy budget. Although β-lactam antibiotics have traditionally been given by intermittent infusion, administration by continuous infusion is gaining popularity because it takes full advantage of the known pharmacodynamics of the β-lactams and potentially consumes the least amount of hospital resources. Other options that will also maintain the time above MIC for the entire dosing interval are the use of antibiotics with longer half-lives or more frequent, larger doses. An advantage of continuous infusion, however, is that it can be given at a lower total daily dose than standard dosing schedules. Although the IV drip method used in the past was cumbersome and inaccurate, today, because of lightweight, portable, and accurate infusion pumps, a continuous infusion is relatively easy and cost-effective to administer. Giving a loading dose prior to starting the continuous infusion will bring the antibiotic concentration into the therapeutic range immediately and minimize any lag time in drug tissue equilibration. Constant infusion of β-lactam antibiotics has the potential for appreciable cost reductions because it may represent the best method to maintain levels above the MIC during the entire dosing interval using the least amounts of drug, labor, and supplies.

A number of in vitro and animal models substantiate the equivalent or superior efficacy of continuous infusion of β-lactams compared to standard dosing. These models have been used extensively to elucidate the pharmacodynamics of β-lactams because they hold a significant advantage over studies in humans: The doses and dosing intervals of antibiotic are easily varied, reducing the interdependence of the pharmacodynamic parameters. Using an in vitro model, investigators have demonstrated that a continuous infusion (CI) at 5 × MIC of *P. aeruginosa* is as efficacious as intermittent dosing (II) using less total daily drug [50,51]. Experiments in animal models have confirmed these in vitro results and demonstrated further that a continuous infusion may be the better dosing strategy if the same total daily dose is used [52,53].

The mouse thigh model has been used to evaluate the difference between neutropenic and nonneutropenic host response [54]. The real difference in efficacy between CI and II shows up in the neutropenic host: Even with a lower total daily dose, CI provides much better efficacy than bolus dosing [55,56]. In neutropenic rats with gram-negative infection, a ceftazidime bolus dose that protects 50% of the animals from death (PD_{50}) had to be 65-fold higher than the PD_{50} dose for a continuous infusion of the same drug. Once again, this experiment confirms that time above MIC correlates to efficacy for the β-lactams, and when host defenses are not present the β-lactam concentration should exceed the MIC of the pathogen for the entire dosing interval [57].

Continuous infusion is a practical way to maintain 100% time above MIC with less total daily drug (e.g., 3 g/24 h CI of ceftazidime versus 1–2 g every 8 h). Although clinical efficacy data are sparse, the pharmacodynamics of continuous infusion are well-characterized in both normal volunteers and critically ill patients, and several small clinical trials have shown the equivalence of continuous infusion and standard dosing [58–62]. In one of the first clinical trials of continuous infusion, Bodey et al. [63] compared the efficacy of cefamandole dosed as either a continuous infusion or an intermittent dose given in combination with carbenicillin. There was no significant difference in clinical cure between the two regimens. By subgroup analysis, patients with persisting, severe neutropenia had a better clinical outcome (65% versus 21%, $p = 0.03$) with continuous infusion [63]. In a study of CI benzylpenicillin versus daily IM procaine penicillin G in 123 patients with pneumococcal pneumonia, there was also no difference in clinical cure rates [64]. A nonrandomized trial of continuous versus intermittent dosing of cefuroxime showed that the CI results in a lower total antibiotic dose. The CI results in equivalent efficacy, shorter length of hospital stay, and overall cost savings to the institution [65].

At Hartford Hospital, there have been two continuous infusion β-lactam clinical studies. The investigators compared cefuroxime given either as a continuous infusion of 1500 mg or intermittently as 750 mg every 8 h ($n = 25$ in each group) to treat hospitalized community-acquired pneumonia (CAP) [66]. Steady state cefuroxime serum concentrations were 13.25 ± 6.29 μg/mL, more than 2–4 times the MIC_{90} of typical CAP pathogens. There was no difference in clinical cure rates, but the CI regimen was associated with a shorter length of treatment, decreased length of stay, lower total cefuroxime dose, and overall cost savings. The average amount of intravenous cefuroxime per patient decreased significantly ($p = 0.04$) from 8.0 ± 3.4 g for intermittent dosing to 5.9 ± 3.2 g for the continuous infusion. The average daily costs (including antibiotics, labor, and supplies) decreased significantly ($p = 0.04$), $63.64 ± 30.95 for the continuous infusion compared with $83.85 ± 34.82 for intermittent dosing.

The second Hartford Hospital study was a prospective, randomized trial of the efficacy and economic impact of ceftazidime given as either a continuous infusion (3 g/day) or intermittent infusion (2 g q8h) plus once-daily tobramycin for the treatment of nosocomial pneumonia in the ICU [67]. The investigators evaluated 35 patients, 17 in the CI group and 18 in the II group. Clinical efficacy did not vary significantly between groups (94% success in CI vs. 83% in II). Number of adverse events, duration of treatment, and total length of hospital stay also did not vary significantly. The continuous infusion regimen used half of the intermittent dose and maintained concentrations above the MIC of the pathogen for 100% of the dosing interval. The intermittent dosing regimen maintained concentrations above the MIC for 76% of the dosing interval. The costs (including drug acquisition, antibiotic preparation and administration, adverse events, and treatment failures) associated with the CI of ceftazidime, $625.69 ± 387.84, were significantly lower ($p \leq 0.001$) than with the II, $1004.64 ± 429.95.

There are some potential disadvantages to giving antibiotics by continuous infusion. For patients with limited IV access, the continuous infusion may require their only IV line. Drug compatibility will be an issue if two drugs must be infused simultaneously through one line. Although the cost of infusion pumps should be considered in any cost-effectiveness analysis of drug delivery by continuous infusion, since most manufacturers will provide the use of the infusion pumps with a supply contract, the cost to the hospital is usually limited to the price of the administration sets. Overall, the advantages of the continuous infusion, both pharmacodynamically and economically, far outweigh the disadvantages. The continuous infusion of β-lactams in place of frequent intermittent dosing is a good example of how the knowledge and application of pharmacodynamic concepts can lead to cost-effective antibiotic therapy.

5 TISSUE PENETRATION

Because of the difficulties associated with measuring tissue concentrations of drugs, we generally use serum concentration as a surrogate marker in pharmacodynamic models. Although most common bacterial pathogens are extracellular, infections occur in the tissues, and it is the pharmacodynamic profile of an antibiotic at the site of infection that ultimately determines its clinical efficacy. Antibiotic concentrations can vary significantly depending on the type of tissue. Drug penetration into tissues depends on the properties of the specific tissue type, the properties of the antibiotic, and the interactions that occur at the tissue/drug interface. Protein binding, tissue permeability, tissue metabolic processes, and drug physiochemical properties such as lipid solubility, pK_a, and molecular weight all influence an antibiotic's movement into human tissues. Only the free fraction (non-protein-bound) of an antibiotic is available to exert a pharmacological effect. For β-lactams, the percent tissue penetration is inversely proportional to the protein binding of the drug. Animal studies show a direct correlation between serum protein binding and penetration into peripheral lymph. The penetration into rabbit lymph of ceftriaxone, a drug that is highly protein bound, is 67.3%. In comparison, the penetration of amoxicillin, a drug with much less serum protein binding, is 97.6% [68].

Methodological problems in obtaining tissue samples are the limiting factor in characterizing antibiotic tissue concentrations. A complete pharmacodynamic picture would include a concentration–time curve for the various tissue compartments. Most studies done in humans to date, however, simply characterize drug penetration into various tissue compartments. In spite of the limitations, these studies have provided important information about the extracellular and intracellular disposition of these drugs. Tissue penetration studies consistently show that penicillins and cephalosporins have rapid and good penetration into interstitial fluid [69–72]. The opposite occurs in relation to intracellular space. There is essentially no uptake of β-lactams into peripheral blood mononuclear cells, polymorphonuclear cells, or alveolar macrophages, thus explaining the ineffectiveness of β-lactams against intracellular pathogens such as *Mycoplasma* or *Chlamydia* [73,74].

Standard methods of characterizing tissue concentrations by using whole tissue homogenates tend to underestimate the interstitial concentration of β-lactams. A promising new technique, currently being developed for studying the pharmacodynamics of drug tissue penetration in both animals and humans, has been applied to the study of β-lactams with some success. Microdialysis is an in vivo sampling technique for the continuous monitoring of drugs or other analytes in the extravascular space. The advantage of microdialysis is that it can be used in a variety of tissue compartments with minimal invasiveness and can therefore be used in subjects that are awake and freely moving. Because it overcomes the limitations of other methods, microdialysis offers a unique opportunity to characterize the pharmacokinetic profile of drugs in tissue compartments such as the interstitial fluid, adipose tissue, muscle, or dermis.

Two microdialysis studies in animals have evaluated the tissue pharmacokinetic profile of various β-lactams. In the rat thigh model, investigators found an excellent correlation between piperacillin and ceftriaxone concentrations in plasma and predicted free levels of drug in the tissue [75,76]. In a separate study using awake and freely moving rats, the investigators measured ceftriaxone and ceftazidime concentrations in two regions of the animal's brain. Interestingly, not only are the half-lives of the antibiotics in the brain different from their respective half-lives in serum, but drug distribution within the brain differs by region and is not homogenous. Based on this study, antibiotic distribution appears to differ by specific tissue compartment and region [77]. Similar differences, by tissue compartment, in equilibration rates and pharmacokinetic profiles have been observed in human subjects [78]. Microdialysis promises to be a useful tool in pharmacodynamic studies of the future.

The central nervous system presents special problems in relation to studying the pharmacodynamics of drugs. The brain is a unique tissue compartment. Tight junctions of endothelial cells and a low rate of transcellular drug transport both act to exclude antibiotics from the CNS. Impaired host defenses and the slow rate of bacterial growth in the CNS decrease the effectiveness of antibiotics. The primary determinants of antibiotic blood-brain barrier penetration are a drug's lipid solubility, degree of protein binding, ionization, and active transport into or out of the CSF [79]. Although highly lipophilic compounds pass readily into the CSF, β-lactams are hydrophilic, weak organic acids, and their penetration is normally less than 10%. This penetration significantly increases during the inflammation associated with meningitis [80–83]. An additional issue in relation to β-lactams is the active transport mechanism that pumps these drugs out of the CSF. Benzylpenicillin has the highest affinity for the transport pump, but other β-lactams are also subject to elimination by this route.

Antibiotic concentrations are especially difficult to measure in the brain due to the invasiveness in obtaining either spinal fluid (CSF) or tissue samples, and relatively few pharmacodynamic studies have examined the activity of β-lactams in the CNS. Although there is limited evidence that antibiotic pharmacodynamics in the brain differ from the dynamics in other tissue compartments, because we cannot easily characterize this in human subjects, antibiotic dosing in CNS infections is still largely empirical. The data we do have, have been obtained from in vitro models or animal studies.

In vitro, for cefotaxime, investigators have shown a limited PAE to *E. coli* of about 0.5 h in pooled human CSF. The same studies do not demonstrate a PAE for cefotaxime to *E. coli* in Mueller-Hinton broth (MHB), indicating that there may be a mechanism for PAE that is unique to the CSF [84,85]. There are conflicting results from animal studies measuring the PAE of β-lactams in the CSF [86]. In one study, adding β-lactamase to the CSF reversed the PAE, indicating that small amounts of residual drug in the CSF may actually be responsible for the in vivo PAE [87].

Although studies in animals have suggested that the β-lactam pharmacodynamic parameter in CSF that correlates to efficacy is actually the peak concentration rather than the time above MIC, the results from these studies are inconclusive [88–90]. Using a rabbit pneumococcal meningitis model to investigate the relationship between CSF penicillin concentration and bactericidal rate of killing, the investigators demonstrated that maximal killing occurred at 10–30 times the minimal bactericidal concentration (MBC) of the pathogen [91]. Unfortunately, they did not also determine the duration of time above MBC. As the concentration of drug increases, the time above MBC in the CSF will also increase and will most likely approach 100% of the dosing interval. When the dose of the antibiotic is high enough to provide 100% time above MIC, the pharmacodynamic parameters of time and concentration cannot be separated to determine which parameter really correlates to efficacy.

In contrast, the one study to examine the relationship between the pharmacodynamic parameters of time above MBC, peak/MBC, and AUC/MBC demonstrated that $T >$ MIC continues to be the important pharmacodynamic parameter for β-lactams, even in the CSF. By varying the doses and dosing intervals of ceftriaxone in a rabbit meningitis model of cephalosporin-resistant *S. pneumoniae* (MIC and MBC = 4.0 μg/mL), the investigators determined that $T >$ MBC is the only pharmacodynamic parameter that independently correlated with ceftriaxone's bactericidal activity. During the first 24 h, the highest rate of bactericidal killing occurred when $T >$ MBC exceeded 95% of the dosing interval. Also, in the first 24 h, twice-daily administration of the same total ceftriaxone dose resulted in longer time > MBC and higher killing rates [92]. On the basis of this study, it appears that the same pharmacodynamic model, time-dependent killing, that defines β-lactam activity in serum and other tissue compartments also defines β-lactam efficacy in the CSF [93].

6 β-LACTAM AND β-LACTAMASE INHIBITOR COMBINATIONS

The incidence of gram-negative bacterial resistance has been on the rise in recent years. *Escherichia coli*, the leading cause of gram-negative bacteremia in both the community and hospital setting, develops resistance to β-lactams by the production of TEM-1 and TEM-2 plasmid-mediated β-lactamases. β-Lactamases are a large family of enzymes, ubiquitous to bacteria, that hydrolyze the β-lactam ring of penicillins and cephalosporins. The incidence of gram-negative bacterial resistance as well as the increasing incidence of nosocomial gram-positive infections (due to bacteria such as *S. aureus* that are intrinsically resistant to β-lactams) have led to the search for new antibiotics. One approach is to combine a β-lactam with a potent β-lactamase inhibitor. Currently in the United States there are three β-lactamase inhibitors on the market (clavulanate, sulbactam, and tazobactam) that are used in combination with a β-lactam antibiotic. The goal of β-lactam–β-lactamase inhibitor combinations is to expand the coverage of the β-lactam to gram-positive bacteria and overcome drug resistance to gram-negative bacteria [94,95].

Strategies for the optimal dosing of β-lactam–β-lactamase inhibitors based on pharmacodynamic principles have not been established or even extensively studied. In addition to the pharmacodynamic issues that relate to the individual β-lactam, several additional pharmacodynamic questions arise in relation to combination drugs. These questions include: Would the sequential dosing of inhibitor and β-lactam affect the bactericidal activity of the combination? Second, is it the ratio of the combination of drugs that matters, or is it the time above the MIC of the component drugs that determines efficacy? Finally, if it is the time above the MIC of each drug that correlates to overall efficacy, what is the optimal time above the MIC for the inhibitor, and how does that affect the time above the MIC required for the β-lactam?

Two pharmacodynamic studies have addressed the issue of sequential dosing. In vitro, the sequential dosing of tazobactam followed by piperacillin does not enhance the bactericidal activity of piperacillin [96]. Similarly, in vivo, as studied in *E. coli* bacteremia in mice, the pharmacodynamics of ampicillin-sulbactam does not depend on whether sulbactam is dosed sequentially or simultaneously with ampicillin [97].

The question of optimal $T >$ MIC is complicated for β-lactam–β-lactamase inhibitor combinations because the turnover rate of both the enzyme and the inhibitor will affect the inactivation of the β-lactamase [98]. The amount and type of enzyme produced by the bacteria have a marked effect on the dynamics of the inhibitor [99]. Subsequently, the amount of inhibitor present determines restoration of susceptibility to the partner drug [100]. Current dosing regimens provide concentrations of inhibitor that exceed the in vitro susceptibility breakpoint for only 2–3 h, not the entire dosing interval. Inasmuch as these drugs have been shown to work clinically, the unique pharmacodynamics of the β-lactam–β-lactamase inhibitor combination is clearly the determining factor [101].

One explanation for the clinical efficacy of these drugs may relate to a post-β-lactamase inhibition effect. In an adaptation of the model used to determine post-antibiotic effect, the effect of tazobactam was evaluated in β-lactamase-producing strains of *E. coli*. Preincubation of bacteria with tazobactam and piperacillin resulted in piperacillin-induced killing during a second exposure to piperacillin alone. Bacteria not initially exposed to tazobactam were not killed by piperacillin during the second exposure [102]. Similarly, other investigators have reported a post-β-lactamase inhibition effect in which regrowth of amoxicillin-resistant bacteria is prevented by amoxicillin alone following exposure to and removal of amoxicillin and clavulanate [103].

In an in vitro study of piperacillin versus piperacillin/tazobactam, as expected, the addition of tazobactam to piperacillin did not alter the killing of an *E. coli* piperacillin-susceptible strain. By adding tazobactam to piperacillin, the killing of an isogenic TEM-3 *E. coli* resistant to piperacillin became equivalent to the killing of the susceptible strain, even though the concentration of tazobactam fell below 4 mg/L (the concentration used in susceptibility testing) at 3 h. As an explanation, the investigators suggest that several hours of an essentially β-lactamase-negative state, during which bacteria must reaccumulate sufficient quantities of β-lactamase to inactivate the drug, follow exposure to high levels of inhibitor. Therefore, the dosing interval of β-lactam–β-lactamase inhibitor combinations can be extended for some finite period of time limited by the re accumulation of β-lactamase by persisting bacteria [104]. On the basis of this small number of in vitro studies, it appears that dosing piperacillin-tazobactam every 8 h instead of every 6 h is a reasonable dosing regimen.

7 CORRELATION TO IN VITRO RESISTANCE

Clinical studies evaluating resistance rates and patient outcomes have been primarily conducted in respiratory tract infections. In comparison to other infection sites, respiratory tract infections are more prevalent and recovery of bacteria is primarily noninvasive, allowing more data to be compiled. A limitation to interpreting these data is that only a handful of the most commonly isolated bacteria are studied, often excluding serious pathogens such as vancomycin-resistant *Enterococcus faecium* (VRE) or methicillin resistant *Staphylococcus aureus* (MRSA), which are not associated with these body sites. Although limited, these studies provide clues for the treatment of other infections that require aggressive antibiotic therapy. The reporting of resistance continues to rise, but the impact on clinical outcomes may not always correlate with microbiological reports.

Using a retrospective review of pneumonia caused by *Streptococcus pneumoniae*, Pallares and colleagues compared cases involving penicillin-nonsensitive strains (MIC $\geq$ 0.12–8 μg/mL) to a matched control group with penicillin-sensitive strains (MIC $\leq$ 0.1 μg/mL) [105]. Of the 24 cases, 14 presented with intermediate-resistant pneumococci (0.12 $\leq$ MIC $\leq$ 1 μg/mL) and the remaining 10 were resistant (MIC $\geq$ 2 μg/mL). A higher mortality rate (54% vs 25%, P = 0.0298) was observed when these cases were compared to the control group. This difference may have been multifactorial because cases also had statistically significant more episodes of pneumonia in the past year ($P = 0.01$), exposure to β-lactam therapy in the past 3 months ($P = 0.0008$), recent hospitalizations ($P = 0.0038$), and nosocomial pneumonia ($P = 0.0032$) and were initially critically ill ($P = 0.0030$). These factors provide evidence that cases with penicillin-nonsensitive strains had more comorbidities. When the authors examined their data, they reported that of the 19 cases that received a β-lactam as treatment, 11 recovered. Furthermore, all eight deaths occurred in patients who were initially critically ill, suggesting that this parameter, not the choice of drug therapy, accounted for mortality differences. Two strains with a higher MIC (4 and 8 μg/mL) resulted in therapeutic failures, providing support that current breakpoints need to be revised upward to correlate with clinical outcomes. The authors concluded that penicillin-resistant strains with MIC ≤ 2 μg/mL responded well to β-lactam therapy if patients were not critically ill at the initial presentation.

As a followup, the same group performed a 10-year prospective study [106]. It was shown that mortality was higher (38% vs. 24%, $P = 0.001$) when a penicillin-resistant *S. pneumoniae* was isolated. As described previously, when all other factors relating to severity were included, no statistical significance was found ($P = 0.32$). The mortality resulting from the administration of penicillin G, ampicillin, ceftriaxone, or cefotaxime was in the range of 19–25% regardless of the susceptibility patterns or agent used. These data suggest that the use of cephalosporin or high dose intravenous penicillin may be effective for treatment even when the MIC of penicillin predicts resistance (≤2 μg/mL).

These studies have since been substantiated by the work of other investigators [107,108]. Gress et al. [107] compared the outcomes of intermediate-resistant and susceptible *S. pneumoniae* and found no difference in length of stay ($P = 0.96$), fever ($P = 0.74$), or mortality ($P = 0.15$). The treatment in this study was penicillin or ampicillin, and the conclusion was that both agents provided adequate serum and tissue concentrations to effectively treat organisms that had an MIC of ≤1 μg/mL. Cabellos et al. [108] confirmed the usefulness of procaine penicillin in the treatment of pneumococcal pneumonia. Fifteen of 16 patients were cured, and the only failure occurred in a patient who had a *S. pneumoniae* with penicillin MIC of 4 μg/mL. The findings were supported with pharmacokinetic and serum bactericidal activity data.

Friedland [109] prospectively studied children with pneumococcal pneumonia and found that after 3 days of therapy, clinical improvement was noted in 70% (12/17) of patients with penicillin-resistant strains, compared to 62% (28/45) of patients with penicillin-susceptible strains [109]. At the day 7 evaluation, 88% (15/17) of patients with a penicillin-resistant strain had improved along with 93% (42/45) in whom a penicillin-susceptible *S. pneumoniae* was isolated. Two deaths occurred in each group and all were treated with intravenous therapy. Every patient treated with oral β-lactam therapy improved, regardless of the penicillin susceptibility profile. These data show poor correlation between penicillin resistance (≤2 μg/mL) and clinical outcome for non-CNS infections caused by *S. pneumoniae*.

Although resistance data for pneumococcal pneumonia do not correlate well with clinical outcomes, studies in acute otitis media (AOM) have produced more predictable outcomes. In a comparative study utilizing either cefuroxime axetil or cefaclor for the treatment of AOM, Dagan et al. [110] found that cefuroxime axetil consistently produced better outcomes. These data showed that increasing penicillin resistance correlated with statistically significant ($P < 0.001$) bacteriological failures despite cephalosporin therapy. The penicillin MIC ranges of <0.1, 0.125–0.25, and 0.38–1 μg/mL resulted in overall failure rates of 6%, 21%, and 64%, respectively. When further stratified to the drug regimens, the failure rate of cefuroxime axetil was 9%, 8%, and 50%, respectively. In these same ranges, the cefaclor failure rate was 4%, 43%, and 80%. The escalating failure rate in these patients probably resulted from poor antibiotic penetration into the middle ear fluid, because the pharmacodynamics was not optimized with these dosage regimens.

Gehanno et al. [111] also reported the diminished activity of cefuroxime axetil as the penicillin MIC increased. When 84 children with *S. pneumoniae* were treated with 30 mg/kg of cefuroxime suspension for 8 days, a clinical success rate of 86% (72/84) was observed for the penicillin MIC range of ≤0.015 to ≥4 μg/mL. The clinical success rate was 92% (39/42) for penicillin-susceptible strains, 90% (9/10) for penicillin-intermediate strains, and 75% (24/32) for penicillin-resistant strains. The conclusion was that cefuroxime axetil was clinically effective for AOM but may not be the drug of choice when resistant strains emerge due to the higher failure rate.

Craig and Andes [112] had predicted this scenario when they evaluated the pharmacokinetics and antimicrobial effects of these agents in AOM. Against penicillin-intermediate and -resistant *S. pneumoniae*, failure was expected with cefaclor because the usual dosage regimen did not produce any appreciable time above the minimal inhibitory concentration ($T >$ MIC) that is required of β-lactams for clinical success. Cefuroxime was more likely to produce a successful outcome because the $T >$ MIC against penicillin-intermediate *S. pneumoniae* ranged from 33% to 53% whereas the $T >$ MIC for penicillin-resistant strains was 0–23%. The $T >$ MIC can be thought of as a surrogate marker for resistance, because as the MIC increases the $T >$ MIC is reduced, predicting failure. In the analysis of AOM, an inverse correlation was observed between resistant strains and clinical outcomes.

The previous examples do not provide a strong correlation between microbiological resistance and clinical outcomes. The primary reason for these discrepancies is that microbiological tests are performed with only bacteria and antibiotics, whereas clinical outcomes include an additional component of host-specific factors. When the host has a functional immune system or is not critically ill, outcomes may be much better than predicted by pharmacodynamic relationships alone. Conversely, a host with comorbidities or situations that compromise the pharmacodynamics can unmask the true effectiveness of an antibiotic. Linden et al. [113] reported that the poor outcomes between vancomycin-resistant and -susceptible *Enterococcus faecium* (VREF vs. VSEF) were multifactorial, with the antibiotic accounting for a partial effect. The effect of reduced antibiotic susceptibility also increased the number of adverse events for patients infected with *Pseudomonas aeruginosa*–resistant isolates [114]. These patients simultaneously presented with additional problems that may have added to their poor outcomes. The in vitro reporting of bacterial resistance should be used as a guide but cannot serve as the sole determinant of therapeutic decision making, because it is the triad of antibiotic, host, and bacteria that determines outcomes.

8 CONCLUSION

β-Lactam antibiotics are time-dependent agents that display bactericidal activity within the therapeutically achievable dosages. Because most agents in this drug class have short half-lives, it is often necessary to administer frequent doses or use novel dosing strategies to optimize their pharmacodynamic and pharmacokinetic properties. The data gathered over the past half century using in vitro, animal, and human studies clearly show their usefulness in the treatment of numerous infections when factors such as tissue penetration, postantibiotic effect, and protein binding are considered.

REFERENCES

1. A Fleming. On the antibacterial action of cultures of a penicillium, with special reference to their use in the isolation of *B. influenzae*. Br J Exp Pathol 1929;10: 226.
2. H Eagle, R Fleischman, AD Musselman. Effect of schedule of administration on therapuetic efficacy of penicillin: Importance of aggregate time penicillin remains at effectively bactericidal levels. Am J Med 1950;9:280–299.
3. PM Shah, W Junghanns, W Stille. Dosis-Wirkuns-Beziehung der Bakterizidie bei *E. coli, K. pneumoniae* und *Staphylococcus aureus*. Dent Med Wochenschr 1976; 101:325–328.
4. H Eagle, R Fleischman, AD Musselman. Effective concentrations of penicillin in vitro and in vivo for streptococci, pneumococci, and *Treponema pallidum*. J Bacteriol 1950;59:625–43.
5. H Eagle, R Fleischman, M Levy. On duration of penicillin action in relation to its concentration in serum. J Lab Clin Med 1953;41:122–132.
6. H Eagle, HJ Magnuson, R Fleischman. Effect of method of administration on thera-

peutic efficacy of sodium penicillin in experimental syphilis. Bull Johns Hopkins Hosp 1946;79:168–89.
7. H Eagle, AD Musselman. The rate of bactericidal action of penicillin in vitro as function of its concentration, and its paradoxically reduced activity at high concentrations against certain organisms. J Exp Med 1948:88:99–131.
8. WMM Kirby. Bacteriostatic and lytic actions of penicillin on sensitive and resistant staphylococci. J Clin Invest 1945;24:165–169.
9. LR Griffiths, HT Green. Paradoxical effect of penicillin in-vivo (letter). J Antimicrob Chemother 1985;15:507–508.
10. RH George, A Dyas. Paradoxical effect of penicillin in vivo (letter). J Antimicrob Chemother 1987;17:684–685.
11. H Eagle, R Fleischman, M Levy. ''Continuous'' vs ''discontinuous'' therapy with penicillin. N Engl J Med 1953;248:481–488.
12. RF Parker, S Luse. Action of penicillin on Staphylococcus: Further observations of effect of short exposure. J Bacteriol 1948;56:75–81.
13. RF Parker, HC Marsh. Action of penicillin on staphylococcus. J Bacteriol 1946; 51:181–186.
14. JW Bigger. Bactericidal action of penicillin on *Staphylococcus pyogenes*. Irish J Med Sci 1944;228:585–595.
15. E Jawetz. Dynamics of the action of penicillin in experimental animals. Arch Intern Med 1946;77:1.
16. LH Schmidt, A Walley, RD Larson. The influence of the dosage regimen on the therapeutic activity of penicillin G. J Pharmacol Exp Ther 1949;96:258–268.
17. LH Schmidt, A Walley. The influence of the dosage regimen on the therapeutic effectiveness of penicillin G in experimental lobar pneumonia. J Pharmacol Exp Ther 1951;103:479–488.
18. H Eagle, R Fleischman, AD Musselman. Bactericidal action of penicillin in vivo: Participation of host, and slow recovery of surviving organisms. Ann Intern Med 1950;33:544–571.
19. H Eagle, AD Musselman. The slow recovery of bacteria from the toxic effects of penicillin. J Bacteriol 1949;58:475–490.
20. GL Drusano. Role of pharmacokinetics in the outcome of infections. Antimicrob Agents Chemother 1988;32:289–297.
21. GR Donowitz, GL Mandell. Beta-lactam antibiotics (part 1). N Engl J Med 1988; 318:419–426.
22. GR Donowitz, GL Mandell. Beta-lactam antibiotics (part 2). N Engl J Med 1988; 318:490–500.
23. M Fassbender, H Lode, T Schaberg, K Borner, P Koeppe. Pharmacokinetics of new oral cephalosporins, including a new carbacephem. Clin Infect Dis 1993;16: 646–653.
24. A Kumar, MB Hay, GA Maier, JW Dyke. Post-antibiotic effect of ceftazidime, ciprofloxacin, imipenem, piperacillin and tobramycin for *Pseudomonas cepacia*. J Antimicrob Chemother 1992;30:597–602.
25. H Hanberger, LE Nilsson,M Nilsson, R Maller. Post-antibiotic effect of β-lactam antibiotics on gram-negative bacteria in relation to morphology, initial killing and MIC. Eur J Clin Microbiol Infect Dis 1991;10:927–934.

26. H Hanberger, E Svensson, LE Nilsson, M Nilsson. Pharmacodynamic effects of meropenem on gram-negative bacteria. Eur J Clin Microbiol Infect Dis 1995;14: 383–390.
27. PJ McDonald, WA Craig, CM Kunin. Persistent effect of antibiotics on *Staphylococcus aureus* after exposure for limited periods of time. J Infect Dis 1977;135: 217–223.
28. RW Bundtzen, AU Gerber, DL Cohn, WA Craig. Postantibiotic suppression of bacterial growth. Rev Infect Dis 1981;3:28–37.
29. F Baquero, E Culebras, C Patron, JC Perez-Diaz, JC Medrano, MF Vicente. Postantibiotic effect of imipenem of gram-positive and gram-negative micro-organisms. J Antimicrob Chemother 1986;18(suppl E):47–59.
30. H Erlendsdottir, S Gudmundsson. The post-antibiotic effect of imipenem and penicillin-binding protein 2. J Antimicrob Chemother 1992;30:231–232.
31. HL Nadler, DH Pitkin, W Sheikh. The postantibiotic effect of meropenem and imipenem on selected bacteria. J Antimicrob Chemother 1989;24(suppl A):225–231.
32. CI Bustamante, GL Drusano, BA Tatem, HC Standiford. Postantibiotic effect of imipenem on *Pseudomonas aeruginosa*. Antimicrob Agents Chemother 1984;26: 678–682.
33. S Gudmundsson, B Vogelman, WA Craig. The in-vivo postantibiotic effect of imipenem and other new antimicrobials. J Antimicrob Chemother 1986;18(suppl E): 67–73.
34. O Cars, I Odenholt-Tornqvist. The post-antibiotic sub-MIC effect in vitro and in vivo. J Antimicrob Chemother 1993;31(suppl D):159–166.
35. PJ McDonald, BL Wetherall, H Pruul. Postantibiotic leukocyte enhancement: increased susceptibility of bacteria pretreated with antibiotics to activity of leukocytes. Rev Infect Dis 1981;3:38–44.
36. B Vogelman, S Gudmundsson, J Turnidge, J Leggett, WA Craig. In vivo postantibiotic effect in a thigh infection in neutropenic mice. J Infect Dis 1988;157:287–298.
37. WA Craig. Post-antibiotic effects in experimental infection models: Relationship to in vitro phenomena and to treatment of infections in man. J Antimicrob Chemother 1993;31(suppl D);149–158.
38. S Gudmundsson, S Einarsson, H Erlendsdottir, J Moffat, W Bayer, WA Craig. The post-antibiotic effect of antimicrobial combinations in a neutropenic murine thigh infection model. J Antimicrob Chemother 1993;31(suppl D):177–191.
39. R Wise. Protein binding of β-lactams: The effects on activity and pharmacology particularly tissue penetration. I. J Antimicrob Chemother 1983;12:1–18.
40. DN Gerding, WH Hall. The penetration of antibiotics into peritoneal fluid. Bull NY Acad Med 1975;51:1016–1019.
41. DJ Merrikin, J Briant, GN Rolinson. Effect of protein binding on antibiotic activity in vivo. J Antimicrob Chemother 1983;11:233–238.
42. R Wise, AP Gillett, B Cadge, SR Durham, S Baker. The influence of protein binding upon tissue fluid levels of six β-lactam antibiotics. J Infect Dis 1980;142:77–82.
43. JE Leggett, WA Craig. Enhancing effect of serum ultrafiltrate on the activity of

cephalosporins against gram-negative bacilli. Antimicrob Agents Chemother 1989; 33:35–40.
44. HF Chambers, J Mills, TA Drake, MA Sande. Failure of a once-daily regimen of cefonicid for treatment of endocarditis due to Staphylococcus aureus. Rev Infect Dis 1984;6:S870–874.
45. WA Craig, SC Ebert. Killing and regrowth of bacteria in vivo: A review. Scand J Infect Dis Suppl 1991;64:63–70.
46. AU Gerber, H-P Brugger, C Fell, T Stritzko, B Stadler. Antibiotic therapy of infections due to Pseudomonas aeruginosa in normal and granulocytopenic mice: Comparison of murine and human pharmacokinetics. J Infect Dis 1986;153:90–97.
47. B Vogelman, S Gudmundsson, J Leggett, J Turnidge, S Ebert, WA Craig. Correlation of antimicrobial pharmacokinetic parameters with therapeutic efficacy in an animal model. J Infect Dis 1988;158:831–847.
48. N Frimodt-Møller, MW Bentzon, VF Thomsen. Experimental infection with *Streptococcus pneumoniae* in mice: Correlation of in vitro activity and pharmacokinetic parameters with in vivo effect for 14 cephalosporins. J Infect Dis 1986;154:511–517.
49. R Roosendaal, IAJM Bakker-Woudenbert, MVDBV Raffe, MF Michel. Continuous versus intermittent administration of ceftazidime in experimental *Klebsiella pneumoniae* pneumonia in normal and leukopenic rats. Antimicrob Agents Chemother 1986;30:403–408.
50. JW Mouton, JG den Hollander. Killing of *Pseudomonas aeruginosa* during continuous and intermittent infusion of ceftazidime in an in vitro pharmaocokinetic model. Antimicrob Agents Chemother 1994;38:931–936.
51. DM Cappelletty, SL Kang, SM Palmer, MJ Rybak. Pharmacodynamics of ceftazidime administered as continuous infusion or intermittent bolus alone and in combination with single daily-dose amikacin against *Pseudomonas aeruginosa* in an in vitro infection model. Antimicrob Agents Chemother 1995;33:1797–1801.
52. JJ Mordenti, R Quintiliani, CH Nightingale. Combination antibiotic therapy: Comparison of constant infusion and intermittent bolus dosing in an experimental animal model. J Antimicrob Chemother 1985;15:313–321.
53. DH Livingston, MT Wang. Continuous infusion of cefazolin is superior to intermittent dosing in decreasing infection after hemorrhagic shock. Am J Surg 1993;165: 203–207.
54. AU Gerber. Impact of the antibiotic dosage schedule on efficacy in experimental soft tissue infections. Scand J Infect Dis 1991;suppl 74:147–154.
55. IAJM Bakker-Woudenberg, JC van den Berg, P Fontijne, MF Michel. Efficacy of continuous versus intermittent administration of penicillin G *in Streptococcus pneumoniae* pneumonia in normal and immunodeficient rats. Eur J Clin Microbiol 1984;3:131–135.
56. K Totsuka, K Shimizu, J Leggett, B Vogelman, WA Craig. Correlation between the pharmacokinetic parameters and the efficacy of combination therapy with an aminoglycoside and a β-lactam. In: Y Ueda, ed. Proceedings of the International Symposium on Netilmicin. Professional Postgraduate Services, Japan, 1985:41–48.
57. R Roosendaal, IAJM Bakker-Woudenberg, M van den Berghe-van Raffe, MF Mi-

chel. Continuous versus intermittent administration of ceftazidime in experimental Klebsiella pneumoniae pneumonia in normal and leukopenic rats. Antimicrob Agents Chemother 1986;30:403–408.

58. DP Nicolau, JC McNabb, MK Lacy, J Li, R Quintiliani, CH Nightingale. Pharmacokinetics and pharmacodynamics of continuous and intermittent ceftazidime during the treatment of nosocomial pneumonia. (in press)
59. DP Nicolau, CH Nightingale, MA Banevicius, Q Fu, R Quintiliani. Serum bactericidal activity of ceftazidime: Continuous infusion versus intermittent injections. Antimicrob Agents Chemother 1996:40:61–64.
60. S Daenen, Z Erjavec, DRA Uges, HG de Vries-Hospers, P de Jonge, MR Halie. Continuous infusion of ceftazidime in febrile neutropenic patients with acute myeloid leukemia. Eur J Clin Microbiol Infect Dis 1995;14:188–192.
61. AS Benko, DM Cappelletty, JA Kruse, MJ Rybak. Continuous infusion versus intermittent administration of ceftazidime in critically ill patients with suspected gram-negative infections. Antimicrob Agents Chemother 1996;40:691–695.
62. H Lagast, F Meunier-Carpenter, J Klastersky. Treatment of gram-negative bacillary septicemia with cefoperazone. Eur J Clin Microbiol 1983;2:554–558.
63. GP Bodey, SJ Ketchel, V Rodriguez. A randomized study of carbenicillin plus cefamandole or tobramycin in the treatment of febrile episodes in cancer patients. Am J Med 1979;67:608–611.
64. A Brewin, L Arango, WK Hadley, JF Murray. High-dose penicillin therapy and pneumococcal pneumonia. JAMA 1974;230:409–413.
65. JA Zeisler, JD McCarthy, WA Richelieu, MB Nichol. Cefuroxime by continuous infusion: A new standard of care? Infect Med 1992;11:54–60.
66. PG Ambrose, R Quintiliani, CH Nightingale, DP Nicolau. Continuous vs. intermittent infusion of cefuroxime for the treatment of community-acquired pneumonia. Infect Dis Clin Prac 1998;7:463–470.
67. DP Nicolau, J McNabb, MK Lacy, J Li, R Quintiliani, CH Nightingale. Pharmacokinetics and pharmacodynamics of continuous and intermittent ceftazidime during the treatment of nosocomial pneumonia. Clin Drug Invest 1999;in press.
68. G Woodnutt, V Berry, L Mizen. Effect of protein binding on penetration of β-lactams into rabbit peripheral lymph. Antimicrob Agents Chemother 1995;39: 2678–2683.
69. DM Ryan, B Hodges, GR Spencer, SM Harding. Simultaneous comparison of three methods for assessing ceftazidime penetration into extravascular fluid. Antimicrob Agents Chemother 1982;22:995–998.
70. T Kalager, A Digranes, T Bergan, CO Solberg. The pharmacokinetics of ceftriaxone in serum, skin blister and thread fluid. J Antimicrob Chemother 1984;13:479–485.
71. R Wise, IA Donovan, MR Lockley, J Drumm, JM Andrews. The pharmacokinetics and tissue penetration of imipenem. J Antimicrob Chemother 1986;18(suppl E): 93–101.
72. JW Mouton, MF Michel. Pharmacokinetics of meropenem in serum and suction blister fluid during continuous and intermittent infusion. J Antimicrob Chemother 1991;28:911–918.
73. H Koga. High-performance liquid chromatography measurement of antimicrobial

concentrations in polymorphonuclear leukocytes. Antimicrob Agents Chemother 1987;31:1904–1908.

74. WL Hand, N King-Thompson, JW Holman. Entry of roxithromycin (RU 965), imipenem, cefotaxime, trimethoprim, and metronidazole into human polymorphonuclear leukocytes. Antimicrob Agents Chemother 1987;31:1553 -1557.
75. A Nolting, TD Costa, R Vistelle, KH Rand, H Derendorf. Determination of free extracellular concentrations of piperacillin by microdialysis. J Pharm Sci 1996;85: 369-372.
76. A Kovar, TD Costa, H Derendorf. Comparison of plasma and free tissue levels of ceftriaxone in rats by microdialysis. J Pharm Sci 1997;86:52–56.
77. L Granero, M Santiago, J Cano, A Machado, JE Peris. Analysis of ceftriaxone and ceftazidime distribution in cerebrospinal fluid of and cerebral extracellular space in awake rats by in vivo microdialysis. Antimicrob Agents Chemother 1995;39: 2728–2731.
78. M Muller, O Haag, T Burgdorff, A Georgopoulos, W Weninger, B Jansen, G Stanek, H Pehamberger, E Agneter, HG Eichler. Characterization of peripheral-compartment kinetics of antibiotics by in vivo microdialysis in humans. Antimicrob Agents Chemother 1996;40:2703–2709.
79. RA Fishman. Blood-brain and CSF barriers to penicillin and related organic acids. Arch Neurol 1966;15:113–124.
80. LJ Strausbaugh, CR Bodem, PR Laun. Penetration of aztreonam into cerebrospinal fluid and brain of noninfected rabbits and rabbits with experimental meningitis caused by *Pseudomonas aeruginosa*. Antimicrob Agents Chemother 1986;30:701–704.
81. E Marmo, L Coppola, R Pempinello, G di Nicuolo, E Lampa. Levels of amoxicillin in the liquor during continuous intravenous administration. Chemotherapy 1982; 28:171–175.
82. R Yogev, WE Schultz, SB Rosenman. Pentrance of nafcillin into human ventricular fluid: Correlation with ventricular pleocytosis and glucose levels. Antimicrob Agents Chemother 1981;19:545–548.
83. DT Mullaney, JF John. Cefotaxime therapy: Evaluation of its effect on bacterial meningitis, CSF drug levels. and bactericidal activity. Arch Intern Med 1983;143: 1705–1708.
84. GG Zhanel, JA Karlowsky, RJ Davidson, DJ Hoban. Effect of pooled human cerebrospinal fluid on the postantibiotic effects of cefotaxime, ciprofloxacin, and gentamicin against *Escherichia coli*. Antimicrob Agents Chemother 1992;36:1136–1139.
85. JA Karlowsky, GG Zhanel, RJ Davidson, SR Zieroth, DJ Hoban. In vitro postantibiotic effects following multiple exposures of cefotaxime, ciprofloxacin, and gentamicin against *Escherichia coli* in pooled human cerebrospinal fluid and Mueller-Hinton broth. Antimicrob Agents Chemother 1993;37:1154–1157.
86. MA Sande, OM Korzeniowski, GM Allegro, RO Brennan, O Zak, WM Scheld. Intermittent or continuous therapy of experimental meningitis due to *Streptococcus pneumoniae* in rabbits: Preliminary observations on the postantibiotic effect in vivo. Rev Infect Dis 1981;3:98–109.
87. MG Tauber, O Zak, WM Scheld, B Hengstler, MA Sande. The postantibiotic effect

in the treatment of experimental meningitis caused by *Streptococcus pneumoniae* in rabbits. J Infect Dis 1984;149:575–583.

88. MG Tauber, S Kunz, O Zak, MA Sande. Influence of antibiotic dose, dosing interval, and duration of therapy on outcome in experimental pneumococcal meningitis in rabbits. Antimicrob Agents Chemother 1989;33:418–423.
89. JM Decazes, JD Ernst, MA Sande. Correlation of in vitro time-kill curves and kinetics of bacterial killing in cerebrospinal fluid during ceftriaxone therapy of experimental *Escherichia coli* meningitis. Antimicrob Agents Chemother 1983;24: 463–467.
90. I Lustar, GH McCracken Jr. IR Friedland. Antibiotic pharmacodynamics in cerebrospinal fluid. Clin Infect Dis 1998;27:1117–1129.
91. MG Tauber, CA Doroshow, CJ Hackbarth, MG Rusnak, TA Drake, MA Sande. Antibacterial activity of β-lactam antibiotics in experimental meningitis due to Streptococcus pneumoniae. J Infect Dis 1984;149:568–574.
92. I Lutsar, A Ahmed, IR Friedland, M Trujillo, L Wubbel, K Olsen, GH McCracken, Jr. Pharmacodynamics and bactericidal activity of ceftriaxone therapy in experimental cephalosporin-resistant pneumococcal meningitis. Antimicrob Agents Chemother 1997;41:2414–2417.
93. I Lustar, A Ahmed, IR Friedland, M Trujillo, L Wubbel, K Olsen, GH McCracken Jr. Pharmacodynamics and bactericidal activity of ceftriaxone therapy in experimental cephalosporin-resistant pneumococcal meningitis. Antimicrob Agents Chemother 1997;41:2414–2417.
94. MR Jacobs, SC Aronoff, S Johenning, DM Shlaes, S Yamabe. Comparative activities of the β-lactamase inhibitors YTR 830, clavulanate, and sulbactam combined with ampicillin and broad-spectrum penicillins against defined β-lactamase-producing aerobic gram-negative bacilli. Antimicrob Agents Chemother 1986;29:980–985.
95. EE Stobberingh. In vitro effect of YTR 830 (tazobactam) in plasmid and chromosomally mediated β-lactamases. Chemotherapy 1990;36:209–214.
96. PD Lister, AM Prevan, CC Sanders. Importance of β-lactamase inhibitor pharmacokinetics in the pharmacodynamics of inhibitor-drug combinations: Studies with piperacillin-tazobactam and piperacillin-sulbactam. Antimicrob Agents Chemother 1997;41:721–727.
97. M Alexov, PD Lister, CC Sanders. Efficacy of ampicillin-sulbactam is not dependent upon maintenance of a critical ratio between components: Sulbactam pharmacokinetics in pharmacodynamic interactions. Antimicrob Agents Chemother 1996: 40:2468–2477.
98. K Bush, C Macalintal, BA Rasmussen, VJ Lee, Y Yang. Kinetic interactions of tazobactam with β-lactamases from all major structural classes. Antimicrob Agents Chemother 1993;37:851–858.
99. KS Thomson, DA Weber, CC Sanders, WE Sanders Jr. β-lactamase production in members of the family Enterobacteriaceae and resistance to β-lactam-enzyme inhibitor combinations. Antimicrob Agents Chemother 1990;34:622–627.
100. DM Livermore. Determinants of the activity of β-lactamase inhibitor concentrations. J Antimicrob Chemother 1993;31(suppl A):9–21.
101. RN Jones, MN Dudley. Microbiologic and pharmacodynamic principles applied

to the antimicrobial susceptibility testing of ampicillin/sulbactam: Analysis of the correlations between in vitro test results and clinical response. Diagn Microbiol Infect Dis 1997;159:5–18.

102. AB Maderazo, DH Gilbert, MN Dudley. Post-exposure inhibition of TEM-3 β-lactamase by high concentrations of tazobactam. In: Program and Abstracts of the 36th Interscience Conference on Antimicrobial Agents and Chemotherapy, San Francisco, 1996, Am Soc Microbiol, Washington, DC, Abstract A95, p 19.
103. CE Thorburn, J Molesworth. The post β-lactamase inhibitor effect: A novel aspect of the activity of clavulanic acid in antibacterial tests. In: Program Abstracts of 32nd Interscience Conference on Antimicrobial Agents and Chemotherapeutics, Abstract 540.
104. AH Strayer, DH Gilbert, P Pivarnik, AA Medeiros, SH Zinner, MN Dudley. Pharmacodynamics of piperacillin alone and in combination with tazobactam against piperacillin-resistant and -susceptible organisms in an in vitro model of infection. Antimicrob Agents Chemother 1994;38:2351–2356.
105. R Pallares, F Gudiol, J Liñares, J Ariza, G Rufi, L Murgui, J Dorga, PF Viladrich. Risk factors and response to antibiotic therapy in adults with bacteremic pneumonia caused by penicillin-resistant pneumococci. N Engl J Med 1987;317:18–22.
106. R Pallares, J Liñares, M Vadillo, C Cabellos, F Manresa, PF Viladrich, R Martin, F Gudiol. Resistance to penicillin and cephalosporin and mortality from severe pneumococcal pneumonia in Barcelona, Spain. N Engl J Med 1995;333:474–480.
107. TW Gress, KW Yingling, RJ Stanek, MA Mufson. Infection with *Streptococcus pneumoniae* moderately resistant to penicillin does not alter clinical outcome. Infect Dis Clin Pract 1996;5:435–439.
108. C Cabellos, J Ariza, B Barreiro, F Tubau, J Liñares, R. Pallarés, F Manresa, F Gudiol. Current usefulness of procaine penicillin in the treatment of pneumococcal pneumonia. Eur J Clin Microbiol Infect Dis 1998;17:265–268.
109. IR Friedland. Comparison of the response to antimicrobial therapy to penicillin-resistant and penicillin-susceptible pneumococcal disease. Ped Infect Dis J 1995; 14:885–890.
110. R Dagan, O Abramson, E Leibovitz, R Lang, S Goshen, D Greenberg, P Yagupsky, A Leiberman, DM Fliss. Impaired bacteriologic response to oral cephalosporins in acute otitis media caused by pneumococci with intermediate resistance to penicillin. Ped Infect Dis J 1996;15:980–986.
111. P Gehanno, G Lenoir, P Berche. In vivo correlates for *Streptococcus pneumoniae* penicillin resistance in acute otitis media. Antimicrob Agents Chemother 1995;39: 271–272.
112. WA Craig, D Andes. Pharmacokinetics and pharmacodynamics of antibiotics in otitis media. Pediat Infect Dis J 1996;15:255–259.
113. PK Linden, AW Pasculle, R Manez, DJ Dramer, JJ Fung, AD Pinna, S Kusne. Differences in outcomes for patients with bacteremia due to vancomycin-resistant *Enterococcus faecium* or vancomycin-susceptible *E. faecium*. Clin Infect Dis 1996; 22:663–670.
114. Y Carmeli, N Troillet, AW Karchmer, MH Samore. Health and economic outcomes of antibiotic resistance in *Pseudomonas aeruginosa*. Arch Intern Med 1999;159: 1127–1132.

6

Aminoglycoside Pharmacodynamics

Myo-Kyoung Kim and David P. Nicolau
Hartford Hospital, Hartford, Connecticut

1 INTRODUCTION

Aminoglycosides are highly potent, broad-spectrum antibiotics that have remained an important therapeutic option for the treatment of life-threatening infections. Since the introduction of this class of agents into clinical practice some five decades ago, the major obstacle to their use is the potential for drug-related toxicity. However, over the last decade new information concerning the pharmacodynamic profile of these agents has been revealed that leads not only to the potential for improved antibacterial effectiveness but also to the minimization of their toxicodynamic profile. As a result of our contemporary understanding of these principles, parenteral dosing techniques for the aminoglycosides have been modified from the administration of frequent small intermittent dosages to once-daily regimens that not only optimize the pharmacodynamic and toxicodynamic profiles but also substantially reduce the expenditure associated with this therapeutic option. Application of these new principles together with the aminoglycosides' in vitro activity, proven clinical effectiveness, and synergistic potential form the rationale for their continued use in the management of serious infections.

2 HISTORY AND MECHANISM OF ACTION OF AMINOGLYCOSIDES

The aminoglycosides include an important group of natural and semisynthetic compounds. The first parenterally administered aminoglycoside, streptomycin, was introduced in 1944 and was followed by a number of other naturally occurring compounds, including neomycin, kanamycin, tobramycin, gentamicin, sisomicin, and paromomycin. Amikacin and netilmicin are semisynthetic derivatives of kanamycin and sisomicin, respectively, whereas isepamicin is a semisynthetic derivative of gentamicin.

Like that of many antibiotics (i.e., macrolides, tetracyclines, streptogramins), the bactericidal activity of the aminoglycosides is thought to be ribosomally mediated. Existing data suggest that their antibacterial activity results from inhibition of protein biosynthesis by irreversible binding of the aminoglycoside to the bacterial ribosome. The intact bacterial ribosome is a 70S particle that consists of two subunits (50S and 30S) that are assembled from three species of rRNA (5S, 16S, and 23S) and 52 ribosomal proteins. The smaller 30S ribosomal submit, which contains the 16S rRNA, has been identified as a primary target for aminoglycoside that ultimately induces mistranslation on prokaryotic ribosomes [1,2].

To reach their cytoplasmic ribosomal target, aminoglycosides must initially cross the outer membrane (in gram-negative organisms) and the cytoplasmic membrane (in gram-negative and gram-positive bacteria). In gram-negative bacteria the initial step involves ionic binding of the highly positively charged aminoglycosides to negatively charged phosphates mainly in lipopolysaccharides on the outer membrane surface; uptake across this membrane is likely due a ''self-promoted uptake'' mechanism [3,4]. The cationic aminoglycosides may act by competitively displacing the divalent cations in the membrane, resulting in the entry of the antibiotic [3]. The rapid initial binding of the aminoglycosides to the cell accounts for the rapid bactericidal activity, which appears to increase with increasing aminoglycoside concentration. This characteristic of concentration- or dose-dependent killing explains in part the recent attention given to administering the entire dose of the aminoglycoside on a once-daily basis in order to maximize bacterial killing.

Aminoglycoside uptake across the cytoplasmic membrane is the result of its electrostatic binding to the polar heads of phospholipids, whereas the driving force for aminoglycoside entry is provided by a cellular transmembrane electrical potential. The combination of these effects is characterized by rapid binding to the ribosome and an acceleration of aminoglycoside uptake across the cytoplasmic membrane.

Aminoglycosides of the gentamicin, kanamycin, and neomycin families induce misreading of mRNA codons during translation and also inhibit translocation [5]. Streptomycin induces misreading of the genetic code in addition to inhibiting translational initiation. By contrast, spectinomycin, an agent with only bacteriostatic activity, does not cause translation errors but inhibits translocation. These findings support the notion that translational misreading is at least partly responsible for the bactericidal activity characteristic of aminoglycosides [5–8].

Although the ribosome has been identified as a primary target for these agents, the precise mechanism by which aminoglycosides exert their bactericidal activity has remained elusive, because these drugs manifest pleiotropic effects on bacterial cells. These effects include, but are not limited to, disruption of the outer membrane, irreversible uptake of the antibiotic, and blockade of initiation of DNA replication [9].

3 MICROBIOLOGIC SPECTRUM

Although the aminoglycosides are highly potent broad-spectrum antibiotics, their in vitro activity is considered to be most notable against a variety of gram-negative pathogens. These pathogens include common clinical isolates of *Acinetobacter* spp., *Citrobacter* spp., *Enterobacter* spp., *Escherichia coli*, *Klebsiella* spp., *Serratia* spp., *Proteus* spp., *Morganella* spp., and *Pseudomonas aeruginosa*. However, although these agents are generally considered active against these microbes, substantial differences in antimicrobial potency exist among the various aminoglycosides. For example, even though the antimicrobial spectra of gentamicin and tobramycin are quite similar, tobramycin is generally more active in vitro against *P. aeruginosa*, whereas gentamicin is more active against *Serratia*.

Although streptomycin has been used extensively for many years, the emergence of resistance against *Mycobacterium tuberculosis* and aerobic gram-negative bacilli and the relatively frequent occurrence of vestibular toxicity combined with the availability of less toxic antibiotics have greatly diminished its clinical utility. The introduction of kanamycin provided a broader spectrum of activity against gram-negative bacilli, including streptomycin-resistant strains, but it was not active against *P. aeruginosa*. As with streptomycin, extensive use of kanamycin quickly led to the emergence and widespread dissemination of kanamycin resistance among Enterobacteriaceae. The development of other agents within the class (i.e., gentamicin, tobramycin, netilmicin, and amikacin) further expanded the spectrum of antimicrobial activity of this class to cover many kanamycin-resistant strains, including *P. aeruginosa*.

Although the aminoglycosides are also active against *Salmonella* spp., *Shigella* spp., *N. gonorrhea*, and *Haemophilus influenzae*, they are not recommended for infections caused by these species because of the wide availability of effective and less toxic drugs. Also, although they are generally active against *Staphylococci*, aminoglycosides are not advocated as single agents for infections due to this genera. However, an aminoglycoside, usually gentamicin, is frequently administered in combination with a cell-wall-active agent to provide synergy in the treatment of serious infections due to *Staphylococci*, *Enterococci*, and *Viridans streptococci.*

4 PHARMACOKINETIC CHARACTERIZATION

Although the focus of this chapter is related to the pharmacodynamics of aminoglycosides and their application in the management of systemic infection, it should be noted that although these agents are poorly absorbed after oral administration the prolonged use of large oral doses in patients with altered renal function may result in detectable aminoglycoside serum concentrations and the development of toxicity. In addition, although they penetrate poorly through intact skin their use as a topical antibacterial for large areas of denuded skin (i.e., thermal injury) may lead to substantial systemic absorption. Similarly, the use of aminoglycosides for local irrigation of closed body cavities may result in considerable systemic accumulation and potential toxicity.

As a consequence of poor oral bioavailability the aminoglycosides must be given parenterally in order to achieve a consistent serum concentration profile. The intramuscular route is well tolerated and results in essentially complete absorption, but intravenous administration is generally preferred because of the rapid and predictable serum profile. The importance of the rapid and reliable attainment of sufficient peak concentrations will be further discussed in subsequent sections of this chapter.

The aminoglycosides are weakly bound to serum proteins and therefore freely distribute into the interstitial or extracellular fluid. The apparent volume of distribution of this class of agents is approximately 25% of the total body weight, which corresponds to the estimated extracellular fluid volume. Although the volume of distribution is generally approximated at 0.25–0.3 L/kg, patients who are malnourished, obese, or pregnant, are in the intensive care unit, or have ascites may have substantial alterations in this parameter that require dosage and/or schedule modifications to maintain the desired serum profile. In general, the concentrations of the aminoglycosides attained in tissue and body fluids are less than that obtained in serum, with the notable exceptions of the kidney, perilymph of the inner ear, and urine. Approximately 20–50% of the serum concentration can be achieved in bronchial, sputum, pleural, or synovial fluid and unobstructed bile. Although low aminoglycoside bronchial fluid concentrations have been reported, the administration of large single daily doses versus conventional dosing substantially improves drug penetration into this fluid while reducing drug accumulation in the renal tissue [10–12]. Compared with other body sites, the penetration into prostate tissue and bone is poor. Penetration of aminoglycosides into cerebral spinal fluid in the presence of inflammation or into the fluid of the eye is inadequate and variable; therefore, direct instillation is often required to provide sufficient concentrations at these sites. Additionally, these agents cross the placenta; therefore the potential risk to the fetus and mother must be considered prior to use.

The kidneys, via glomerular filtration, are responsible for essentially all aminoglycoside elimination from the body. As a result, there is a proportional relationship between drug clearance and glomerular filtration rate, which is routinely used to assist with aminoglycoside dosage modification [13]. In adults and children older than 6 months with normal renal function, the elimination half-life is approximately 2–3 h. In premature or low birth weight infants less than 1 week old, the half-life is 8–12 h, whereas the half-life decreases to 5 h for neonates whose birth weight exceeds 2 kg. As a result of the primary renal elimination, it should be expected that substantial increases in the half-life would be observed in patients with renal dysfunction.

5 PHARMACODYNAMIC OVERVIEW

Over the last several decades new data emerged that extended our understanding of the complex interactions that take place among the pathogen, drug, and host during the infection process. Much of the focus has been on the influence of drug concentration on bacterial cell death. The pharmacodynamic properties or the correlation of drug concentration and the clinical effect (e.g., bacterial killing) of a specific antibiotic class are therefore an integration of two related areas, one being microbiological activity and the other pharmacokinetics (refer to Chapter 2 for a more complete review of this topic). Distinct pharmacodynamic profiles exist for all antimicrobials, because the influence of drug concentration on the rate and extent of bactericidal activity differs among the various classes of drugs.

The pharmacodynamic profile of the aminoglycosides has been characterized both in vitro and in vivo. Utilization of both static (i.e., time-kill studies) and dynamic (i.e., pharmacokinetic modeling) in vitro techniques has provided fundamental information concerning the pharmacodynamic profile of the aminoglycosides. These data indicate that a general pharmacodynamic division among antimicrobials occurs between agents whose rate and extent of bactericidal activity is dependent upon drug concentration (aminoglycosides and fluoroquinolones) and agents such as the β-lactams whose bactericidal activity is independent of drug concentration when their concentration exceeds four times the minimum inhibitory concentration (MIC) [14–17].

Figure 1 depicts these principles as illustrated with ciprofloxacin, tobramycin, and ticarcillin. In this experiment bacteria are exposed to various multiples of the MIC in vitro and, as shown with ticarcillin, little difference in the rate of bactericidal activity is noted when its concentration exceeds 4 times the MIC. Therefore, this type of killing, which is characteristic of β-lactams, is termed concentration- or dose-independent bactericidal activity (refer to Chapter 5 for a more complete discussion of β-lactam pharmacodynamics).

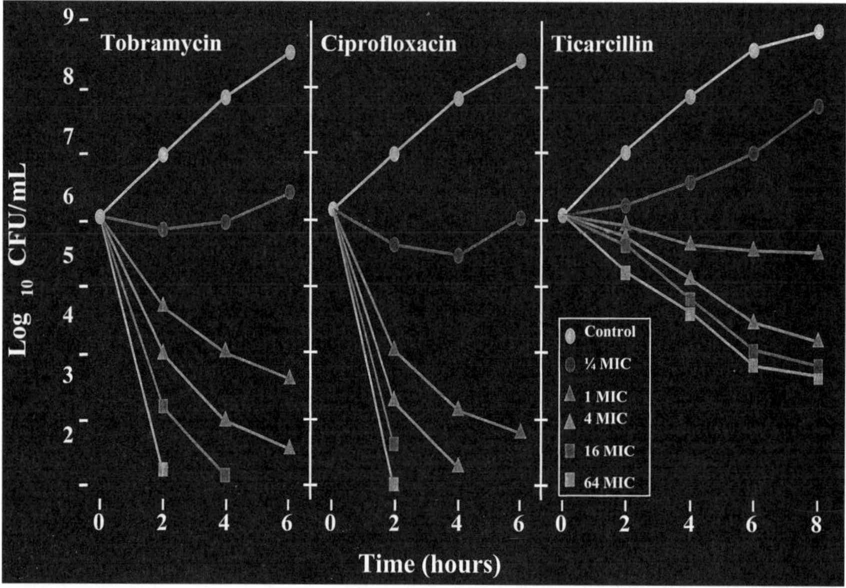

FIGURE 1 Influence of drug concentration on the bactericidal activity of tobramycin, ciprofloxacin, and ticarcillin against *Pseudomonas aeruginosa*. (From Ref. 15.)

By contrast, when the same multiples of the MIC are studied with tobramycin and ciprofloxacin, the number of organisms is seen to decrease more rapidly with each rising MIC interval. Because these agents eliminate bacteria more rapidly when their concentrations are appreciably above the MIC of the organism, their killing activity is referred to as concentration- or dose-dependent bactericidal activity [15]. These in vitro data indicate that optimum bactericidal activity for the aminoglycosides is achieved when the exposure concentration is approximately 8–10 times the MIC [14,15,18,19]. In addition to maximal bactericidal activity, Blaser et al. [20] demonstrated that the peak/MIC ratio of 8 : 1 is correlated with a decrease in the selection and regrowth of resistant subpopulations occurring during treatment with netilmicin.

Antimicrobial activity in vivo is a complex and multifactorial process. As described elsewhere in this text, to be effective an antimicrobial must reach and maintain adequate concentrations at the target site and interact with the target site for a period of time so as to interrupt the normal functions of the cell. In vivo this description of the interaction between the pathogen and the drug (i.e., microbiological activity) is influenced by the drug disposition or pharmacokinetic profile of the host species. As a result of the complex interactions occurring among the pathogen–drug–host triad, in vivo pharmacodynamic characterization of compounds is required.

Because we are not yet able to measure drug concentrations at the site of action (i.e., ribosome for the aminoglycosides) we commonly employ a microbiological parameter (i.e., the MIC) as the critical value in the interpretation of these in vivo pharmacodynamic relationships. When integrating the microbiological activity and pharmacokinetics, several parameters appear to be significant constituents of drug efficacy. The pharmacokinetic parameters, AUC (area under the concentration–time curve), maximum observed concentration (C_{max} or peak), and half-life, are often integrated with the MIC of the pathogen to produce pharmacodynamic parameters such as the AUC/MIC, peak/MIC, and the time for which the drug concentration remains above the MIC ($T >$ MIC). For the aminoglycosides the AUC/MIC, peak/MIC, and $T >$ MIC have all been shown to be pharmacodynamic correlates of efficacy [14,20,21]. However, it is not surprising that several pharmacodynamic parameters have been related to efficacy with these agents, because all of these parameters are related (Fig. 2). Therefore, since the amount of drug delivered against the pathogen is proportional to the amount of drug delivered to the host (AUC), the AUC is the primary pharmacokinetic

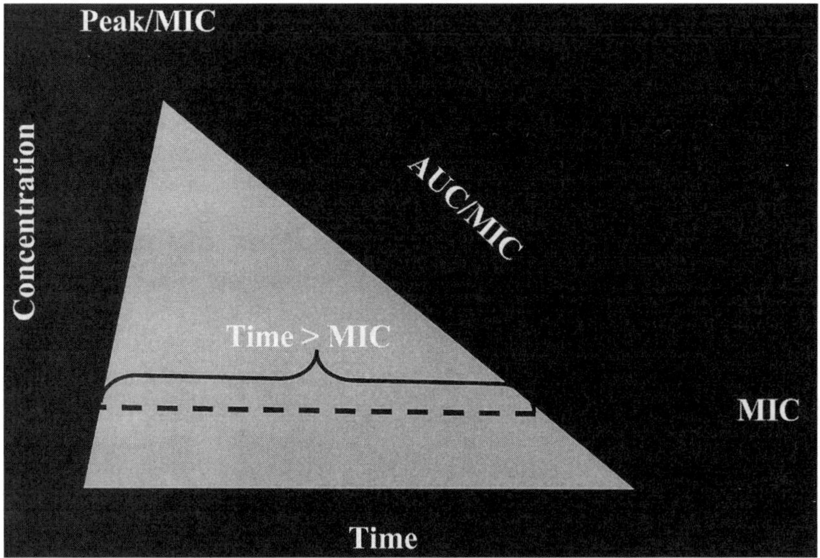

Figure 2 Antimicrobial pharmacodynamics: integration of microbiological potency and selected pharmacokinetic parameters.

parameter associated with efficacy. However, because the AUC is a product of concentration and time under certain conditions, the influence of concentration will appear to be a predominant factor, whereas under a different set of conditions the exposure to the drug or the time above the MIC may assume a larger role in bacterial eradication. In the case of the aminoglycosides, which display concentration-dependent killing and a relatively long PAE, the influence of the time above the MIC is small compared to the influence of peak concentration. As a result the pharmacodynamic parameter that is believed to best characterize the profile of the aminoglycosides in vivo is the peak/MIC ratio.

In support of the concentration-dependent bactericidal activity of the aminoglycosides displayed in in vitro studies and animal models of infection, several studies in humans have also demonstrated the importance of achieving sufficient peak/MIC ratios as related to defined treatment success. Aminoglycoside concentrations have been associated with treatment success in a three studies reported by Moore and colleagues [22–24]. In the first report by this group, higher C_{max} concentrations were associated with improved outcomes in gram-negative pneumonia, whereas in the second report, higher concentrations were associated with improved survival in gram-negative bacteremia [22,23]. Results of these studies suggest the importance of achieving adequate and early aminoglycoside concentrations in severely ill patients with gram-negative infection. Their last study, published in 1987, evaluated the relationship between the ratio of the peak concentration to MIC and clinical outcome through data collection from four randomized, double-blind, controlled clinical trials that used gentamicin, tobramycin, or amikacin for the treatment of gram-negative bacterial infections [22]. For the purposes of the study, the maximal peak concentration (C_{max}) was defined as the highest concentration determined during therapy, and the mean peak concentration was calculated as the average of all C_{max} values during the course of treatment. The investigators demonstrated that ratios of high maximal and mean peak aminoglycoside concentrations (8.5 ± 5.0 μg/mL and 6.6 ± 3.9 μg/mL, respectively) to MIC were significantly ($p < 0.00001$ and $p < 0.0001$, respectively) correlated with clinical response. Of the 188 patients who had a clinical response to therapy, the C_{max}/MIC average value was 8.5 ± 5.0 μg/mL, whereas the 48 nonresponders had a ratio of 5.5 ± 4.6 μg/mL ($p < 0.00001$). Although these studies used fixed dosing intervals and were not designed to assess the in vivo pharmacodynamic parameters and their relationship to outcome, the data provide the backbone for our commitment to the value of the peak/MIC ratio in clinical practice. Deziel-Evans et al. [25] demonstrated that a 91% cure rate was observed in patients with peak/MIC ratios greater than 8, whereas only a 12.5% cure rate was observed for patients with ratios of ≤4 in a retrospective study with 45 patients. In a study by Keating et al. [26], response rates of 57%, 67%, and 85% were observed in neutropenic patients with mean serum aminoglycoside concentration/MIC ratios of 1–4, 4–10, and >10, respectively. Williams et al.

[27] have also reported that C_{max}/MIC ratios correlated significantly with cure in 42 patients undergoing amikacin treatment who could be evaluated for clinical outcome [27]. Additionally, Fiala and Chatterjee [28] noted that infection was cured more frequently in patients with severe gram-negative infections who achieved higher peak/MIC ratios. The association of high peak/MIC ratios with improved outcomes has also been noted in orthopedic patients receiving gentamicin, and recently a similar relationship was noted for 61 febrile neutropenic patients with hematological malignancies [29,30]. Other investigators have also observed beneficial correlations between serum concentrations or pharmacodynamic parameters and therapeutic outcomes in patients treated with aminoglycosides [31–33].

More recently, Kashuba et al. [34,35] reported that achieving an aminoglycoside peak/MIC of $\geq$10 within 48 h of initiation of therapy for gram-negative pneumonia resulted in a 90% probability of therapeutic response by day 7 of therapy. They also note that aggressive aminoglycoside dosing (initial dose of 7 mg/kg) followed by individualized pharmacokinetic monitoring should maximize the rate and extent of response in this patient population.

Additionally, many once-daily aminoglycoside trials and their meta-analysis studies (which will be described in a later section in this chapter) also proved the importance of the correlation between the peak/MIC ratio and clinical outcome.

6 POSTANTIBIOTIC EFFECT

The postantibiotic effect (PAE) is defined as the persisting suppressive activity against bacterial growth after limited exposure of bacteria to an antibiotic. In order to measure the in vitro PAE of aminoglycosides, after a 1–2 h exposure of an antibiotic or a combination antibiotics to bacteria the drug is removed rapidly by dilution, drug inactivation [e.g., cellulose phosphate powder or tobramycin-acetylating enzyme AAC (3)-II and acetyl coenzyme A], or filtration (0.45 μm pore size filters). After this drug elimination process, viable counts (CFU/mL) at each time point are required to develop viability curves. The in vitro PAE is calculated with the equation $PAE = T - C$, where T is the time required for the count of CFUs in the test culture to increase by 1 $\log_{10}$ above the count observed immediately after drug removal and C is the time needed for the count of CFUs in an untreated control culture to increase by 1 $\log_{10}$ above the count observed immediately after the same procedure used on the test culture for drug removal [36].

Like quinolones, aminoglycosides represent a antibiotic class that has a clinically meaningful PAE; however, several factors may affect the presence and duration of the PAE. A range of 0.5–7.5 h has been reported for the PAE of aminoglycosides [36,37]. Major factors influencing PAE include organism, concentration of antibiotic, duration of antimicrobial exposure, and antimicrobial combinations. Minor factors include size of the inoculum, growth phase of the organism at the time of exposure, mechanical shaking of the culture, type of medium, pH and temperature of the medium, and the effect of re-exposure [36].

The examples below illustrate how the above factors affect the presence and duration of the PAE. Unlike β-lactam antibiotics with PAEs against only gram-positive organisms, aminoglycosides exhibit a PAE on both gram-positive and gram-negative organisms [37,38]. However, the PAE duration depends on the type of bacterium. For example, the duration of the PAE following exposure of *Pseudomonas aeruginosa* to gentamicin and tobramycin is 2.2 h and 2.1 h, respectively, whereas that of *Escherichia coli* is 1.8 h and 1.2 h, respectively [36]. Additionally, it has been shown that there is a positive correlation between subsequent dose or concentration of aminoglycosides and duration of the PAE [39–42]. The maximum concentration to exert the maximal PAE effect of aminoglycosides is difficult to determine because most bacteria are completely and rapidly killed at high drug concentrations. In contrast, the PAE of penicillin G gradually increases up to a point of maximal effect at a concentration 8–16 times the MIC [42–44]. The same theory also applies to duration of exposure.

The duration of PAE also varies depending on concurrently applied antibiotics when they are tested as a combination therapy. The combined effect of aminoglycosides and cell wall inhibitors on the duration of the PAE was studied by several researchers [45–48]. In general, these combinations produced additive effects (i.e., similar to the sum of PAEs for individual drugs) or synergistic effects (i.e., at least 1 h longer than the sum of PAEs for individual drugs) in *Staphylococcus aureus* and various streptococci. The effects of antibiotic combinations against gram-negative bacilli were mainly additive or indifferent (i.e., no different from the longest of the individual PAEs). As an exception, the addition of tobramycin to rifampin, which can achieve prolonged PAEs in gram-negative bacilli showed synergism of the PAE in *P. aeruginosa, E. coli*, and *K. pneumonia*.

However, there are unavoidable limitations in this in vitro determination of the PAE duration. One major drawback is that bacteria undergo a single exposure for a short period of time to a fixed concentration of a testing antimicrobial agent. However, in a clinical setting the antimicrobial agent should be used multiple times. In addition, it should maintain the concentration above the MIC for a relatively longer time period than that which occurs during PAE testing, and the concentration should decline continuously throughout the dosing interval. Karlowsky et al. [49,50] demonstrated that multiple exposures of *E. coli* and *P. aeruginosa* to aminoglycosides significantly decreased the duration of PAE along with attenuating bacterial killing activity. McGrath et al. [51] suggested that the reasons for this phenomenon may be adaptive resistance or the selection of drug-resistant variants. Li et al. [52] demonstrated that *P. aeruginosa* organism exposed to constant tobramycin concentrations have a longer PAE than those exposed to exponentially decreasing tobramycin concentrations at similar AUCs above the MIC. These studies suggest that conventional testing yields an overestimate of the PAE in comparison to the PAE presented in a clinical situation with continuously changing concentrations.

Furthermore, the duration of PAE significantly varies depending on the testing environment; important factors influencing the testing environment include inoculum concentration, temperature, pH, oxygen tension, and free cation (Ca^{2+}, Mg^{2+}) content [53–57]. The other obstacle to applying this in vitro PAE duration to clinical practice is that the PAE does not consider host immunity. However, some effort has been undertaken to include host immunity by using other terminology such as postantibiotic leukocyte enhancement (PALE) and postantibiotic sub-MIC effect. PALE describes the phenomenon that pathogens in the PAE phase are more susceptible to the antimicrobial effect of human leukocytes than non-PAE controls. The postantibiotic sub-MIC effect illustrates the additive effects of PAE and the bactericidal effects when the drug is still present, only in sub-MIC levels.

Despite some of the limitations involved in predicting the exact duration of PAE, the general consensus is that PAE is an important factor to be considered in the development of a drug regimen. The precise mechanisms of the PAE are largely unknown. However, several hypotheses have been suggested. They include limited persistence of antibiotic at the site of action, recovery from nonlethal damage to cell structures, and the time required for synthesis of new proteins or enzymes before growth. Drug-induced nonlethal damage due to the irreversible binding to bacterial ribosomes represents a feasible mechanism of the PAE of aminoglycoside [42,59]. In a study measuring the rate of [^{3}H]-adenosine incorporation, Gottfredsson et al. [60] showed that DNA synthesis by *P. aeruginosa* after exposure to tobramycin was markedly affected during the PAE phase. However, in a study that used cumulative radiolabeled nucleoside precursor uptake in a clinical strain of *E. coli*, Barmada et al. [61] showed that DNA and RNA synthesis resumed almost immediately after exposure to tobramycin, whereas protein synthesis did not recover until 4 h later. Therefore the duration of PAE produced by aminoglycosides against *E. coli* seems to be better correlated with inhibition of protein synthesis than with inhibition of DNA or RNA synthesis [61]. Even if the rationale for this difference is unknown, it may be due to a discrepancy in the mechanisms of action of two species. Theoretically, provided that a certain threshold of growth suppression to restrain DNA synthesis is attained, greater accumulation or entrapment of intracellular tobramycin in *P. aeruginosa* may account for this disagreement [60,61].

Although numerous data are available on the in vitro PAE, there is less in vivo information. Six animal models have been developed to evaluate the in vivo PAE: thigh infection in mice, pneumonia in mice, infected subcutaneous threads in mice, meningitis in rabbits, infected tissue cages in rabbits, and endocarditis in rats [36]. Among these models, the mice thigh infection model is commonly used to evaluate the PAE of aminoglycosides, although the pneumonia model is also adopted for them [62–65]. The endocarditis rat model has been used to evaluate the in vivo PAEs of aminoglycosides when they are added to penicillin or imipenem [40,66]. In these models, antibiotic is administered to achieve a concentration that exceeds the MIC during the first 1–2 h. Next, bacterial loads from tissue are counted at various time points and drug concentrations of plasma are measured simultaneously. After graphing the bacterial growth curve, in vivo PAE can be calculated by the equation

$$\mathrm{PAE} = T - C - M$$

where M is the length of time serum concentration exceeds the MIC, T is the time required for the counts of CFU in tissue to increase by 1 $\log_{10}$ above the count at the time closest to but not less than time M, and C is the time required for the counts of CFU in tissue of untreated control to increase by 1 $\log_{10}$ above the count at time zero [36].

Major factors affecting the in vivo PAE include the infection site, type of organism, type of antimicrobial agent, the drug dose, simulation of human pharmacokinetics, and the presence of leukocytes [36,37]. For example, the in vivo PAEs for 15 clinical isolates of Enterobacteriaceae following administration of gentamicin (8 mg/kg) ranged from 1.4 to 7.3 h [67]. Like the in vitro PAE, higher doses of drugs are correlated with longer in vivo PAEs [36]. The PAEs of single doses of 4, 12, and 20 mg/kg tobramycin in the thighs of neutropenic mice infected with *P. aeruginosa* were 2.2 h, 4.8 h, and 7.3 h, respectively. Generally, the combinations of aminoglycoside and β-lactam lengthened the PAE for *S. aureus* and *P. aeruginosa* by 1.0–3.3 h, compared to the longest PAE of the individual drugs. However, no difference was observed against *E. coli* and *K. pneumoniae* [65]. The adoption of a different infection model also may influence the duration of the in vivo PAE. PAEs with amikacin against *Klebsiella pneumoniae* in the mouse pneumonia model was roughly 1.5–2.5 times as long as that observed in the mouse thigh model at the corresponding dose [65]. Furthermore, other environmental conditions also influence the in vivo PAE [67].

The in vivo PAE can be used to incorporate the effect of host immunity in conjunction with the PAE. The duration of the in vivo PAE of aminoglycosides was prolonged 1.9–2.7-fold by the presence of leukocytes [67]. In addition, neutrophils are also proven to prolong the in vivo PAEs for aminoglycosides against a standard strain of *K. pneumoniae* [68]. The other benefit of the in vivo PAE is that the half-life of some antimicrobials can be prolonged to simulate human pharmacokinetics by inducing transient renal impairment in mice with uranyl nitrite. The in vivo PAE in the renally impaired mice was approximately 7 h longer than that observed in normal mice, with large doses inducing a similar effect. This difference is likely due to sub-MIC levels that persist for a longer time with renal impairment than with normal renal function [36].

In spite of the lack of an ideal method to apply the PAE to clinical practice, the PAE has a major impact on antimicrobial dosing regimens. For antibiotics with longer PAEs, dosing may be less frequent than that of antibiotics with shorter PAEs. Therefore, PAE may be one of the rationales for the implementation of once-daily aminoglycoside dosing.

7 RESISTANCE AND SYNERGY

Although this chapter primarily concerns the pharmacodynamic profile of the aminoglycosides and its implications for clinical practice, it is important to realize that the development of antimicrobial resistance is often the rate-limiting step for a compound's clinical utility. Not unlike other antimicrobials, the aminoglycosides face similar issues regarding resistance. Although this topic is beyond the scope of this chapter, it should be noted that at least three mechanisms confer resistance to the aminoglycosides: impaired drug uptake, mutations of the ribosome, and enzymatic modification of the drug. Intrinsic resistance is often due to impaired uptake, whereas acquired resistance usually results from acquisition of transposon- and plasmid-encoded modifying enzymes [69]. To this end the pharmacodynamic implications regarding resistance are that one should select a regimen that maximizes the rate and extent of killing. If this approach is universally endorsed, it will likely minimize the development of resistance in vivo, because the pharmacodynamic optimization of aminoglycosides has been shown to have this effect in vitro [20,70]. Additionally, adaptive resistance and refractoriness to aminoglycosides has been demonstrated in vitro and in a neutropenic murine model by exposing *Pseudomonas aeruginosa* to concentrations below or at the MIC of the organism [71–73]. Exposure to an aminoglycoside without a drug-free period leads to decreased bacterial killing. Therefore, longer dosing intervals which can be achieved with the pharmacodynamically based once-daily aminoglycoside dosing approach allow for a drug-free period in which the bacteria are not exposed to an aminoglycoside; yet they still preserve the antibacterial activity of these agents after multiple doses.

Aminoglycosides exhibit synergistic bactericidal activity when given in combination with cell-wall-active agents such as β-lactams and vancomycin [74,75]. For example, enterococcal endocarditis should be treated with a combination of an aminoglycoside plus a penicillin or vancomycin because by itself neither agent is sufficiently bactericidal. However, when combination therapy is advocated to achieve synergy for gram-negative organisms, maximally effective doses of both agents should be maintained, because synergy does not occur universally for all pathogens to all β-lactam–aminoglycoside combinations [74,76]. It should also be noted that combination exposure may also prolong the in vitro and in vivo PAE observed with the aminoglycosides (see Sect. 6) although the clinical relevance of this effect is not fully understood.

8 TOXICODYNAMICS

Since the introduction of aminoglycosides into clinical practice a variety of adverse events have been reported during aminoglycoside therapy; however, most (e.g., gastrointestinal) are mild and resolve when the drug is discontinued. The aminoglycosides rarely produce hypersensitivity reactions, and despite direct injection into the central nervous system and the eye, local adverse events (i.e., seizures, hypersensitivity reactions) are generally not observed. Although infrequent in contemporary clinical practice, the aminoglycosides have the potential to cause or exacerbate neuromuscular blockade. Despite the concern for increased risk with the administration of the high doses routinely used in once-daily dosing protocols, this adverse event has not been observed [77,78]. However, although they are generally well tolerated, the major obstacle that has curtailed the use of aminoglycosides is the potential for ototoxicity and nephrotoxicity.

Although ototoxicity has long been recognized as a potential complication of aminoglycoside therapy, questions still remain regarding the full delineation of risk factors and a universally accepted definition. As a result of discrepancies in both the definition of ototoxicity and the sensitivity of testing, the reported incidence of ototoxicity has spanned a wide range (2–25%). Two distinct forms of ototoxicity—auditory and vestibular—have been reported and may occur alone or simultaneously. The precise mechanism of injury remains elusive; however, ototoxicity is believed to result from the destruction of the sensory hair cells in the cochlea and the vestibular labyrinth [79].

Auditory toxicity often occurs at frequencies that are higher than that required for conversation, and thus patient complaints that usually manifest as tinnitus or a feeling of fullness in the ear are usually voiced after considerable auditory damage has already been done [80]. Like the progression of auditory loss, the initial symptoms of vestibular toxicity often go unrecognized due to the nonspecific nature of its initial presentation (i.e., nausea, vomiting, cold sweats, nystagmus, vertigo, and dizziness) [81]. Although considered to be less frequent than auditory toxicity, these vestibular effects are by and large irreversible and therefore may have a profound impact on the daily function status. Owing to the lack of well controlled comparative trials with sufficient power to detect differences in ototoxicity among aminoglycosides and the generally poor risk factors analysis, it is difficult if not impossible to substantiate that a particular agent may preferentially result in one form of ototoxicity rather than another.

Although serum concentration data may be useful to ensure an adequate pharmacodynamic profile, these data cannot accurately predict the development of ototoxicity. Recently acquired data suggest that toxicity is related to drug accumulation within the ear, not peak concentrations, which supports the concept of saturable transport and reinforces the belief that higher peak concentrations should not result in increased ototoxicity [82]. For these reasons the once-daily administration techniques may minimize drug accumulation and therefore drug-related toxicity [83,84].

Although nephrotoxicity has been reported in more than half of patients receiving aminoglycoside therapy, the broad range of definitions and the poor risk factor assessment of the affected patient population often make the true incidence difficult, if not impossible, to determine. Considered by many to be a noteworthy event, toxicity is nevertheless generally mild and reversible, and few patients have progressive toxicity severe enough to warrant dialysis [85]. At present it is thought that this toxicity is due to aminoglycoside accumulation in the lysosomes of the renal proximal tubule cells, which results in necrosis of the tubular cells, and the clinical presentation of acute tubular necrosis manifested by nonoliguric renal failure within a week [86].

Several investigators have reported that advanced age, pre-existing renal dysfunction, hypovolemia, shock, liver dysfunction, obesity, duration of therapy, use of concurrent nephrotoxic agents, and elevated peak/trough aminoglycoside concentrations are risk factors for development of nephrotoxicity [87–90]. Additionally, in the last-cited study [90], multiple logistic regression analysis also revealed that trough concentration, duration of therapy, advanced age, leukemia, male gender, decreased albumin, ascites, and concurrent clindamycin, vancomycin, piperacillin, or cephalosporins were independent risk factors for nephrotoxicity. Similar risk factors were identified in patients receiving once-daily aminoglycosides [91].

Similar to that previously described in the inner ear, a saturable aminoglycoside transport system has been used to describe the uptake of drug in the kidney. Therefore, less frequent single daily dose administration may minimize accumulation and nephrotoxicity [10,92]. In this regard, once-daily regimens have been reported to lessen the incidence of nephrotoxicity [78,84,93].

Although the risk of these toxicities cannot be completely eliminated, recognition of risk factors and the implementation of regimens that minimize drug accumulation will lead to optimal therapeutic outcomes and minimize toxicity.

9 CLINICAL USE AND APPLICATION OF PHARMACODYNAMICS

The parenteral aminoglycosides, particularly gentamicin, tobramycin, and amikacin, have long been used empirically for treatment of the febrile neutropenic patient or of patients with serious nosocomial infection. Although aminoglycoside utilization has generally been declining owing to the introduction of parenteral fluoroquinolones, emergence of fluoroquinolone-resistant *P. aeruginosa* will likely result in resurgence in clinical use of the aminoglycosides. To this point it is also apparent that the antipseudomonal β-lactams should not be given alone to treat systemic pseudomonal infections, because this organism often develops resistance under therapy. Thus the aminoglycosides play an important role in combination therapy for gram-negative infections.

As discussed earlier, the aminoglycosides are also commonly used with a cell-wall-active agent for synergistic purposes for gram-positive infections. In this situation gentamicin is frequently administered to provide synergy in the treatment of serious infections due to *Staphylococci*, *Enterococci*, and *Viridans streptococci*.

In the current era of aminoglycoside utilization, two predominant intravenous administration techniques are employed in clinical practice. The older of the two approaches is the administration of multiple doses, usually 1.7–2 mg/kg every 8 h for gentamicin and tobramycin, whereas amikacin was frequently dosed using regimens of 5 mg/kg every 8 h or 7.5 mg/kg every 12 h (Fig. 3). Using this technique, maintenance of concentrations within the therapeutic range for patients with alterations in elimination or volume of distribution was achieved with the use of a nomogram or by individualized pharmacokinetic dosing methods based on the patient-specific aminoglycoside disposition. Of the nomogram-based methods, the scheme of Sarubbi and Hull [94] appears to have gained the widest acceptance. By this method, a loading dose of 1–2 mg/kg gentamicin or tobramycin and of 5–7.5 mg/kg amikacin based on ideal body weight was given to adults with renal impairment. After the loading dose, subsequent doses were

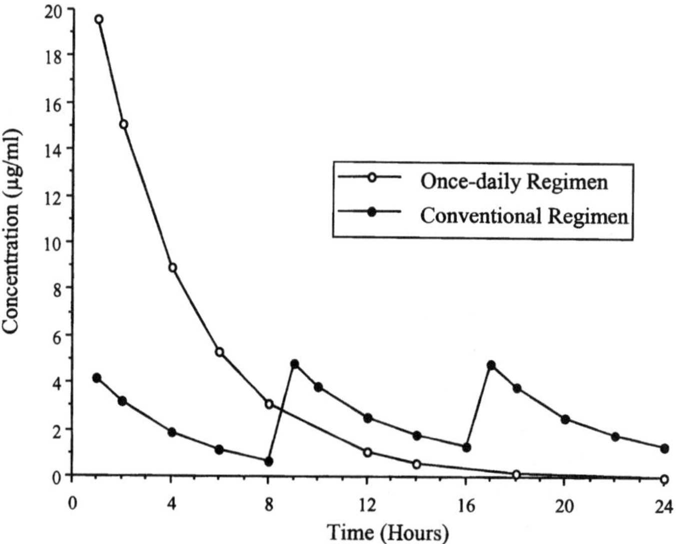

FIGURE 3 Concentration–time profile comparison of (●) conventional q8h intermittent dosing versus (○) the once-daily daily administration technique.

selected as a percentage of the chosen loading dose according to the desired dosing interval and the estimated creatinine clearance of the patient (Table 1). Alternatively, one-half the loading dose may be given at intervals equal to that of the estimated half-life. Although the nomogram approach has been utilized frequently, the preferred method of dosage adjustment is to individualize the regimen by using the standard pharmacokinetic dosing principles when aminoglycoside concentrations are available [95,96].

The second method has been referred to as the once-daily, single-daily, or extended interval dosing method (Fig. 3). Although the potential benefits of this second method were not well described until the early 1990s, this administration technique has now become the standard of practice in the United States; three of every four hospitals surveyed in 1998 used it [97,98]. For this reason and the wide availability of tertiary text references concerning the dosing of aminoglycosides using the more frequent intermittent approach, the remainder of this section will focus on the once-daily dosing methodology.

When considering the pharmacodynamic profile of aminoglycosides as described earlier in this chapter, four distinct advantages of using extended dosing

Table 1 Selection of Aminoglycoside Maintenance Dosing Using the Method of Sarubbi and Hull

Creatinine clearance (mL/min)	Half-life (hs)	Dose interval		
		8 h	12 h	24 h
90	3.1	84%	—	—
80	3.4	80	91%	—
70	3.9	76	88	—
60	4.5	71	84	—
50	5.3	65	79	—
40	6.5	57	72	92%
30	8.4	48	63	86
25	9.9	43	57	81
20	11.9	37	50	75
17	13.6	33	46	70
15	15.1	31	42	67
12	17.9	27	37	61
10	20.4	24	34	56
7	25.9	19	28	47
5	31.5	16	23	41
2	46.8	11	16	30
0	69.3	8	11	21

Source: Ref. 94.

intervals are readily apparent [99]. As stated previously, giving aminoglycosides as a single daily dose, as opposed to conventional strategies, provides the opportunity to maximize the peak concentration/MIC ratio and the resultant bactericidal activity (Fig. 3). Second, this administration technique should minimize drug accumulation within the inner ear and kidney and therefore minimize the potential for toxic effects to these organs. Third, the PAE may also allow for longer periods of bacterial suppression during the dosing interval. Finally, this aminoglycoside dosing approach may prevent the development of bacterial resistance.

Once-daily aminoglycoside therapy has been evaluated in several large clinical studies with a total study population of 100 or more patients [100–109]. Compared with multidose aminoglycoside regimens, the once-daily regimen was shown to be as efficacious as or superior to traditional dosing for the treatment of a wide variety of infections. Toxicity evaluations showed that there were no differences between the two dosing methods for either nephrotoxicity or ototoxicity. These toxicity data have been supported by other recent observations from investigators in Detroit [84,93]. In addition, clinical experience at our own institution in a large patient population who received 7 mg/kg of either gentamicin or tobramycin indicates a reduced potential for nephrotoxicity [78].

Studies have also been conducted in pediatrics [110,111] and pregnant populations [112] for determination of serum concentrations as well as clinical efficacy. Several recently published meta-analyses evaluating once-daily dosing with standard dosing regimens also demonstrate that increased bacterial killing and trends for decreased toxicity are actually borne out in clinical practice when the extended interval dosing is used [113–121].

At present, the strategy for once-daily dosing has not been consistent in the literature, as doses for gentamicin, tobramycin, and netilmicin have ranged from 3 to 7 mg/kg, whereas the usual amikacin dose is 15–20 mg/kg. Dosing regimens that use doses of less than 6 mg/kg for gentamicin, tobramycin, and netilmicin have arrived at the dose by converting the conventional mg/kg dose to a dose that is then administered once daily. At present there appear to be four commonly advocated methods for the once-daily administration of aminoglycosides. Although these approaches differ somewhat with regard to dose and/or interval, all reflect the need for dosage modification in the patient with renal disease. As of yet, no method has been shown to be superior to any of the others. Concerns about the extended intervals and possible risk of increased toxicity in patients with reduced drug clearance should be mentioned, but they should be no greater than those encountered with conventional dosing based on our current understanding of aminoglycoside-induced toxicity.

The first method of once-daily dosage determination was proposed and implemented on the basis of the pharmacokinetic and pharmacodynamic profiles of these agents. This method, which was developed at our institution, is intended to optimize the peak/MIC ratio in the majority of clinical situations by administering a dose of 7 mg/kg of either gentamicin or tobramycin [78]. Like conventional regimens, once-daily protocols require modification for patients with renal dysfunction in order to minimize drug accumulation. In the Hartford Hospital program this is accomplished by administering a fixed dose with dosing interval adjustments for patients with impaired renal function [78]. Due to the high peak concentrations obtained and the drug-free period at the end of the dosing interval, it is no longer necessary to draw standard peak and trough samples; rather a single random blood sample is obtained between 6 and 14 h after the start of the aminoglycoside infusion. This serum concentration is used to determine the dosing interval based on a nomogram for once-daily dosing (Fig. 4). Although Demczar et al. [122] suggested that the nomogram may be inappropriate for the monitoring of therapy, based on their assessment of aminoglycoside distribution in 11 healthy subjects, a subsequent population pharmacokinetic analysis using data derived from more than 300 patients receiving 7 mg/kg of tobramycin further supports the clinical utility of the original nomogram [123].

As a result of low toxicity, the short duration of therapy, and the excellent renal function of most patients, criteria have been developed to withhold the initial random concentration (which is obtained after the first or second dose) in patients (1) receiving 24 h dosing, (2) without concurrently administered nephrotoxic agents (e.g., amphotericin, cyclosporine, vancomycin), (3) without exposure

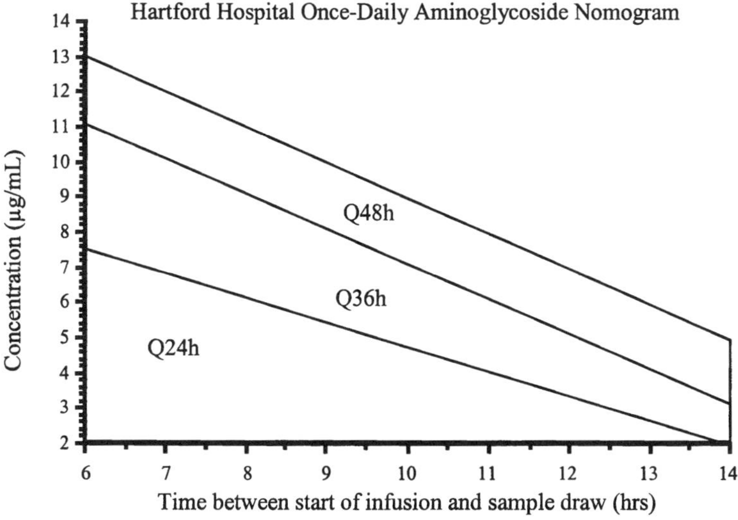

FIGURE 4 Once-daily aminoglycoside nomogram for the assessment of dosing interval using a 7 mg/kg dose of gentamicin or tobramycin. (From Ref. 78.)

to contrast media, (4) neither quadriplegic nor amputee, (5) not in the intensive care unit, and (6) less than 60 years of age [78]. Even though the initial random concentration may be withheld in eligible patients, monitoring of the serum creatinine should continue to occur at 2–3 day intervals throughout the course of therapy. For patients who continue on the once-daily regimen for 5 or more days, a random concentration is obtained on the fifth day and weekly thereafter. Even though an initial random concentration may no longer be necessary in many patients, for those experiencing rapidly changing creatinine clearances or those in whom the creatinine clearance is significantly reduced (i.e., ≤30 mL/min) it may be necessary to obtain several samples to adequately structure the administration schedule to maximize efficacy and minimize toxicity. The 7 mg/kg dosage regimen has also been advocated by other investigators to rapidly obtain sufficient aminoglycoside exposures [34,124].

The second method proposed by Gilbert uses a 5 mg/kg gentamicin or tobramycin dose in patients without renal dysfunction [99,125]. If dosage adjustment is required to compensate for diminished renal function, the dose and/or dosing interval may be modified to optimize therapy and minimize drug accumulation (Table 2). A similar scheme for dosage modification was advocated by

Table 2 Suggested Once-Daily Dosage Requirements for Patients with Altered Renal Function

Aminoglycoside	Creatinine clearance (ml/min)	Dosage interval (h)	Dose (mg/kg)
Gentamicin/tobramycin	>80	24	5.0
	70	24	4.0
	60	24	4.0
	50	24	3.5
	40	24	2.5
	30	24	2.5
	20	48	4.0
	10	48	3.0
	Hemodialysis[a]	48	2.0
Amikacin	>80	24	15
	70	24	12
	50	24	7.5
	30	24	4.0
	20	48	7.5
	10	48	4.0
	Hemodialysis[a]	48	5.0

[a] Administered post-hemodialysis.
Source: Adapted from Ref. 125.

Prin et al. [126] for patients with renal dysfunction. Finally, Begg et al. [127] suggested two methods to optimize once-daily dosing. The first, suggested for patients with normal renal function, uses a graphical approach with target AUC values. The second method, for patients with renal dysfunction, uses two aminoglycoside serum concentrations and a target AUC value based on the 24 h AUC that would result with multiple-dose regimens for dosage modifications.

Although all the above-noted once-daily methodologies have used fixed doses, subsequent dosage adjustments may be guided by individualized pharmacokinetic methods similar to that used for the conventional multiple-dose approach. On the other hand, although individualization of therapy can be accomplished, no data are available to support the assumption that these manipulations will improve outcomes or minimize toxicity further than the fixed dose methodologies.

At the time of once-daily implementation, the methodology was introduced into clinical practice to further optimize the clinical outcomes of patients receiving these agents for serious infections. However, in addition to meeting this goal and reducing the incidence of drug-induced adverse events, this approach has also substantially reduced expenditures associated with the initiation of aminoglycoside therapy compared to traditional dosing techniques [128–130].

10 SUMMARY

The pharmacodynamic profile of aminoglycosides is maximized when high dose, extended interval aminoglycoside therapy is employed. The use of this aminoglycoside administration technique has considerable in vitro and in vivo scientific support, which justifies its wide-scale use within this country. The implementation of such programs should maximize the probability of clinical cure and minimize toxicity and may help to avoid the development of resistance. Although such dosing is not appropriate for all patients, this strategy appears to be useful in the majority of patients requiring aminoglycoside therapy and can be successfully employed as a hospital-wide program.

REFERENCES

1. Cundliffe E. Antibiotics and prokaryotic ribosomes: Action, interaction and resistance. In: WE Hill, A Dahlberg, RA Garrett, PB Moore, D Schlessinger, JR Warner, eds. Ribosomes. Am Soc Microbiol, Washington, DC, 1990:479–490.
2. Davies JE. Resistance to aminoglycosides: Mechanisms and frequency. Rev Infect Dis 1983;5:S261–S266.
3. Hancock REW. Aminoglycoside uptake and mode of action: With special reference to streptomycin and gentamicin. J Antimicrob Chemother 1981;8:249–276.
4. Hancock REW, Farmer SW, Li Z, Poole K. Interaction of aminoglycosides with

the outer membranes and purified lipopolysaccharide and OmpF porin of *Escherichia coli.* Antimicrob Agents Chemother 1991;35:1309–1314.
5. Gale EF, Cundliffe E, Reynolds PE, Richmond MH, Waring MJ. The Molecular Basis of Antibiotic Action. Wiley, London, 1981.
6. Davis BD, Tai PC, Wallace BJ. Complex interactions of antibiotics with the ribosome. In: M. Nomura, A Tissieres, P Lengyel, eds. Ribosomes. Cold Spring Harbor Laboratory, Cold Spring Harbor, NY, 1974:771–789.
7. Gorini L. Streptomycin and misreading of the genetic code. In: M Nomura, A Tissieres, P Lengyel, eds. Ribosomes. Cold Spring Harbor Laboratory, Cold Spring Harbor, NY, 1974:791–803.
8. Ruusala T, Kurland CG. Streptomycin preferentially perturbs ribosomal proofreading. Mol Gen 1984;198:100–104.
9. Matsunaga K, Yamaki H, Nishimura T, Tanaka N. Inhibition of DNA replication initiation by aminoglycoside antibiotics. Antimicrob Agents Chemother 1986;30: 468–474.
10. De Broe ME, Verbist L, Verpooten GA. Influence of dosage schedule on renal cortical accumulation of amikacin and tobramycin in man. J Antimicrob Chemother 1991;27(suppl C):41–47.
11. Santre C, Georges H, Jacquier JM, Leroy O, Beuscart C, Buguin D, Beaucaire G. Amikacin levels in bronchial secretions of 10 pneumonia patients with respiratory support treated once daily versus twice daily. Antimicrob Agents Chemother 1995; 39:264–267.
12. Valcke YJ, Vogelaers DP, Colardyn FA, Pauwels RA. Penetration of netilmicin in the lower respiratory tract after once-daily dosing. Chest 1992;101:1028–1032.
13. Zarowitz BJ, Robert S, Peterson EL. Prediction of glomerular filtration rate using aminoglycoside clearance in critically ill medical patients. Ann Pharmacother 1992; 26:1205–1210.
14. Begg EJ, Peddie BA, Chambers ST, Boswell DR. Comparison of gentamicin dosing regimens using an in-vitro model. J Antimicrob Chemother 1992;29:427–433.
15. Craig WA, Ebert SC. Killing and regrowth of bacteria in vitro: A review. Scand J Infect Dis 1991;suppl 74:63–70.
16. Drusano GL, Johnson DE, Rosen M, Standiford HC. Pharmacodynamics of a fluoroquinolone antimicrobial agent in a neutropenic rat model of Pseudomonas sepsis. Antimicrob Agents Chemother 1993;37:483–490.
17. Dudley MN. Pharmacodynamics and pharmacokinetics of antibiotics with special reference to the fluoroquinolones. Am J Med 1991;91(suppl 6A):45S–50S.
18. Davis BD. Mechanism of the bactericidal action of the aminoglycosides. Microbiol Rev 1987;51:341–350.
19. Ebert SC, Craig WA. Pharmacodynamic properties of antibiotic: Application to drug monitoring and dosage regimen design. Infect Control Hosp Epidemiol 1990; 11:319–326.
20. Blaser J, Stone B, Groner M, et al. Comparative study with enoxacin and netilmicin in a pharmacodynamic model to determine importance of ratio of antibiotic peak concentration to MIC for bactericidal activity and emergence of resistance. Antimicrob Agents Chemother. 1987;31:1054–1060.
21. Leggett JE, Ebert S, Fantin B, Craig WA. Comparative dose-effect relationships

at several dosing intervals for β-lactam, aminoglycoside and quinolone antibiotics against gram-negative bacilli in murine thigh-infection and pneumonitis models. Scan J Infect Dis 1991;74:179–184.

22. Moore RD, Smith CR, Lietman PS. Association of aminoglycoside plasma levels with therapeutic outcome in gram-negative pneumonia. Am J Med 1984;77:657–662.
23. Moore RD, Smith CR, Lietman PS. The association of aminoglycoside plasma levels with mortality in patients with gram-negative bacteremia. J Infect Dis 1984; 149:443–448.
24. Moore RD, Lietman PS, Smith CR. Clinical response to aminoglycoside therapy: Importance of the ratio of peak concentration to minimal inhibitory concentration. J Infect Dis 1987;155:93–99.
25. Deziel-Evans L, Murphy J, Job M. Correlation of pharmacokinetic indices with therapeutic outcomes in patients receiving aminoglycoside. Clin Pharm. 1986;5: 319–324.
26. Keating MF, Bodey GP, Valdivieso M, Rodriguez V. A randomized comparative trial of three aminoglycosides: Comparison of continuous infusions of gentamicin, amikacin, and sisomicin combined with carbenicillin in the treatment of infections in neutropenic patients with malignancies. Medicine 1979;58:159–170.
27. Williams PJ, Hull JH, Sarubbi FA, Rogers JF, Wargin WA. Factors associated with nephrotoxicity and clinical outcome in patients receiving amikacin. J Clin Pharmacol 1986;26:79–86.
28. Fiala M, Chatterjee SN. Antibiotic blood concentrations in patients successfully treated with tobramycin. Postgrad Med 1981;57:548–551.
29. Berirtzoglou E, Golegou S, Savvaidis I, Bezirtzoglou C, Beris A, Xenakis T. A relationship between serum gentamicin concentrations and minimal inhibitor concentration. Drugs Exp Clin Res 1996;22:57–60.
30. Binder L, Schiel X, Binder C, Menke CF, Schuttrumpf S, Armstrong VW, Unterhalt M, Erichsen N, Hiddemann W, Oellerich M. Clinical outcome and economic impact of aminoglycoside peak concentrations in febrile immuocompromised patients with hematologic malignancies. Clin Chem 1998;44:408–414.
31. Anderson ET, Young LS, Hewitt WL. Simultaneous antibiotic levels in ''breakthrough'' gram-negative rod bacteremia. Am J Med 1976;61:493–497.
32. Noone P, Parsons TMC, Pattison JR, Slack RCB, Garfield-Davies D, Hughes K. Experience in monitoring gentamicin therapy during treatment of serious gram-negative sepsis. Br Med J 1974;1:477-481.
33. Reymann MT, Bradac JA, Cobbs CG, Dismukes WE. Correlation of aminoglycoside dosage with serum concentrations during therapy of serious gram-negative bacillary disease. Antimicrob Agents Chemother 1979;16:353–361.
34. Kashuba ADM, Bertino JS Jr, Nafziger AN. Dosing of aminoglycosides to rapidly attain pharmacodynamic goals and hasten therapeutic response by using individualized pharmacokinetic monitoring of patients with pneumonia caused by gram-negative organism. Antimicrob Agents Chemother 1998;42:1842–1844.
35. Kashuba ADM, Nafziger AN, Drusano GL, Bertino JS Jr. Optimizing aminoglycoside therapy for nosocomial pneumonia caused by gram-negative bacteria. Antimicrob Agents Chemother 1999;43:1623–1629.

36. Craig W, Gunmundsson S. Postantibiotic effect. In: V. Lorian, ed. Antibiotics in Laboratory Medicine. 4th ed. Williams & Wilkins, Baltimore, 1987:296–329.
37. Zhanel G, Hoban D, Harding G. The postantibiotic effect: a review of in vitro and in vivo data. Ann Pharmacother 1991;25:153–163.
38. Bundtzen R, Gerber A, Cohn D, et al. Postantibiotic suppression of bacterial growth. Rev Infect Dis 1981;3:28–37.
39. Vogelman B, Gudmundsson S, Turnidge J, et al. In vivo postantibiotic effect in a thigh infection in neutropenic mice. J Infect Dis 1988;157:287–298
40. Hessen M, Pitsakis P, Levison M. Postantibiotic effect of penicillin plus gentamicin versus Enterococcus faecalis in vitro and in vivo. Antimicrob Agents Chemother 1989;33:608–611.
41. McGrath B, Marchbanks C, Gilbert D, et al. In vitro postantibiotic effect following exposure to imipenem, temafloxacin, and tobramycin. Antimicrob Agents Chemother 1993;37:1723–1725.
42. Vogelman B, Craig W. Postantibiotic effects. J Antimicrob Chemother 1985; 15(suppl A):37–46.
43. Odenholt-Tornqvist I. Pharmacodynamics of beta-lactam antibiotics: Studies on the paradoxical effect and postantibiotic effects in vitro and in an animal model. Scand J Infect Dis 1989;58(suppl):1–55.
44. Craig W, Leggett K, Totsuka K, et al. Key pharmacokinetic parameters of antibiotic efficacy in experimental animal infections. J Drug Dev 1998;1(suppl 3):7–15.
45. Dornbusch K, Henning C, Linden E. In-vitro activity of the new penems FCE 22101 and FCE 24362 alone or in combination with aminoglycosides against streptococci isolated from patients with endocarditis. J Antimicrob Chemother 1989;23(suppl C):109–117.
46. Fuursted K. Comparative killing activity and postantibiotic effect of streptomycin combined with ampicillin, ciprofloxacin, imipenem, piperacillin, or vancomycin against strains of Streptococcus faecalis and Streptococcus faecium. Chemotherapy 1988;34:229–234.
47. Winstanley T, Hastings J. Penicillin-aminoglycosides synergy and post-antibiotic effect for enterococci. J Antimicrob Chemother 1989;23:189–199.
48. Gudmundsson S, Erlendsdottir H, Gottfredsson M, et al. The postantibiotic effect induced by antimicrobial combinations. Scand J Infect Dis 1991;74:80–93.
49. Karlowsky J, Zhanel G, Davidson R, et al. Postantibiotic effect in Pseudomonas aeruginosa following single and multiple aminoglycoside exposures in vitro. J Antimicrob Chemother 1994;33:937–947.
50. Karlowsky J, Zhanel G, Davidson R, et al. In vitro postantibiotic effects following multiple exposures of cefotaxime, ciprofloxacin, and gentamicin against Escherichia coli in pooled human cerebrospinal fluid and Mueller-Hinton broth. Antimicrob Agents Chemother 1993;37:1154–1157.
51. McGrath B, Marchbanks C, Gilbert D, et al. In vitro postantibiotic effect following repeated exposure to imipenem, temafloxacin, and tobramycin. Antimicrob Agents Chemother 1993;37:1723–1725.
52. Li R, Zhu Z, Lee S, et al. Antibiotic exposure and its relationship to postantibiotic effect and bactericidal activity: Constant versus exponentially decreasing tobra-

mycin concentrations against Pseudomonas aeruginosa. Antimicrob Agents Chemother 1997;41:1808–1811.
53. Rescott D, Nix D, Holden P, et al. Comparison of two methods for determining in vitro postantibiotic effects of three antibiotics on Escherichia coli. Antimicrob Agents Chemother 1998;32:450–453.
54. Fuursted K. Postexposure factors influencing the duration of postantibiotic effect: Significance of temperature, pH, cations, and oxygen tension. Antimicrob Agents Chemother 1997;41:1693–1696.
55. Gudmundsson A, Erlendsdottir H, Gottfredsson M, et al. The impact of pH and cationic supplementation on in vitro postantibiotic effect. Antimicrob Agents Chemother 1991;35:2617–2624.
56. Park MK, Myers R, Marzella L. Hyperoxia and prolongation of aminoglycoside-induced postantibiotic effect in Pseudomonas aeruginosa: Role of reactive oxygen species. Antimicrob Agents Chemother 1993;37:120–122.
57. Hanberger H, Nilsson L, Maller R, et al. Pharmacodynamics of daptomycin and vancomycin on Enterococcus faecalis and Staphylococcus aureus demonstrated by studies of initial killing and postantibiotic effect and influence of Ca^{2+} and albumin on these drugs. Antimicrob Agents Chemother 1991;35:1710–1716.
58. Cars O, Odenholt-Tornqvist I. The postantibiotic sub-MIC effect in vitro and in vivo. J Antimicrob Chemother 1993;31(suppl D):159–166.
59. Craig W, Vogelman B. The postantibiotic effect. Ann Intern Med. 1987;106:900–902.
60. Gottfredsson M, Erlendsdottir H, Gudmundsson, et al. Different patterns of bacterial DNA synthesis during the postantibiotic effect. Antimicrob Agents Chemother 1995;39:1314–1319.
61. Barmada S, Kohlhepp S, Leggett J, et al. Correlation of tobramycin-induced inhibition of protein synthesis with postantibiotic effect in Escherichia coli. Antimicrob Agents Chemother 1993;37:2678–2683.
62. Minguez F, Izquierdo J, Caminero M, et al. In vivo postantibiotic effect of isepamicin and other aminoglycosides in a thigh infection model in neutropenic mice. Chemotherapy 1992;38:179–184.
63. Vogelman B, Gudmundsson S, Turnidge J, et al. In vivo postantibiotic effect in a thigh infection in neutropenic mice. J Infect Dis 1988;157:287–298.
64. Gudmundsson S, Einarsson S, Erlendsdottir H. The post-antibiotic effect of antimicrobial combinations in a neutropenic murine thigh infection model. J Antimicrob Chemother 1993;31(suppl D):177–191.
65. Craig W, Redington J, Ebert S. Pharmacodynamics of amikacin in vitro and in mouse thigh and lung infections. J Antimicrob Chemother 1991;27(suppl C):29–40.
66. Hessen M, Pitsakis P, Levison M. Absence of a postantibiotic effect in experimental Pseudomonas endocarditis treated with imipenem, with or without gentamicin. J Infect Dis 1998;158:542–548.
67. Craig W. Post-antibiotic effects in experimental infection model: relationship to in-vitro phenomena and to treatment of infection in man. J Antimicrob Chemother 1993;31(suppl D):149–158.

68. Fantin B, Craig W. Factors affecting duration of in vivo postantibiotic effect for aminoglycosides against gram-negative bacilli. Antimicrob Agents Chemother 1991;27:829–836.
69. Mingeot-Leclercq MP, Glupczynski Y, Tulkens PM. Aminoglycosides: Activity and resistance. Antimicrob Agents Chemother 1999;43:727–737.
70. Karlowsky JA, Zhanel GG, Davidson RJ, Hoban DJ. Once-daily aminoglycoside dosing assessed by MIC reversion time with *Pseudomonas aeruginosa*. Antimicrob Agents Chemother 1994;38:1165–1168.
71. Daikos GL, Jackson GG, Lolans V, Livermore DM. Adaptive resistance to aminoglycoside antibiotics from first-exposure down-regulation. J Infect Dis 1990;162:414–420.
72. Daikos GL, Lolans VT, Jackson GG. First-exposure adaptive resistance to aminoglycoside antibiotics in vivo with meaning for optimal clinical use. Antimicrob Agents Chemother 1991;35:117–123.
73. Gerber AU, Vastola AP, Brandel J, Craig WA. Selection of aminoglycoside-resistant variants of *Pseudomonas aeruginosa* in an in vivo model. J Infect Dis 1982;146:691–697.
74. Owens RC Jr, Banevicius MA, Nicolau DP, Nightingale CH, Quintiliani R. In vitro synergistic activities of tobramycin and selected β-lactams against 75 gram-negative clinical isolates. Antimicrob Agents Chemother 1997;41:2586–2588.
75. Marangos MN, Nicolau DP, Quintiliani R, Nightingale CH. Influence of gentamicin dosing interval on the efficacy of penicillin containing regimens in experimental *Enterococcus faecalis* endocarditis. J Antimicrob Chemother 1997;39:519–522.
76. Hallander HO, Donrbusch K, Gezelius L, Jacobson K, Karlsson I. Synergism between aminoglycosides and cephalosporins with anti-pseudomonal activity: Interaction index and killing curve method. Antimicrob Agents Chemother 1982;22:743–752.
77. Gilbert DN. Once-daily aminoglycoside therapy. Antimicrob Agents Chemother 1991:35:399–405.
78. Nicolau DP, Freeman CD, Belliveau PP, Nightingale CH, Ross JW, Quintiliani R. Experience with a once-daily aminoglycoside program administered to 2,184 adult patients. Antimicrob Agents Chemother 1995;39:650–655.
79. Hutchin T, Cortopassi G. Proposed molecular and cellular mechanism for aminoglycoside ototoxicity. Antimicrob Agents Chemother 1994;38:2517–2520.
80. Fausti SA, Henry JA, Scheffer HI, Olson DJ, Frey RH, McDonald WJ. High-frequency audiometric monitoring for early detection of aminoglycoside ototoxicity. J Infect Dis 1992;165:1026–1032.
81. Federspil P. Drug-induced sudden hearing loss and vestibular disturbances. Adv Otorhinolaryngol 1981;27:144–158.
82. Beaubien AR, Ormsby E, Bayne A, Carrier K, Crossfield G, Downes M, Henri R, Hodgen M. Evidence that amikacin ototoxicity is related to total perilymph area under the concentration-time curve regardless of concentration. Antimicrob Agents Chemother 1991;35:1070–1074.
83. Proctor L, Petty B, Lietman P, Thakor R, Glackin R, Shimizu H. A study of potential vestibulotoxicity effects of once daily versus thrice daily administration of tobramycin. Laryngoscope 1987;97:1443–1449.

84. Rybak MJ, Abate BJ, Kang SL, Ruffing MJ, Lerner SA, Drusano GL. Prospective evaluation of the effect of an aminoglycoside dosing regimen on rates of observed nephrotoxicity and ototoxicity. Antimicrob Agents Chemother 1999;43:1549–1555.
85. Garrison MW, Zaske DE, Rotschafer JC. Aminoglycosides: Another perspective. DICP: Ann Pharmacother 1990;24:267–272.
86. Mingeot-Leclercq MP, Tulkens PM. Aminoglycosides: Nephrotoxicity. Antimicrob Agents Chemother 1999;43:1003–1012.
87. Moore RD, Smith CR, Lietman PS. Risk factors for nephrotoxicity in patients treated with aminoglycosides. Ann Intern Med 1984;100:352–357.
88. Sawyers CL, Moore RD, Lerner SA, Smith CR. A model for predicting nephrotoxicity with aminoglycosides. J Infect Dis 1986;153:1062–1068.
89. Whelton A. Therapeutic initiatives for avoidance of aminoglycoside toxicity. J Clin Pharmacol 1985;25:67–81.
90. Bertino JS Jr, Booker LA, Franck PA, Jenkins PL, Nafziger AN. Incidence and significant risk factors for aminoglycoside-associated nephrotoxicity in patients dosed by using individualized pharmacokinetic monitoring. J Infect Dis 1993;167:173–179.
91. Nodoushani M, Nicolau DP, Hitt CH, Quintiliani R, Nightingale CH. Evaluation of nephrotoxicity associated with once-daily aminoglycoside administration. J Pharm Tech 1997;13:258–262.
92. Verpooten GA, Giuliano RA, Verbist L, Eestermans G, De Broe ME. Once daily dosing decreases the accumulation of gentamicin and netilmicin. Clin Pharmacol Ther 1989;45:22–27
93. Murray KR, McKinnon PS, Mitrzyk B, Rybak MJ. Pharmacodynamic characterization of nephrotoxicity associated with once-daily aminoglycoside. Pharmacotherapy 1999;19:1252–1260.
94. Sarubbi FA Jr, Hull JH. Amikacin serum concentrations: Prediction of levels and dosage guidelines. Ann Intern Med 1978;89:612–618.
95. Sawchuk RJ, Zaske DE. Pharmacokinetics of dosing regimens which utilize multiple intravenous infusions: Gentamicin in burn patients. J Pharmacokinet Biopharm 1976;4:183–195.
96. Sawchuk RJ, Zaske DE, Cipolle RJ, Wargin WA, Strate RG. Kinetic model for gentamicin dosing with the use of individual patient parameters. Clin Pharmacol Ther 1977;21:362–369.
97. Schumock GT, Raber SR, Crawford SY, Naderer OJ, Rodvold KA. National survey of once-daily dosing of aminoglycoside antibiotics. Pharmacotherapy 1995;15:201–209.
98. Chuck SK, Raber SR, Rodvold KA, Areff D. National survey of extended-interval aminoglycoside dosing. Clin Infect Dis 2000;30:433–439.
99. Gilbert DN. Once-daily aminoglycoside therapy. Antimicrob Agents Chemother 1991;35:399–405.
100. DeVries PJ, Verkooyen RP, Leguit P, Verbrugh HA. Prospective randomized study of once-daily versus thrice-daily netilmicin regimens in patients with intraabdominal infections. Eur J Clin Microbiol Infect Dis 1990;9:161–168.
101. Mauracher EH, Lau WY, Kartowisastro H, et al. Comparison of once-daily and

thrice-daily netilmicin regimens in serious systemic infections: A multicenter study in six asian countries. Clin Ther 1989;11:604–613.
102. Maller R, Ahrne H, Eilard T, et al. Efficacy and safety of amikacin in systemic infections when given as a single daily dose or in two divided doses. J Antimicrob Chemother 1991;27(suppl C):121–128.
103. Maller R, Ahrne H, Holmen C, et al. Once- versus twice-daily amikacin regimen: efficacy and safety in systemic gram-negative infections. J Antimicrob Chemother 1993;31:939–948.
104. Prins JM, Buller HR, Kuijper EJ, Tange RA, Speelman P. Once versus thrice daily gentamicin in patients with serious infections. Lancet 1993;341:335–339.
105. Rozdzinski E, Kern WV, Reichle A, et al. Once-daily versus thrice-daily dosing of netilmicin in combination with β-lactam antibiotics as empirical therapy for febrile neutropenic patients. J Antimicrob Chemother 1993;31:585–598.
106. TerBraak EW, DeVries PJ, Bouter KP, et al. Once-daily dosing regimen for aminoglycoside plus β-lactam combination therapy of serious bacterial infections: Comparative trial with netilmicin plus ceftriaxone. Am J Med 1990;89:58–66.
107. International Antimicrobial Therapy Cooperative Group of the EORTC. Efficacy and toxicity of single daily doses of amikacin and ceftriaxone versus multiple daily doses of amikacin and ceftazidime for infection in patients with cancer and granulocytopenia. Ann Intern Med 1993;119:584–593.
108. Beaucaire G, Leroy O, Beuscart C, et al. Clinical and bacteriological efficacy, and practical aspects of amikacin given once daily for severe infections. J Antimicrob Chemother 1991;27(suppl C):91–103.
109. Prins JM, Buller HR, Kuijper EJ, Tange RA, Speelman P. Once-daily gentamicin versus once-daily netilmicin in patients with serious infections: A randomized clinical trial. J Antimicrob Chemother 1994;33:823–835.
110. Marik PE, Lipman J, Kobilski S, Scribante J. A prospective randomized study comparing once- versus twice-daily amikacin dosing in critically ill adult and paediatric patients. J Antimicrob Chemother 1991;28:753–764.
111. Nicolau DP, Quintiliani R, Nightingale CH. Once-a-day aminoglycoside therapy. Rep Ped Infect Dis 1997;7:28.
112. Bourget P, Fernandez H, Delouis C, Taburet AM. Pharmacokinetics of tobramycin in pregnant women: Safety and efficacy of a once-daily dose regimen. J Clin Pharm Ther 1991;16:167–176.
113. Galoe AM, Graudal N, Christensen HR, Kampmann JP. Aminoglycosides: Single or multiple daily dosing? A meta-analysis on efficacy and safety. Eur J Clin Pharmacol 1995;48:39–43.
114. Freeman CD, Strayer AH. Mega-analysis of meta-analysis: An examination of meta-analysis with an emphasis on once-daily aminoglycoside comparative trials. Pharmacotherapy 1996;16:1093–102.
115. Hatala R, Dinh T, Cook D. Once-daily aminoglycoside dosing in immunocompetent adults: A meta-analysis. Ann Intern Med 1996;124:717–725.
116. Barza M, Ioannidis JP, Cappelleri JC, Lau J. Single or multiple doses of aminoglycosides: A meta-analysis. Br Med J 1996;312:338–345.
117. Munckhof WJ, Grayson JL, Turnidge JD. A meta-analysis of studies on the safety

and efficacy of aminoglycosides given with once daily or as divided doses. J Antimicrob Chemother 1996;37:645–663.

118. Ferriols-Lisart R, Alos-Alminana M. Effectiveness and safety of once-daily aminoglycosides: A meta-analysis. Am J Health-Syst Pharm 1996;53:1141–1150.
119. Bailey TC, Little JR, Littenberg B, Reichley RM, Dunagan WC. A meta-analysis of extended-interval dosing versus multiple daily dosing of aminoglycosides. Clin Infect Dis 1997;24:786–795.
120. Ali MZ, Goetz MB. A meta-analysis of the relative efficacy and toxicity of single daily dosing versus multiple daily dosing of aminoglycosides. Clin Infect Dis 1997; 24:796–809.
121. Hatala R, Dinh TT, Cook DJ. Single daily dosing of aminoglycosides in immunocompromised adults: A systematic review. Clin Infect Dis 1997;24:810–815.
122. Demczar DJ, Nafziger AN, Bertino JS Jr. Pharmacokinetics of gentamicin at traditional versus high doses: Implications for once-daily aminoglycoside dosing. Antimicrob Agents Chemother 1997;41:1115–1119.
123. Xuan D, Lu JF, Nicolau DP, Nightingale CH. Population pharmacokinetics study of tobramycin after once-daily dosing in hospitalized patients. Int J Antimicrob Agents 2000;15:185–191.
124. Konrad F, Wagner R, Neumeister B, Rommel H, Georgieff M. Studies on drug monitoring in thrice and once daily treatment with aminoglycosides. Intensive Care Med 1993;19:215–220.
125. Gilbert DN, Bennett WM. Use of antimicrobial agents in renal failure. Infect Dis Clin North Am 1989;3:517–531.
126. Prins JM, Koopmans RP, Buller HR, Kuijper EJ, Speelman P. Easier monitoring of aminoglycoside therapy with once-daily dosing schedules. Eur J Clin Microbiol Infect Dis 1995;14:531–535.
127. Begg EJ, Barclay ML, Duffull SB. A suggested approach to once-daily aminoglycoside dosing. Br J Clin Pharmacol 1995;39:605–609.
128. Nicolau DP, Wu AHB, Finocchiaro S, Udeh E, Chow MSS, Quintiliani R, Nightingale CH. Once-daily aminoglycoside dosing: Impact on requests for therapeutic drug monitoring. Thera Drug Mon 1996;18:263–266.
129. Hitt CM, Klepser ME, Nightingale CH, Quintiliani R, Nicolau DP. Pharmacoeconomic impact of a once-daily aminoglycoside administration. Pharmacotherapy 1997;17810–17814.
130. Parker SE, Davey PG. Once-daily aminoglycoside administration in gram-negative sepsis: Economic and practical aspects. PharmacoEconomics 1995;7:393–402.

7

Pharmacodynamics of Quinolones

Robert C. Owens, Jr.
Maine Medical Center, Portland, Maine, and University of Vermont College of Medicine, Burlington, Vermont

Paul G. Ambrose
Cognigen Corporation, Buffalo, New York

1 INTRODUCTION

"We know everything about antibiotics except how much to give," Maxwell Finland once stated. With the proliferation of pharmacodynamics as a science, we are finally addressing the question of how much to give. We are watching the pendulum swing from an era of more-or-less arbitrary dosage selection toward the present-day science that integrates both pharmacokinetic and microbiologic data to determine optimal dosing strategies and to set perhaps more clinically meaningful breakpoints. It is conceivable that body-site-specific susceptibility breakpoints based on the pharmacodynamic profiles of antimicrobial agents will exist in the not-too-distant future, replacing the *one breakpoint fits all* approach that we have historically endured. Pharmacodynamics is central to the idea of optimizing antimicrobial therapy. Figure 1 illustrates the relationship between pharmacodynamics and the optimal selection, dosing, and duration of antimicrobial therapy. A comprehensive review by Ron Polk [1] provides, in great detail, the various aspects of the optimal use of antibiotics.

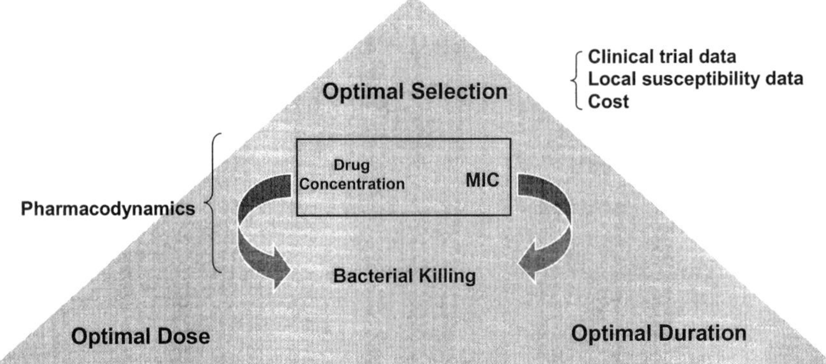

FIGURE 1 Pharmacodynamics is central to the optimization of antimicrobial therapy. (Courtesy of Robert Owens, Pharm.D.)

During the three decades since nalidixic acid was first introduced, thousands of related quinolone compounds have been synthesized, and most have been abandoned prior to development for a variety of reasons. A better understanding of structure–activity and structure–toxicity relationships has allowed chemists to modify the adaptable basic quinolone structure to enhance or limit the extent of antimicrobial activity and to improve various other product attributes such as the pharmacokinetic profile, tolerability, drug interaction potential, and toxicity of each new agent. The quinolones have undergone a ''structural evolution'' that began in 1962 upon the inadvertent discovery of nalidixic acid, and the pilgrimage continues today with the search for the perfect compound [2].

For some time now, clinicians have been familiar with antibiotic classes categorized by generations (e.g., cephalosporins, quinolones, macrolides). Certain schemes have been based upon pharmacodynamics [2–5] (Table 1), rather than relying on simply microbiological susceptibility data or merely the date a compound was licensed for use. Classifying quinolones by generations allows one to realize the pharmacokinetic and microbiological evolution of the quinolones as a direct result of structural changes. To this day, the fluoroquinolones remain the prototypical class of antibiotics because they are available in both oral and parenteral dosage forms, have excellent oral bioavailability, are active against a wide range of bacteria, achieve therapeutic concentrations both intracellularly and extracellularly, distribute widely into organ tissue and secretions, and are rapidly bactericidal. It is for these reasons that the fluoroquinolones have revolutionized transitional therapy as well as other aspects of the treatment of modern infectious diseases.

Table 1 Quinolone Generations (Pharmacodynamic Classification)

First generation	Second generation		Third generation	Fourth generation
Nalidixic acid, oxolinic acid, cinoxacin	Lomefloxacin (Maxaquin), norfloxacin (Noroxin), enoxacin (Penetrex)	Ofloxacin (Floxin), ciprofloxacin[a] (Cipro)	Levofloxacin (Levaquin), sparfloxacin[a] (Zagam), grepafloxacin[a] (Raxar)	Trovafloxacin[a] (Trovan), gatifloxacin (Tequin), moxifloxacin[a] (Avelox), gemifloxacin[a] (Factive), sitafloxacin (DU 6859a)
		Microbiological activity		
Enterobacteriaceae	Enterobacteriaceae + *P. aeruginosa*	Enterobacteriaceae + Atypicals *P. aeruginosa*	Enterobacteriaceae *P. aeruginosa* (+/−) Atypicals + Streptococci	Enterobacteriaceae *P. aeruginosa* (+/−) Atypicals Streptococci + Anaerobes
		Site of infection		
Urine only	Urine only	Systemic + Urine	Systemic ± Urine	Systemic ± Urine

[a] Dual elimination pathways exist.
Source: Courtesy of Robert Owens, Pharm. D.

2 PHARMACODYNAMIC CONCEPTS

Since the dawn of the antibiotic era in the late 1930s, controversy has existed as to the most appropriate method to administer and dose antibiotics to maximize the killing of microorganisms while minimizing toxicity. Harry Eagle, a half-century ago, pioneered the first pharmacodynamic studies using penicillin in streptococcal and syphylitic animal models of infection [6–8]. It was at this time that dosing methods (e.g., continuous infusion versus intermittent injection) as well as the dose of penicillin employed in relation to the minimum inhibitory concentration (MIC) were evaluated for their ability to impact in vivo outcome. Following a long respite, the science known as pharmacodynamics reemerged as Shah et al. [9] classified antimicrobial agents on the basis of their patterns of bactericidal activity. One of the two patterns described was a concentration-dependent killing effect, where an increase in the rate and extent of bacterial killing occurred with increasing drug concentrations in relation to the MIC of the bacteria. Agents that demonstrated concentration-dependent bactericidal activity included the aminoglycosides (and now include the fluoroquinolones and most likely metronidazole) (see Fig. 2).

The second pattern, now known as time-dependent killing, exhibited a saturable concentration-dependent increase in the rate and extent of bacterial killing, occurring at approximately 2–4 times the MIC of the pathogen. In essence, these agents proceeded to kill bacteria most efficiently when the concentration of drug remained in excess of the MIC of the pathogen for a specified length of time, rather than when doses were employed that provided high serum concentrations

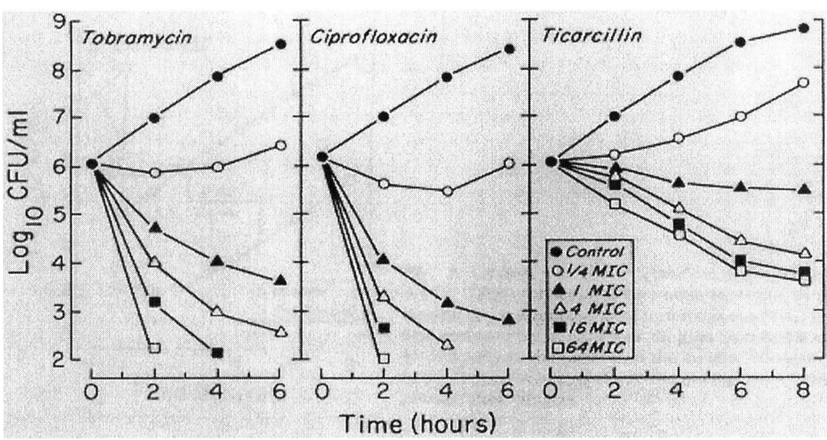

FIGURE 2 Concentration-dependent versus time-dependent bactericidal activity. (From Ref. 20.)

(relative to the MIC), because the latter did not result in enhanced bacterial killing. β-Lactams (e.g., penicillins, cephalosporins, monobactams, carbapenems), lincosamides (e.g., clindamycin), macrolides (e.g., erythromycin, clarithromycin), and oxazolidinones (e.g., linezolid) best fit this pattern of bactericidal activity. For the purposes of this chapter, we will focus on the quinolones and concentration-dependent bacterial killing.

Historically, the MIC has been used by the practicing clinician to select drug therapy for a particular infection. The lower the MIC, the better the drug must be, and the choice has been traditionally made accordingly and sometimes still is today. Unfortunately, the MIC has many shortcomings and therefore cannot be used alone to predict the outcome for a given infection. The MIC is a measure of a drug's potency against a particular organism. It should be remembered that the MIC is an artificial value, and is further subject to a one-tube dilution standard error if broth dilution techniques are used. This can translate into a considerable difference in actual MIC values (e.g., is the MIC 8 μg/mL or 16 μg/mL, or somewhere in between?). The MIC does not describe the rate and extent of bacterial killing or persistent antimicrobial effects such as the post-antibiotic effect (PAE) or the more clinically relevant sub-MIC effect (SME). The PAE and SME are used to describe the continued suppression of bacterial growth despite either complete removal of the antimicrobial agent from the organism's milieu or concentrations of the agent that are below the MIC value for the particular organism, respectively. Also, the MIC does not describe the impact of increasing drug concentrations or increased time of exposure of the drug on bacteriological outcome. MIC testing does not account for protein binding; although somewhat controversial, this has historically misled clinicians to choose therapies with confidence based solely on in vitro data. For example, the use of oxacillin for the treatment of enterococcal endocarditis (despite MIC values in the susceptible range) has led to clinical and microbiological failures in humans; similarly, the use of cefonicid and teicoplanin for the treatment of staphylococcal infections has led to treatment failures, some so extensive that clinical trials were terminated sooner than planned [10–12]. Fortunately, these weaknesses can be overcome or a drug selection can be modified if the appropriate pharmacokinetic aspects of the antimicrobial agent are also factored into the equation.

Bacterial killing can be characterized mathematically. For example, the product of concentration and time ($C \times t$) may be reflected by the pharmacokinetic term "area under the concentration–time curve" (AUC). Hence, bacterial killing is a function of a drug's AUC when it is indexed to the MIC. The 24 h AUC/MIC ratio is the pharmacodynamic correlate that can be used to describe the time course of antimicrobial activity and to predict clinical or microbiological outcome and perhaps the development of resistance.

Under certain circumstances, one of the terms of the product (either concentration or time) makes a small or negligible contribution to the killing process and can therefore be ignored. The pharmacodynamic parameter can be simplified to the peak concentration (peak)/MIC ratio or the length of time the serum concentration remains above the MIC (t > MIC). How this simplification occurs depends on the pattern of bactericidal activity demonstrated by the antimicrobial agent in question (e.g., concentration-dependent killing or time-dependent killing). For concentration-dependent killing agents (e.g., aminoglycosides, quinolones), the 24 h AUC/MIC ratio and peak/MIC ratio have been used to correlate in vivo outcome. For the time-dependent killing agents (e.g., β-lactams), t > MIC has best correlated with efficacy.

3 CLINICAL PHARMACODYNAMIC TARGETS

For the quinolones, as one might expect, both the peak/MIC ratio and the 24 h AUC/MIC ratio have been correlated with outcome. The magnitude of the peak/MIC ratio that has been associated with improved outcomes is 10–12 [13]. In addition, the peak/MIC ratio has been suggested to be the parameter of choice when resistant subpopulations of bacteria exist [26]. Unfortunately, increasing the amount of drug given in excess of standard doses for many agents in this class also increases the probability of unwanted adverse events, so unless the pathogen is relatively susceptible this ratio may not always be the best parameter to optimize.

When a peak/MIC ratio of at least 10:1 is not possible, one can no longer ignore the contribution of the time of exposure (Fig. 3). Under these circum-

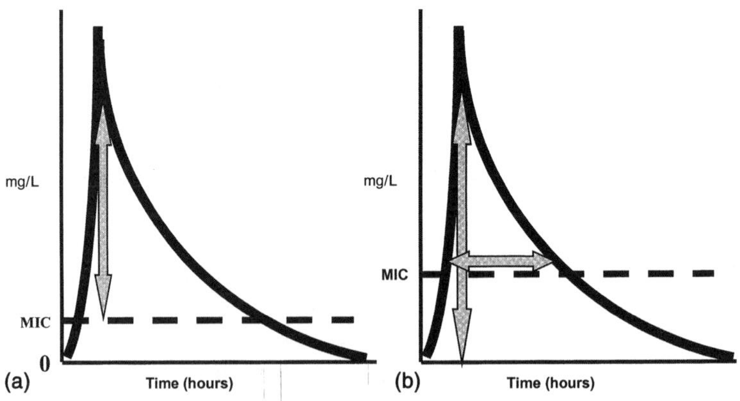

Figure 3 Pharmacodynamic relationships of (a) peak/MIC ratio and (b) 24 h AUC/MIC ratio. (Courtesy of Robert Owens, Pharm. D.)

stances, the parameter that best correlates with efficacy defaults to the 24 h AUC/MIC ratio.

The optimal pharmacodynamic targets are pathogen-specific. Data obtained from animal models of sepsis, *in vitro* pharmacodynamic experiments and clinical outcome studies indicate that the magnitude of the 24 h AUC/MIC ratio can be used to predict clinical response. Forrest et al. [14] demonstrated that a 24 h AUC/MIC ratio of ≥125 was associated with the best clinical cure rates in the treatment of infections caused by gram-negative enteric pathogens and *P. aeruginosa.* However, for gram-positive bacteria, data collected in humans by Drusano and colleagues [13] and Ambrose et al. [15] suggest that the 24 h AUC/MIC ratio can be appreciably lower. For infections caused by anaerobic pathogens, the optimal pharmacodynamic correlate for efficacy remains to be determined. However, the likely 24 h AUC/MIC ratio target will again be below 125. The 24 h AUC/MIC ratio for trovafloxacin ranged from 50 to 100 [16], similar to that of metronidazole, and was successful within this range. One must also remember that free drug concentrations should be considered, so taking into account that trovafloxacin is 75% protein-bound, a free drug 24 h AUC/MIC ratio required to predict success against anaerobic pathogens may in fact be as low as 15–25. Pharmacodynamic studies evaluating quinolones against anaerobic pathogens are needed considering that most newer agents (e.g., gatifloxacin, moxifloxacin, gemifloxacin, sitafloxacin) have in vitro activity against these organisms.

4 PHARMACOKINETICS OF FLUOROQUINOLONES

The pharmacokinetic profiles for the newer and some older fluoroquinolones are listed in Table 2. Once a standard of care for most infections, the appeal of parenteral therapy has lost significant ground to newer, equally potent, and pharmacokinetically equivalent oral dosing formulations. Although bacteria have become quite sophisticated, they are still unable to discriminate between the routes by which an antibiotic is delivered to the infection site. The fluoroquinolones have revolutionized the treatment of modern infectious diseases for a variety of reasons, none perhaps more important than their pharmacokinetic characteristics. Whether administered intravenously or orally, similar pharmacodynamic relationships can be achieved because of their high degree of bioavailability, which is consistent among the newer generation agents. Protein binding is one characteristic that is highly variable among the quinolones. The degree of protein binding not only influences penetration into tissues but also determines the amount of drug that is capable of interacting with bacteria at the site of infection [17]. The exact role of protein binding is often more controversial than not, but clearly, the pharmacokinetic parameter used in pharmacodynamic analyses should reflect *free drug* (active drug) rather than *total drug* concentrations.

TABLE 2 Pharmacokinetic Profiles of Various Fluoroquinolones

Parameter	Norfloxacin	Ciprofloxacin	Levofloxacin	Sparfloxacin	Gatifloxacin	Moxifloxacin	Trovafloxacin	Gemifloxacin
Dose (mg)	400	750	500	200	400	400	200	320
Bioavailability (%)	50	70	99	92	96	90	88	80
% Protein-bound	15	25	30	40	20	55	75	59
Peak (μg/mL)	1.5	3.5	6	1.3	4.3	4.5	2.3	1.48
Free peak (μg/mL)	1.3	2.6	4.2	0.8	3.4	2.0	0.6	0.6
$AUC_{(0-24)}$(μg · h/mL)	13.6	64	47.5	17.7	51.3	48	31.2	9.3
Free $AUC_{(0-24)}$(μg · h/mL)	11.6	48	33.3	10.6	41.0	21.6	7.8	3.8
$T_{1/2}$	3.3	4	6	20	9	12	12	7.4
% Renal elimination (active drug)	40	60	95	10	85	20	6	30

Courtesy of Robert Owens, Pharm. D.

5 OUTCOME DATA

5.1 Animal Models and In-Vitro Models of Infection

In 1991, Leggett et al. [18] published data evaluating ciprofloxacin in neutropenic murine thigh and pulmonary infection models using strains of *P. aeruginosa* and *K. pneumoniae*, respectively. The manipulation of the dosing intervals in these studies minimally affected the extent of bacterial killing, suggesting that the AUC/MIC ratio may be most closely associated with this endpoint.

Drusano et al. [26] evaluated lomefloxacin in the neutropenic rat model of *Pseudomonas* sepsis. Doses were administered in a variety of regimens to study the effect of different pharmacodynamic indices associated with outcome. The peak/MIC ratio was significantly associated with reduced mortality, compared with the AUC/MIC ratio and the time > MIC. The doses used in this study provided peak/MIC ratios of approximately 20:1 and <10:1. The reason for the clear association between the index of the peak/MIC ratio and survival was stated to be the increased inoculum size used (1×10^9) in the study. These findings demonstrated that with a higher burden of organisms, one is more likely to encounter resistant subpopulations, and in such settings the peak/MIC ratio becomes the more appropriate pharmacodynamic index that predicts outcome.

Several studies have been recently published or presented evaluating the pharmacodynamic relationships of quinolones against gram-positive pathogens, particularly *S. pneumoniae*. Onyeji et al. [19] compared the efficacy of ciprofloxacin and levofloxacin in a murine model of peritoneal sepsis. Clinical isolates of *S. pneumoniae* were used that displayed a variety of susceptibilities to penicillin, and MIC values for ciprofloxacin (1 and 2 μg/mL) and levofloxacin (1 and 2 μg/mL) were reflective of those also seen clinically. Dosing regimens were varied such that concentrations of drug measured in the animals simulated those in humans. Five-day survival rates between ciprofloxacin (2–6%) and levofloxacin (7–9%) groups were negligible ($p > 0.05$), perhaps because the 24 h AUC/MIC ratios were not very different from those seen in humans. For ciprofloxacin, 24 h AUC/MIC ratios ranged between 17.5 and 35, and for levofloxacin values ranged between 22 and 44. Neither ciprofloxacin nor levofloxacin achieved a desirable peak/MIC ratio of at least 10, as expected.

Studies evaluating the impact of protein binding have been conducted. Craig and Andes [20] studied six fluoroquinolones in the classic nonneutropenic murine thigh infection model in an effort to determine optimal AUC/MIC ratios in terms of survival and bactericidal activity, using both free and total drug concentrations. After being infected with *S. pneumoniae*, mice were treated with ciprofloxacin, levofloxacin, sitafloxacin, moxifloxacin, gemifloxacin, or gatifloxacin. Serum concentrations and protein binding were determined using microbiological assay and ultrafiltration, respectively. The E_{max} model was used to correlate 24 h AUC/MIC values using both free and total drug concentrations with colony forming units in the thigh on day 1 and survival on day 5. Results indicated that the 24 h AUC/MIC ratio correlated with survival on day 5 and the extent of bacterial killing on day 1 ($p < 0.001$). Additionally, free drug better correlated with survival on day 5 than did total drug concentrations ($R^2 = 82\%$ and 74%, respectively) (see Fig. 4). Survival (90% of animals) was predicted with an 24 h AUC/MIC ratio of 34 ± 4, and a similar value predicted a 2.5 $\log_{10}$ kill after one day of treatment. Again, agreement existed among all quinolones tested as to the pharmacodynamic breakpoint required for endpoints of survival and the extent of bacterial killing (24 h AUC/MIC somewhere between 25 and 35), and unbound drug was better correlated with these effects than total drug concentrations.

Similarly, for *S. pneumoniae*, in vitro models of infection have demonstrated that for levofloxacin and ciprofloxacin a 24 h AUC/MIC ratio of approximately 30 was associated with a 4 log kill, whereas values less than 30 were associated with a significantly reduced extent of bacterial killing and in some instances bacterial regrowth [21,22]. These observations are supported by data from nonneutropenic animal models of infection, where maximal survival was associated with a 24 h AUC/MIC ratio of 25 against the pneumococcus [23]. Clinically, there have been a significant number of treatment failures and superinfections involving meningeal seeding from *S. pneumoniae* in patients receiving ciprofloxacin, where the 24 h AUC/MIC ratio is approximately 12 [24]. Conversely, similar treatment failures or superinfections have not occurred with quin-

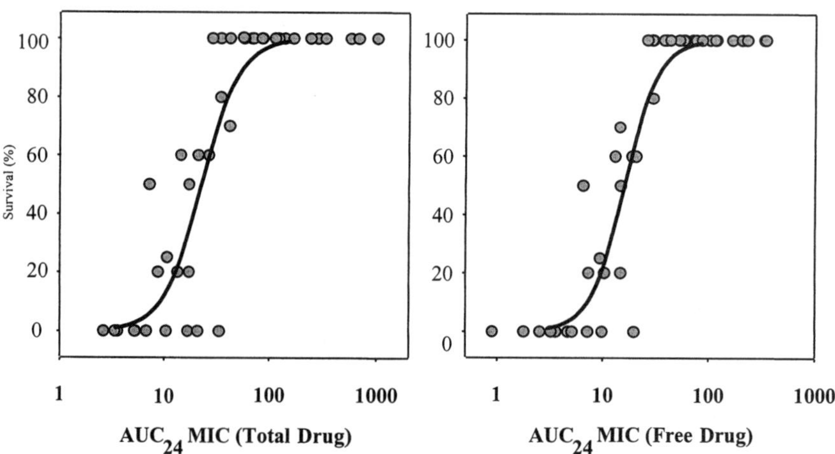

Figure 4 Correlation between survival and (a) free-drug concentration ($R^2 =$ 74) and (b) total drug concentrations ($R^2 = 82$). (From Ref. 20.)

olones for which the 24 h AUC/MIC ratios against this bacterium are greater than 30–40 [15].

5.2 Human Studies

Some of the first data to correlate pharmacodynamics and response in humans were published by Peloquin et al. [25]. Intravenous ciprofloxacin was evaluated in the treatment of lower respiratory tract infections in seriously ill patients hospitalized in the intensive care unit. A relationship between time of exposure and outcome was established. Interestingly, against *P. aeruginosa*, a low peak/MIC ratio (<10:1) was observed and resulted in the development of resistance in 10 of 13 pathogens. Although the researchers concluded that the time duration of exposure was the important determinant of outcome, against difficult to treat and less susceptible pathogens (e.g., *P. aeruginosa*), failure to obtain an optimal peak/MIC ratio resulted in the emergence of resistance. This is consistent with findings from the animal model of infection reported by Drusano et al. [26], further emphasizing the importance of the peak/MIC ratio when dealing with resistant subpopulations. Eventually, after the addition of 24 new patients, Forrest et al. [14] in 1993 published their reanalyzed data from the 1989 publication (see Fig. 5). Multivariate analysis and logistic regression showed that the 24 h AUC/MIC ratio predicted outcome best, rather than the time of exposure as previously reported.

A relationship also exists between the 24 h AUC/MIC ratio and the liklihood of developing resistance while on therapy. Thomas et al. [27] described this relationship in 107 hospitalized patients being treated for bacterial pneumonia. Patients were treated with a variety of dosing regimens involving a fluoroquinolone (ciprofloxacin, 200 mg q12h to 400 mg q8h) or a cephalosporin (cefmenoxime, 1–2 g q4-6h or ceftazidime, 1–2 g q8-12h), providing a wide range of exposures. Gram-negative pathogens predominated, as expected in nosocomial pneumonia, accounting for over 90% of the organisms isolated. Gram-positive pathogens such as *S. aureus* and *S. pneumoniae* were infrequently isolated. With the exception of Bush group 1 β-lactamase elaborating organisms (e.g., *Enterobacter* spp.) treated with a β-lactam, a pharmacodynamic breakpoint was established. If a 24 h AUC/MIC ratio of at least 100 was achieved, the potential to develop resistance was <10%. In contrast, the probability of developing a resistant strain during therapy was greater than 80% if the 24 h AUC/MIC was <100. Because the majority of pathogens encountered were gram-negative bacilli, most of which were *P. aeruginosa*, it is difficult to generalize this identified pharmacodynamic relationship to gram-positive pathogens. More information is clearly needed here.

Ciprofloxacin, a second-generation fluoroquinolone, remains the most potent antipseudomonal quinolone in terms of in vitro microbiological activity. For

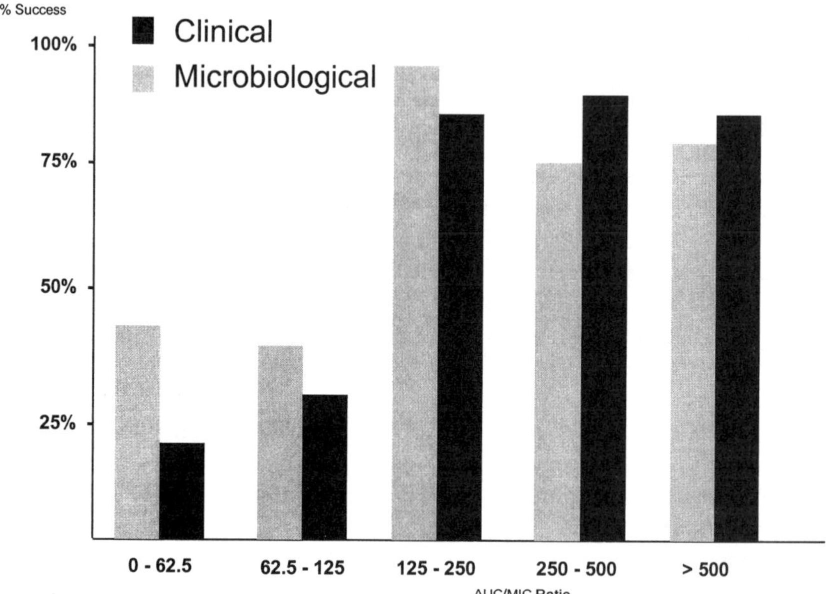

FIGURE 5 Pharmacodynamic correlates of efficacy for gram-negative pathogens. (From Ref. 14.)

instance, ciprofloxacin is consistently 4–8 times as active against *Pseudomonas aeruginosa* in vitro as trovafloxacin and levofloxacin. Along these lines, ciprofloxacin is also pharmacodynamically superior to other available fluoroquinolones against *P. aeruginosa* in terms of an achievable 24 h AUC/MIC ratio when dosed appropriately. Unfortunately none of the currently available fluoroquinolones routinely achieve a target 24 h AUC/MIC ratio against *P. aeruginosa* of at least 125, which is one reason combination therapy is always recommended for the treatment of infection outside of the lower urinary tract when a quinolone is employed.

One must consider, however, that ciprofloxacin's strength against *P. aeruginosa* is counterbalanced by its poor pharmacodynamic profile against many gram-positive microorganisms. For instance, ciprofloxacin, even when dosed at 750 mg every 12 h, does not reach a pharmacodynamic goal of approximately 30 for *S. pneumoniae*. This poor pharmacodynamic profile is consistent with numerous reports of failures and superinfections when ciprofloxacin has been used in community-acquired infection due to *S. pneumoniae* [24,28–33].

With the advent of newer generation fluoroquinolones (e.g., temafloxacin) with significantly greater potency against the pneumococcus in the early 1990s and the recent observations of increasing β-lactam resistance among pneumococci, it is not surprising that Daniel Musher in 1992 stated, ''Those of us who, a few years ago, scoffed at the notion of using a quinolone for treatment of pneumococcal pneumonia may be just doing that in the not-too-distant future.''

Newer generation fluoroquinolones are filling the ever-widening niche being created by pneumococci that are now demonstrating widespread resistance to multiple drug classes, including the β-lactams, macrolides and azalides, sulfonamides, and tetracyclines. In fact, with respect to the treatment of community-acquired pneumonia, Marvin Turck has widely been quoted as saying ''*a fluoroquinolone for your mother or a β-lactam for your mother-in-law*''. Despite their high degree of activity against most strains of *S. pneumoniae*, the fluoroquinolones, particularly less active agents such as ciprofloxacin, ofloxacin, and levofloxacin, are showing elevated rates (albeit small percentages) of resistance [34,35]. Some newer generation fluoroquinolones (e.g., moxifloxacin, gatifloxacin, gemifloxacin) are also affected, but to a lesser degree [34,36]. The fluoroquinolones do have the potential for overuse because of their convenience and agent-specific low side effect profiles. Appropriate use of these compounds, and the selection of those agents with optimized pharmacodynamic profiles, will most likely reduce the selective pressure being placed on pneumococci.

Preston et al. [13] evaluated the association between levofloxacin's pharmacodynamic profile and clinical as well as microbiological outcomes. In this study, concentrations of levofloxacin in serum were obtained from patients being treated for urinary tract, pulmonary, and skin/soft-tissue infections after they had been given standard doses appropriate for the site of infection. Of the initial 313 patients, 116 had sufficient pharmacokinetic, microbiological, and outcome data for evaluation. Patients in whom a peak/MIC ratio of >12.2 was achieved had a 100% chance of a eradicating the infecting organism from the site of infection. Conversely, if the peak/MIC ratio was <12.2, the liklihood of successful eradication was 80.8%. Although there was significant covariation between the peak/MIC and 24 h AUC/MIC indices on outcome predictability, the peak/MIC ratio reached statistical significance for all pathogens and infection sites. A recent reanalysis of the infections caused by *S. pneumoniae*, however, revealed that a 24 h AUC/MIC ratio of >30 was associated with favorable outcomes [37]. These data are consistent with the previous work conducted by Drusano's group which demonstrated that when a peak/MIC ratio of at least 10:1 could not be achieved, the index most closely associated with outcome was the 24 h AUC/MIC ratio.

Most recently Ambrose and Grasela [15] reported a correlation between the free-drug 24 h AUC/MIC ratio and microbiological eradication of *S. pneumoniae* in patients enrolled in phase III, double-blinded, randomized trials in North America. Of the initial 778 patients enrolled in these studies involving community-acquired pneumonia and acute bacterial exacerbations of chronic bronchitis, 376 patients had sufficient clinical and microbiological data for evalu-

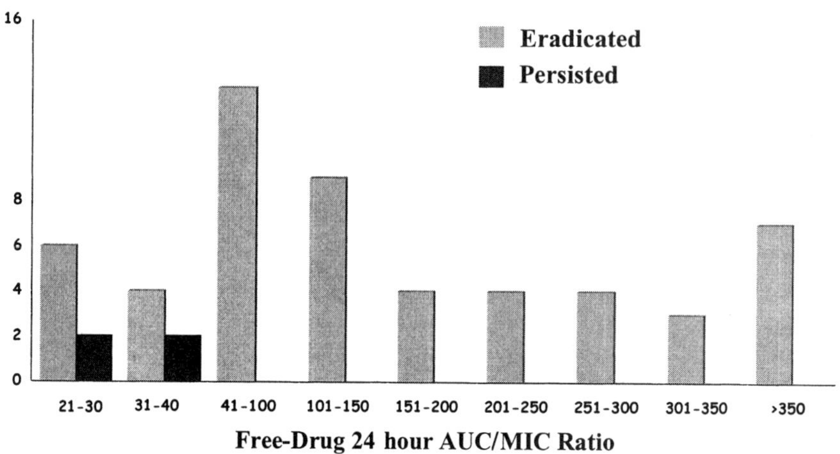

FIGURE 6 Pharmacodynamic correlates of efficacy for *Streptococcus pneumoniae*. (Courtesy of Paul Ambrose.)

ation. Of these patients, 58 were infected with *S. pneumoniae* that was isolated from either blood or sputum. These data established that for gatifloxacin and levofloxacin a 24 h AUC/MIC ratio of at least 33 correlated with the eradication of *S. pneumoniae* in patients being treated for pneumococcal pulmonary infections (Fig. 6). Although not every patient with an 24 h AUC/MIC ratio that did not reach this pharmacodynamic breakpoint failed therapy, these patients certainly had a high probability of failure.

In the clinic, we are now seeing what has already been predicted pharmacodynamically [38]. As MICs continue to increase gradually for older fluoroquinolones, the pharmacokinetics of these agents can no longer compensate for this decrease in activity. Davidson et al. [39] reported recently well documented clinical failures that could be traced back to the inability of a less active fluoroquinolone to eradicate *S. pneumoniae*. When pulse field gel electropheresis and PCR were performed on the pretherapy and post-therapy isolates, it was evident that the organisms were in fact the same and resistance had developed during therapy. Pretherapy isolates in both cases were susceptible to the agent, and after receiving levofloxacin for the treatment of community-acquired pneumococcal pneumonia, the strains had acquired resistance via *gyr*A and *par*C mutations. A likely explanation for these findings are the propensity to select for resistant strains secondary to reduced concentrations at the end of the dosing interval. There are differences among the newer generation fluoroquinolones in their ability to select for resistant strains. The rank order, in terms of most likely to least likely to select for resistance among pneumococci, is as follows: ciprofloxacin > levofloxacin > gatifloxacin = moxifloxacin [40–43].

Finally, various pharmacodynamic targets for predicting higher probabilities for successul outcomes in humans now exist. For quinolones against gram-negative enteric bacilli and *P. aeruginosa*, a 24 h AUC/MIC ratio of 125 may be targeted for the treatment of infections by these pathogens. For preventing the emergence of resistance, primarily for non-Bush group 1 β-lactamase-elaborating gram-negative bacilli, a 24 h AUC/MIC ratio of at least 100 has been suggested. And for gram-positive pathogens such as *S. pneumoniae*, an AUC/MIC ratio of at least 30 has been associated with higher probabilities of successful eradication of these organisms. More data are clearly needed to assess the effect of these pharmacodynamic indices on newly emerging mechanisms of resistance and for anaerobic pathogens.

6 PHARMACODYNAMIC ANALYSES

Once data have become available demonstrating an association between a pharmacodynamic relationship and outcome, one can predict the efficacy of certain compounds using available pharmacokinetic and microbiological data individualized toward specific patient and pathogen populations. This can be quite useful to the clinician in the assessment of newer agents in the formulary decision process, particularly when they are being compared to other, newer agents as well as more traditional anti-infectives. The methodology of such analyses should be viewed with a certain amount of skepticism, as these analyses have now become popular among the marketing departments of the pharmaceutical industry. Moreover, clinicians should be careful when performing these analyses to ensure that the data are generalized to appropriate patient populations. Ultimately, this approach would be most useful when performed individually at the bedside, using patient-specific data, in an effort to optimize treatment in real time.

6.1 Single-Point Analyses

Because of the recent interest in pharmacodynamics and its ability to distinguish anti-infective agents, it has become popular to perform so-called single point pharmacodynamic analyses. These analyses are popular because they are both convenient and easy to perform. They rely primarily on the selection of mean pharmacokinetic values (e.g., 24 h AUC) collected in healthy volunteers which can be readily gleaned from product package inserts. In addition to the mean pharmacokinetic parameters, MIC_{90} values are obtained most often from large national surveillance studies. By integrating these data, one can calculate 24 h AUC/MIC ratios for various quinolone–pathogen combinations very quickly. At best, these evaluations convey what is *possible* rather than what is *probable*. At worst, they are meaningless to the practicing clinician [44]. Unfortunately, many hazards exist with these evaluations. For instance, significant variability exists in both pharmacokinetic data and MIC values; local resistance trends are not represented when national susceptibility data are used, and significant bias is often introduced into the analysis.

Considerable variability exists when fixed doses of drug are administered to populations of individuals with varying weights, heights, and organ function. Additionally, healthy volunteers must be discriminated from clinically sick patients. Mean 24 h AUC values cannot adequately reflect the range of possibilities.

Similarly, the MIC_{90} value of a given drug versus a specific organism, although perhaps useful for comparing susceptibility data from different locations, cannot possibly be used alone to simulate the range of potential susceptibilities encountered clinically. In fact, most strains encountered would have MIC values far less than the MIC_{90} value they are labeled with. By the same token, how do we accommodate for the 10% of organisms whose MICs are in excess of the MIC_{90} value?

Because of this rather arbitrary method for conducting a pharmacodynamic analysis, one can also foresee the introduction of bias. With the availability of a variety of surveillance studies, one is left to decide which MIC value to select. A twofold variance in MIC can lead to the resulting 24 h AUC/MIC ratio being either below or above the desired pharmacodynamic target, with the agent being deemed either unfavorable or favorable, respectively. As an example, for levofloxacin, if one selects an MIC_{90} of 1.0 or 2.0 μg/mL, keeping the mean 24 h AUC value fixed (500 mg dose administered orally, 24 h AUC = 47.5 μg · h/mL), the conclusions are dramatically different. If an MIC_{90} of 1.0 μg/mL is used, the resulting 24 h AUC/MIC ratio is 47.5; whereas if 2.0 μg/mL is used, the 24 h AUC/MIC ratio is 23.75. Keeping in mind that the 24 h AUC/MIC ratio pharmacodynamic target of 30 is desirable for *S. pneumoniae*, the seemingly minute one-dilution difference in MIC resulted in two discordant conclusions. One can clearly see that although this approach might seem convenient, the results may equate to ''garbage in, garbage out.''

6.2 Monte Carlo Analysis

A departure from a past paradigm involves a novel method for conducting pharmacodynamic analyses. The use of a certain methodology has received considerable attention lately. This methodology, termed *Monte Carlo* analysis, accounts for individual variability across a wide range of input variables. The results of Monte Carlo analyses estimate what is *probable*, rather than defining what is *possible* [45–48]. Monte Carlo simulations are sampling experiments for estimating the distribution of an outcome that is dependent on multiple probabilistic input variables. For example, MIC values obtained from an institution or region

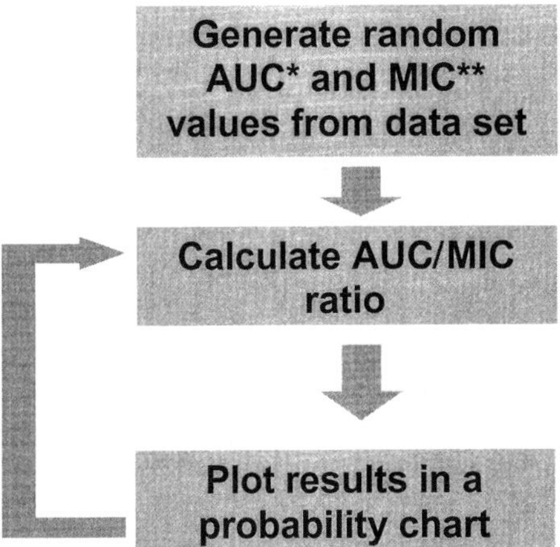

FIGURE 7 Pharmacodynamics and the use of Monte Carlo methodology. *Individual AUC values obtained from patients (clinical trials). **Individual MIC values derived from local or national surveillance data.

and the 24 h AUC values from patients are considered as input variables. Random values across input variables that conform to their probabilities are generated, and then an output is calculated (e.g., AUC/MIC ratio) (see Fig. 7). Each individual output that is calculated is then plotted in a probability chart. Monte Carlo methodology demonstrates the range of possible outcomes and the probability associated with each.

In a recent study, we characterized the pharmacodynamics of levofloxacin, gatifloxacin, and moxifloxacin using pharmacokinetic parameters and local clinical isolates of *Streptococcus pneumoniae* [47]. Clinical isolates of *Streptococcus pneumoniae* were collected consecutively over the 1999–2000 respiratory infection season by our laboratory ($n = 100$). Pharmacokinetic data were obtained from patients enrolled in a variety of trials for levofloxacin (172 acutely ill adult patients with community-acquired infections enrolled in multicenter clinical trials treated intravenously [mean AUC ± SD = 50.8 ± 35.8 μg/(mL · h)]) [13], gatifloxacin (64 acutely ill adult patients with community-acquired infections enrolled in a multicenter trial treated intravenously [mean AUC ± SD = 41 ± 16.3 μg/mL · h)]) [46], and moxifloxacin (286 adult volunteers in phase I and II trials that received oral moxifloxacin were used [mean AUC ± SD = 18.5 ± 4.5 μg/mL · h)]) [49]. Twenty-four-hour AUC values were corrected for protein binding based on the following: levofloxacin 30% protein-bound, gatifloxacin 20%, and moxifloxacin 50% protein bound. Monte Carlo simulation (1000 subjects × 3) was used to estimate the probability of attaining a free-drug 24 h

AUC/MIC ratio of at least 30. *Streptococcus pneumoniae* susceptibility testing results were as follows: gatifloxacin, $MIC_{50/90}$ 0.25/0.25, range 0.125–12.0; levofloxacin, $MIC_{50/90}$ 0.75/1.0, range 0.125 to >32; moxifloxacin, $MIC_{50/90}$ 0.125/0.19, range 0.023 to 6.0. The probabilities (mean % ± SD) of achieving a 24 h AUC/MIC ratio of at least 30 against *S. pneumoniae* isolates were as follows: gatifloxacin, 98.8 ± 0.23%; moxifloxacin, 97.9 ± 0.75%; and levofloxacin, 81.1 ± 1.44%.

Our results indicated that in our region of the country, gatifloxacin and moxifloxacin were associated with high probabilities of reaching a target 24 h AUC/MIC ratio of 30 over a wide range of actual AUCs and MICs compared with levofloxacin. The results of our regional pharmacodynamic analysis were similar to those previously presented using similar pharmacokinetic data and the national SENTRY database of 1977 isolates of *S. pneumoniae* [46]. A limitation of our analysis is that the 24 h AUC values for moxifloxacin were obtained from individuals enrolled in phase I and II trials rather than from infected patients. However, because moxifloxacin is considered to have a dual route of elimination (e.g., urinary, hepatobiliary elimination), the AUC values would not be expected to be dramatically influenced by moderate renal or hepatic impairment [49]. Also, 24 h AUC values for gatifloxacin and levofloxacin were measured after intravenous administration, whereas moxifloxacin AUC values were obtained after oral dosing. Nevertheless, because of the high degree of bioavailability of all three compounds, it is not likely that this fact would change the results of the analysis significantly [49].

The implications of more sophisticated pharmacodynamic analyses are wide ranging, but from a practical viewpoint we have been able to use these data for formulary evaluation of new antimicrobial agents where sufficient data exist to correlate findings with clinical outcome. Furthermore, clinicians practicing at institutions that perform such analyses will have an opportunity to select agents that demonstrate optimal pharmacodynamic profiles against specific pathogens such as, in this case, the pneumococci.

7 SUMMARY

Over the last several years an amalgam of information has become available to clinicians and researchers alike, illustrating the importance of pharmacodynamics and its role in optimizing drug selection and dosing. Once of putative value, recent developments in pharmacodynamics have provided insight into far more than the basic understanding of how antimicrobial agents actually kill bacteria more efficiently. In terms of the fluoroquinolones, new pharmacodynamic breakpoints have been discovered and validated in humans. Twenty-four-hour AUC/MIC ratios of 125 and around 25–35 have been established for many gram-negative and gram-positive pathogens, respectively. More data are needed to assess anaerobic breakpoints in patients to clarify outcome determinants.

Pharmacodynamic data have provided insight into the determination of new, clinically meaningful breakpoints germane to patient care for other drug classes as well. One day, clinicians may not ask why their patients with pulmonary infections caused by penicillin-resistant *S. pneumoniae* still, in fact, respond to penicillin. Pharmacodynamics will provide the backbone of such a monumental shift in both theory and practice.

REFERENCES

1. Polk R. Optimal use of modern antibiotics: Emerging trends. Clin Infect Dis 1999; 29:264–274.
2. Owens RC Jr, Ambrose PG. Clinical use of the fluoroquinolones. Med Clin N Am 2000;84:1447–1469.
3. Ambrose PG, Owens RC Jr, Quintiliani R, Nightingale CH. New generation quinolones. Conn Med 1997;61:269–272.
4. Owens RC Jr, Ambrose PG, Quintiliani R, Nightingale CH. Classifying quinolone anti-infective agents by generation: A pharmacodynamic approach to rational drug selection. Antibio Clin 1997;1:70–74.
5. Ambrose PG, Owens RC Jr. New antibiotics in pulmonary and critical care medicine: Focus on advanced generation quinolones and cephalosporins. Semin Respir Crit Care Med 2000; 21:19–32.
6. Eagle H, Fleischman R, Levy M. Continuous vs discontinuous therapy with penicillin. N Engl J Med 1953;238:481–486.
7. Eagle H. Effect of schedule of administration on therapeutic efficacy of penicillin: Importance of aggregate time penicillin remains at effectively bactericidal levels. Am J Med 1950;9:280–299.
8. Eagle H, Fleischman R, Mussleman AD. Effective concentrations of penicillin in vitro and in vivo for streptococci and pneumococci and Treponema. J Bacteriol 1950; 59:625–643.
9. Shah PM, Junghanns W, Stille W. Dosis-Wirkungs-Beziehung der Bakterizidie bei E. coli, K. pneumoniae und Staphylococcus aureus. Deut Med Wochenschr 1976; 101:325–328.
10. Eliopoulos GM, Moellering RC Jr. Antibiotic synergism and antimicrobial combinations in clinical infections. Rev Infect Dis 1982;4:282–293.
11. Calain P, Krause K-H, Vadaux P, et al. Early termination of a prospective, randomized trial comparing teicoplanin and flucloxacillin for treating severe staphylococcal infections. J Infect Dis 1987;155:187–191.
12. Chambers HF, Mills J, Drake TA, Sande MA. Failure of a once-daily regimen of cefonicid for treatment of endocarditis due to Staphylococcus aureus. Rev Infect Dis 1984;6(suppl. 4):S870–S874.
13. Preston SL, Drusano GL, Berman AL, Fowler CL, Chow AT, Dornseif B, Reichl V, Natarajan J, Corrado M. Pharmacodynamics of levofloxacin. J Am Med Assoc 1998;279:125–129.

14. Forrest A, Nix DE, Ballow CH, Schentag J. Pharmacodynamics of intravenous ciprofloxacin in seriously ill patients. Antimicrob Agents Chemother 1993;37:1073–1081.
15. Ambrose PG, Grasela DM, Grasela TH, et al. Pharmacodynamics of fluoroquinolones against Streptococcus pneumonia: Analysis of phase III clinical trials. In: Program and Abstracts of the 40th Interscience Conference on Antimicrobial Agents and Chemotherapy, Sept 17–21, 2000, Toronto, Canada.
16. Quintiliani R, Owens RC Jr, Grant ED. Clinical role of fluoroquinolones in patients with respiratory tract infections. Infect Dis Clin Pract 1999;8(suppl. 1):S28–S41.
17. Craig WA, Ebert SC. Protein binding and its significance in antibacterial therapy. Infect Dis Clin N Am 1989;3:407–414.
18. Leggett JE, Ebert S, Fantin B, et al. Comparative dose-effect relations several dosing intervals for β-lactam, aminoglycoside, and quinolone antibiotics against gram-negative bacilli in murine thigh-infection and pneumonitis models. Scand J Infect Dis 1991;74:179–184.
19. Onyeji CO, Bui KQ, Owens RC Jr, Nicolau DP, Quintiliani R, Nightingale CH. Comparative efficacies of levofloxacin and ciprofloxacin against Streptococcus pneumoniae in a mouse model of experimental septicemia. Int J Antimicrob Agents 1999;12:107–114.
20. Craig WA, Andes DR. Correlation of the magnitude of the AUC_{24}/MIC for 6 fluoroquinolones against Streptococcus pneumoniae with survival and bactericidal activity in an animal model. In: Program and Abstracts of the 40th Interscience Conference on Antimicrobial Agents and Chemotherapy, Sept 17–21, 2000, Toronto, Canada.
21. Lacy MK, Lu W, Xu X, Nicolau DP, Quintiliani R, Nightingale CH. Pharmacodynamic comparison of levofloxacin, ciprofloxacin and ampicillin against Streptococcus pneumoniae in an in vitro model of infection. Antimicrob Agents Chemother 1999;43:672–677.
22. Lister PD, Sanders CC. Pharmacodynamics of levofloxacin and ciprofloxacin against Streptococcus pneumoniae. J Antimicrob Chemother 1999;43:79–86.
23. Vesga O, Craig WA. Activity of levofloxacin against penicillin-resistant Streptococcus pneumoniae in normal and neutropenic mice. In: Program and Abstracts of the 36th Annual Interscience Conference on Antimicrobial Agents and Chemotherapy. New Orleans, LA, September 1996.
24. Lee BL, Padula AM, Kimbrough RC. Infectious complications with respiratory pathogens despite ciprofloxacin therapy. N Engl J Med 1991;325:520–521.
25. Peloquin CA, Cumbo TJ, Nix DE, et al. Evaluation of intravenous ciprofloxacin in patients with nosocomial lower respiratory tract infections. Arch Intern Med 1989; 149:2269–2273.
26. Drusano GL, Johnson DE, Rosen M, et al. Pharmacodynamics of a fluoroquinolone antimicrobial agent in a neutropenic rat model of *Pseudomonas* sepsis. Antimicrob Agents Chemother 1993;37:483–490.
27. Thomas JK, Forrest A, Bhavnani SM, et al. Pharmacodynamic evaluation of factors associated with the development of bacterial resistance in acutely ill patients during therapy. Antimicrob Agents Chemother 1998;42:521–527.
28. Gordon JJ, Kauffman CA. Superinfections with Streptococcus pneumoniae during therapy with ciprofloxacin. Am J Med 1990;89:383–384.

29. Perez-Trallero E, Garcia-Arenzana JM, Jimenez JA, et al. Therapeutic failure and selection of resistance to quinolones in a case of pneumococcal pneumonia treated with ciprofloxacin. Eur J Clin Microbiol Infect Dis 1990;9:905–906.
30. Righter J. Pneumococcal meningitis during intravenous ciprofloxacin therapy. Am J Med 1990;88:548.
31. Frieden TR, Mangi RJ. Inappropriate use of oral ciprofloxacin. J Am Med Assoc 1990;264:1438–1440.
32. Giamarrellou H. Activity of quinolones against gram-positive cocci: Clinical features. Drugs 1995;49(suppl. 2):58–66.
33. Cooper B, Lawlor M. Pneumococcal bacteremia during ciprofloxacin therapy for pneumococcal pneumonia. Am J Med 1989;87:475.
34. Chen DK, McGeer A, DE Azavedo JC, et al. Decreased susceptibility of *Streptococcus pneumoniae* to fluoroquinolones in Canada. N Engl J Med 1999;341:233–239.
35. Linares J, De La Campa AG, Palleres R. Fluoroquinolone resistance in *Streptococcus pneumoniae*. N Engl J Med 1999;341:1546–1547.
36. Applebaum PC. Microbiological and pharmacodynamic considerations in the treatment of infection due to antimicrobial-resistant Streptococcus pneumoniae. Clin Infect Dis 2000;31(suppl. 2):S29–S34.
37. Woodnut G. Pharmacodynamics to combat resistance. J Antimicrob Chemother 2000;46:25–31.
38. Fishman NO, Suh B, Weigel LM, Lorber B, Gelone S, Truant AL, Gootz TD, Christie JE, Edelstein PH. Three levofloxacin treatment failures of pneumococcal respiratory tract infections. In: Program and Abstracts of the 39th Interscience Conference on Antimicrobial Agents and Chemotherapy, San Francisco, CA, September 1999.
39. Davidson RJ, De Azavedo J, Bast D, et al. Levofloxacin treatment failure of pneumococcal pneumonia and development of resistance during therapy. In: Programs and Abstracts of the 40th International Conference on Antimicrobial Agents and Chemotherapy, Toronto, Canada, 2000.
40. Hooper DC. Mechanisms of action and resistance of older and newer fluoroquinolones. Clin Infect Dis 2000;31(suppl. 2):S24–S28.
41. Pestova E, Millichap JJ, Noskin GA, Peterson LR. Intracellular targets of moxifloxacin: A comparison with other fluoroquinolones. J Antimicrob Chemother 2000;45:583–590.
42. Fukuda J, Hiramatsu K. Primary targets of fluoroquinolones in Streptococcus pneumoniae. Antimicrob Agents Chemother 1999;43:410–412.
43. Zhao X, Xu C, Domagala J, Drlica K. DNA topoisomerase targets of the fluoroquinolones: A strategy for avoiding bacterial resistance. Proc Natl Acad Sci USA 1997;94:13991–13996.
44. Ambrose PG, Quintiliani R. Limitations of single point pharmacodynamic analyses. Pediatr Infect Dis J 2000;19:769.
45. Drusano GL, Preston SL, Hardalo CJ, et al. A model using population pharmacokinetics of ziracin with Monte Carlo simulation for preliminary MIC breakpoint selection and dose selection decision support. In: Program and Abstracts of the 39th Annual Interscience Conference on Antimicrobial Agents and Chemotherapy, Sept 26–29, 1999, San Francisco, CA.
46. Ambrose PG, Grasela DM. The use of Monte Carlo simulation to examine pharma-

codynamic variance of drugs: fluoroquinolone pharmacodynamics against *Streptococcus pneumoniae*. Diagn Microbiol Infect Dis 2000; in press.
47. Owens RC Jr, Ambrose PG, Piper D, Thomas S. Pharmacodynamic comparison of new fluoroquinolones against Streptococcus pneumoniae using Monte Carlo analysis. In: Program and Abstracts of the 40th Interscience Conference on Antimicrobial Agents and Chemotherapy, Sept 17–21, 2000, Toronto, Canada.
48. Dudley MN, Ambrose PG. Pharmacodynamics in the study of drug resistance and establishing in vitro susceptibility breakpoints: Ready for prime time. Curr Opinion Microbiol 2000;3:515–521.
49. Stass H, Kubitza D. Pharmacokinetics and elimination of moxifloxacin after oral and intravenous administration in man. J Antimicrob Chemother 1999;43(suppl. B): 83–90.

8

Glycopeptide Pharmacodynamics

Gigi H. Ross and David H. Wright
Ortho-McNeil Pharmaceutical, Raritan, New Jersey

John C. Rotschafer and Khalid H. Ibrahim
University of Minnesota, Minneapolis, Minnesota

1 INTRODUCTION

Pharmacodynamics represents a blending of pharmacokinetic parameters with a measure of bacterial susceptibility, the minimum inhibiting concentration (MIC). As such, there is a prerequisite that the pharmacokinetic parameters of the antibiotic be adequately defined prior to exploring the drug's pharmacodynamic properties. This in itself has not been an easy task with a drug such as vancomycin, which has undergone several different formulation changes to remove impurities and increase the drug's purity.

Measuring vancomycin concentrations by any method other than microbiological assay was not possible until the late 1970s when a radioimmunoassay was introduced. Microbiological assays were technically challenging, were accurate at best to $\pm 10\%$ [1], and often could not be performed if patients were receiving other antibiotics.

Pharmacokinetically, vancomycin, the only commercially available glycopeptide in the United States, has been characterized using one-, two-, and three-compartment models as well as noncompartmentally. As a result, there is model-dependent variability in the reporting of vancomycin pharmacokinetic parameters. Thus, getting to a point where clinically applicable pharmacodynamic parameters could be identified and quantified has not been easy. Even today, there are extremely limited in vitro, animal, and human data characterizing vancomycin's performance against only a few bacteria. Clearly, the characterization and quantification of vancomycin pharmacodynamics remains a work in progress. The purpose of this review is to examine the microbiology, pharmacology, and pharmacokinetics of vancomycin so as to build on the data presently available for describing the pharmacodynamics of the drug.

1.1 History of Vancomycin

Vancomycin was first introduced in 1956, with widespread clinical use by 1958 [2]. Originally, the drug was isolated from the actinomycete *Streptomyces orientalis*; however, its structure and molecular weight were not identified until 1978. The compound consists of a seven-membered peptide chain and two chlorinated β-hydroxytyrosine moieties with a molecular weight of 1449 [2]. Clinical use of the drug was highly prevalent in the late 1950s due to the emergence of penicillinase-producing strains of staphylococcus, but it soon lost favor with the introduction of methicillin. Impurities in early vancomycin formulations led to an unacceptable incidence of infusion-related reactions. Subsequently, for 20 years, vancomycin was used exclusively for the treatment of serious staphylococcal infections in patients with severe penicillin allergies. The current Eli Lilly formulation, marketed in 1986, is estimated to be 93% pure factor B (vancomycin) and is the result of several production changes and improved separation techniques [2]. With the enhancement in purity and the heightened frequency of methicillin-resistant staphylococci and ampicillin-resistant enterococci, clinical use of vancomycin has significantly increased. Today, approximately 800,000 patients receive vancomycin each year, accounting for 14,000 kg of drug worldwide [3].

1.2 Antimicrobial Spectrum

Vancomycin is primarily effective against gram-positive cocci, including staphylococcus, streptococcus, and enterococcus, and is considered to be bactericidal (MBC/MIC ≤ 4) against most gram-positive pathogens with the exception to enterococci, limited numbers of tolerant (MBC/MIC > 32) *S. pneumoniae*, and tolerant staphylococci. The National Committee for Clinical Laboratory Standards has established minimum inhibitory concentration (MIC) standards of susceptibility for vancomycin against staphylococci and enterococci [4]. Sensitive strains have MICs of $\leq$4 mg/L, intermediate isolates have MICs of 8–16 mg/

L, and resistant strains have MICs >32 mg/L. *Staphylococcus aureus* and *Staphylococcus epidermidis*, including both methicillin-susceptible and methicillin-resistant strains, are usually sensitive with MIC_{90} values of ≤2 mg/L [5]. All strains of *Streptococcus* are sensitive to vancomycin, regardless of penicillin susceptibility, with MIC_{90} values less than 1 mg/L [4]. A recent report, however, claims that approximately 2% of *S. pneumoniae* isolates have developed tolerance to vancomycin [6]. *Enterococcus faecalis* organisms are typically susceptible to vancomycin with MIC_{50} ≤1 mg/L, whereas *Entercoccus faecium* are generally nonsusceptible with MIC_{50} ≥16 mg/L [5]. Vancomycin is also effective against other Streptococcus spp., *Listeria monocytogenes, Bacillus* spp., Corynebacteria, and anaerobes such as diphtheroids and *Clostridium* spp., including *C. perfringens* and *C. difficile*. Vancomycin has no activity against gram-negative organisms, atypical pathogens, fungi, or viruses.

2 PHARMACOLOGY

Vancomycin has multiple mechanisms of action: preventing the synthesis and assembly of a growing bacterial cell wall, altering the permeability of the bacterial cytoplasmic membrane, and selectively inhibiting bacterial RNA synthesis [7]. Vancomycin prevents polymerization of the phosphodisaccharide–pentapeptide–lipid complex of the growing cell wall at the D-alanyl-D-alanine end of the peptidoglycan precursor during the latter portion of biosynthesis [7–8]. By tightly binding the free carboxyl end of the cross-linking peptide, vancomycin sterically prevents binding to the enzyme peptidoglycan synthetase. This activity occurs at an earlier point and at a separate site from that of penicillins and cephalosporins [8]. Therefore, no cross resistance or competition of binding sites occurs between the classes. Vancomycin, like β-lactams, does require actively growing bacteria in order to exert its bactericidal effect. However, vancomycin's bactericidal activity is restricted to gram-positive organisms because the molecule is too large to cross the outer cell membrane of gram-negative species.

Many factors appear to impede vancomycin's bactericidal activity: the absence of environmental oxygen, the size of the bacterial inoculum, and the phase of bacterial growth. The antibiotic appears to kill bacteria more effectively under aerobic conditions than under anaerobic conditions [9]. The fact that many gram-positive pathogens, including streptococcus and staphylococcus, can grow under aerobic and anaerobic conditions could prove problematic in clinical situations. Vancomycin activity was reduced by 19% and 99% with increases in inoculum size from 10^6 CFU/mL to 10^7 and 10^8 CFU/mL, respectively [10–11]. When vancomycin was evaluated against growing and nongrowing *Staphylococcus epidermidis* cells, the drug was found to be effective only against actively growing cultures [12]. Finally, activity is relatively unaffected by extremes in pH but is maximal at pH 6.5–8.0 [10,11,13].

3 PHARMACOKINETICS

The pharmacokinetics of vancomycin are highly dependent upon the modeling method used to characterize the parameters. Data can be found in the literature that characterize vancomycin using one-, two-, three-compartment and noncompartmental pharmacokinetic models that employ different serum sampling schemes and vary in the duration of study. As a result the literature varies in the reporting of vancomycin pharmacokinetic parameters.

Absorption is complete only when the drug is given intravenously, because oral absorption is poor and intramuscular administration is both erratic and painful. Vancomycin is readily absorbed after intraperitoneal administration also [14].

The distribution of vancomycin is a complex process and is best characterized by using a multicompartmental approach. Vancomycin has a large volume of distribution, varying from 0.4 to 0.6 L/kg in patients with normal renal function and up to 0.9 L/kg in patients with end stage renal disease [13,15,16]. Distribution includes ascitic, pericardial, synovial, and pleural fluids as well as bone and kidney. Penetration into bile, however, is generally considered poor. Cerebral spinal fluid concentrations are minimal unless sufficient inflammation is present where 10–15% of serum concentrations can be obtained [13,15]. Approximately 10–50% of vancomycin is protein-bound, primarily to albumin, providing a relatively high free fraction of active drug [13,17]. Studies attempting to measure the effect of other serum proteins have reported virtually no binding to the reactive protein, α-1 glycoprotein, but have noted binding to IgA [17].

Drug elimination is almost exclusively via glomerular filtration, with 80–90% of the vancomycin dose appearing unchanged in the urine within 24 h in patients with normal renal function [13,15,16]. The remainder of the dose is eliminated via biliary and hepatic means. Vancomycin, when taken orally, is excreted primarily in the feces. Vancomycin is not significantly removed by conventional hemodialysis or peritoneal dialysis owing to its large molecular weight (~2000), however, high-flux dialyzers can remove vancomycin and other molecules with molecular weights of less than 20,000 [18].

The elimination of vancomycin is multicompartmental, with an alpha, or distribution, half-life of 0.6–3 h and a beta, or elimination, half-life of 4–8 h with normal renal function [15,16]. Renal insufficiency can prolong the terminal half-life to as much as 7–12 days. Due to the complexity of this biexponential decay, attempts to utilize various modeling techniques are difficult. A one-compartment model inappropriately characterizes the distribution phase by formulating a regression line that is a hybrid of the alpha and beta phases. The pharmacokinetic parameters produced are accordingly mythical values that may or may not relate to the actual parameters. The extrapolated peak concentration and the half-life can be greatly underestimated depending upon the sampling scheme used. Generally, pairing a serum concentration obtained early in the distribution phase with a serum concentration late in the elimination phase results in the greatest error. Because one compartment modeling also underestimates the area under the serum concentration–time curve, this error is passed along in the calculation of both distribution volume and drug clearance.

For a concentration-independent or time-dependent antibiotic, vancomycin has an almost ideal pharmacokinetic profile. The drug has a large volume of distribution, low serum protein binding, and a long terminal half-life. Additionally, due to modest hepatic metabolism, vancomycin-drug interactions are limited. As such, vancomycin can be used effectively and conveniently to treat infections in most body sites.

4 GLYCOPEPTIDE RESISTANCE

Vancomycin has been in clinical use for over 40 years without the emergence of resistance. The multiple modes of action of vancomycin necessitate significant alterations in bacterial wall synthesis in order for the intrinsically susceptible organisms to develop resistance. Thus, the rarity of acquired vancomycin resistance led to predictions that such resistance is unlikely to occur on any significant scale [19,20].

The first reports of vancomycin-resistant enterococci, however, began to appear in Europe in the mid-1980s [19]. How the enterococci were able to develop resistance to vancomycin is unclear. However, several hypotheses have been elucidated, ranging from the overuse of antibiotics to the incorporation of glycopeptide antibiotics into animal feed.

Enterococci are normal gut flora, and the emergence of resistance has been linked to vancomycin overuse in the treatment of *Clostridium difficile* enterocolitis [20]. Additionally, the parenteral use of vancomycin has steadily increased since the late 1970s and may have played a role in the development of vancomycin-resistant enterococci (VRE) [21]. The agricultural use of avoparcin, a related glycopeptide, may have been important in Europe, but this drug has not been used in the United States. In any case, the enterococci were the first class of organisms to acquire vancomycin resistance, and vancomycin resistance are now problematic in both Europe and the United States [20].

The genetic basis for glycopeptide resistance in enterococci is complex and is characterized by several different phenotypes. Resistance-conferring genes encode a group of enzymes that enable the enterococci to synthesize cell wall precursors generally ending in D-alanine-D-lactate rather than the usual D-alanine D-alanine vancomycin binding site [22–23]. The affinity of vancomycin and teicoplanin for D-alanine-D-lactate is 1,000-fold less than that for D-alanine-D-alanine [20].

The most frequently encountered resistance phenotype, *vanA*, consists of high level vancomycin resistance (MIC $\geq$ 32 mg/L) accompanied by high level resistance to teicoplanin [22]. The resistance found on *vanA* strains is vancomycin- and/or teicoplanin-inducible. The genes encoding *vanA* resistance are relatively easily transferred to other enterococcal species via conjugation [22,23]. Significant concern has been expressed in both the lay and professional literature that this plasmid mediated form of resistance could be passed on not only to other enterococci but also to gram-positive organisms, such as staphylococci, which could lead to catastrophic consequences worldwide. Although this event has not been realized naturally, the *vanA* plasmid has been successfully introduced into staphylococci in the laboratory, raising concerns that given enough time vancomycin-resistant staphylococci will eventually become a clinical problem [24].

Enterococci with *vanB* phenotypic resistance have variable levels of vancomycin resistance and are susceptible to teicoplanin. The *vanB* phenotype is inducible by vancomycin but not teicoplanin, and vancomycin exposure produces teicoplanin resistance. Genes that encode *VanB* are more commonly chromosomal but can be transferred by conjugation [22,25].

The *vanC* resistance phenotype consists of relatively low levels of vancomycin resistance (MIC = 8–16 mg/L) and is devoid of teicoplanin resistance. Resistance to *vanC* is chromosomally produced by encoded genes found in all strains of *Enterococcus flavescens*, *Enterococcus casseliflavus*, and *Entercoccus gallinarum*. Genes encoded with *vanC* are not transferable [20]. In 1996 Perichon et al. [26] described a fourth phenotype, *vanD*, similar to *vanB*, found in a rare strain of *Enterococcus faecium* [26].

Following a steady increase of VRE prevalence in the United States over the past 10 years, almost 15% of enterococci in hospital intensive care units (participating in the National Nosocomial Infections Surveillance surveys) exhibit vancomycin resistance [23,27]. Similarly rapid increases in VRE prevalence have also been observed outside the intensive care units in U.S. hospitals [23]. Approximately 70% of VRE found in the United States exhibit the *vanA* resistance phenotype with the remaining 25% mostly constituted by the *vanB* resistance phenotype [28].

Evidence exists for both clonal dissemination of resistant strains and rapid transfer of vancomycin resistance genes among species of hospital enterococci [29–30]. With the transfer of resistance genes, multiple different enterococcal subtypes carry the same vancomycin resistance genes, suggesting a possible ''plasmid or transposon VRE epidemic'' [20]. Considerable heterogeneity in the genetic sequence of vancomycin resistance genes found in the United States further suggest that these genes are being modified as they spread among the various enterococcal strains [31].

The greatest threat VRE pose is the potential that they could transfer their resistance encoding genes to other more pathogenic gram-positive bacteria. Vancomycin resistance has been transferred from enterococci to streptococci, listeria, and *S. aureus* in vitro [24,32]. Also, the recent description of a naturally occurring vancomycin-resistant strain of *Streptococcus bovis* harboring the *vanB* resistance phenotype is of significant concern [33].

Low-level vancomycin resistance was reported in clinical isolates of coagulase-negative staphylococci in the late 1980s and early 1990s [34–36]. Although troubling, these reports were not terribly feared due to the relative lack of virulence associated with the coagulase-negative staphylococci. In vitro studies, however, demonstrated that both coagulase-negative staphylococci and *S. aureus* isolates, when exposed to increasing levels of glycopeptides, demonstrated the ability to select for resistant subpopulations [37,38]. Given these findings and the spread of VRE, for which excessive use of vancomycin was identified as an important control measure, the prudent use of vancomycin was suggested by the CDC as critical to prevent the emergence of resistance among staphylococci [39].

In May 1996 a methicillin-resistant *Staphylococcus aureus* (MRSA) clinical isolate that had reduced susceptibility to vancomycin (MIC = 8 mg/L) was isolated from a 4 month-old boy with a sternal surgical incision site [40,41]. This isolate has been referred to as Mu50 by the investigators who isolated the organism. By current NCCLS standards, this *S. aureus* clinical isolate is classified as having intermediate resistance to vancomycin. In August 1997, the first MRSA isolate intermediately susceptible to vancomycin was reported in Michigan and New Jersey [42,43]. Since these reports, the organism has been identified in New York and England. The two U.S. isolates exhibited different antimicrobial susceptibility patterns, suggesting that these strains are developing de novo secondary to vancomycin exposure. All of these decreased susceptibility strains were isolated from patients who had received multiple extended courses of vancomycin therapy.

The exact mechanism of resistance for these glycopeptide intermediate susceptibility *S. aureus* (GISA) strains remains largely unknown. None of the GISA strains isolated to date have carried the *vanA* or *vanB* genes as judged by PCR DNA amplification. Changes in the GISA cell wall structure have been noted, however, and may be in part responsible for the decreased sensitivity to vancomycin. This is inferred from three findings: The cell wall appeared twice as thick as the wall of control strains on electron microscopy; there was a three fold increase in cell wall murein precursor production compared with vancomycin-susceptible MRSA strains; and there was a threefold increase in the production of penicillin-binding protein (PBP) 2 and PBP2′ [40,41].

To date, there is no evidence that vancomycin resistance genes have been naturally transferred to the staphylococci or pneumococci, however, that does not preclude this event from happening in the future. If such a transfer of vancomycin resistance were to occur, particularly if the *S. aureus* strain is already methicillin-resistant, the result would be an especially terrifying pathogen.

5 PHARMACODYNAMICS

5.1 Introduction to Basic Principles

Evaluations of serum peak/MIC ratios, the ratio of the area under the serum concentration–time curve for 24 h to the MIC (AUC/MIC_{24}), and the length of time for which antibiotic concentration exceeds the MIC of the infecting organism ($T >$ MIC) have been employed as surrogate markers of the bactericidal effects of antibiotics. Pharmacodynamic indices for vancomycin have been poorly characterized, and therefore most dosing strategies have been based on extrapolations from aminoglycoside studies. By modifying aminoglycoside dosing models, specific peak and trough concentrations have been proposed with the assumption that similar clinical outcomes will be produced, high peak concentrations being essential for bacterial killing and definitive trough concentration ranges minimizing drug-related toxicity.

On the basis of limited in vitro studies, $T >$ MIC appears to most closely predict efficacy of vancomycin. Therefore, the length of time the antibiotic concentration exceeds the MIC of the offending organism and not the height of the peak above the MIC, as in aminoglycosides, should be considered the goal of the dosing of vancomycin. Although higher serum concentrations of vancomycin may be helpful in driving the drug to relatively inaccessible sites of infection such as endocardial vegetation or cerebrospinal fluid, they are unlikely to improve the rate of bacterial kill. Attempting to push the dose of vancomycin for serious but relatively accessible infections will likely only expose patients to an increased risk of adverse reactions; it is unlikely this approach will alter bacterial response.

Investigations of other pharmacodynamic parameters, including postantibiotic effect (PAE), sub-MIC effect (SME), and postantibiotic sub-MIC effect (PA SME), have also been undertaken to create a more informative depiction of vancomycin bactericidal activity than MICs allow alone. The PAE, or the continued suppression of microbial growth after limited antibiotic exposure of vancomycin against gram-positive bacteria, can persist for several hours depending on the organism and the initial antibiotic concentration [44,45]. This effect may inhibit regrowth when antibiotic concentrations fall below the MIC of the infecting organism, and may be important to consider when dosing vancomycin because of the extended half-life and prolonged dosing intervals. The postantibiotic effect of vancomycin was evaluated against *Staphylococcus epidermidis* by Svensson et al. [12]. The PAE was dependent upon concentration, as drug concentration increased from 0.5 to 8 times the MIC of the organism, the PAE increased from 0.2 h to 1.9 h. Another study found PAEs ranging from 0.6–2.0 h for *S. aureus* to 4.3–6.5 h for *S. epidermidis* [46].

Because patients receiving antibiotics will always have some amount of drug remaining in the body after dosing and elimination, PAEs are typically studied in vitro. SMEs and PA SMEs are parameters studied in vivo. Generally all of these effects are longer when measured in vivo than when mesaured in vitro. SMEs characterize the inhibition of bacterial regrowth following initial sub-MIC concentrations of antibiotic [46]. Postantibiotic SMEs, on the other hand, illustrate microbial suppression following bacterial exposure to supra-MIC concentrations that have declined below the MIC. This phenomenon is important clinically where patients given intermittent boluses will experience gradually lowered serum and tissue levels that will expose bacteria to both supra- and sub-MICs during the dosing interval [46].

5.2 In Vitro Studies

In vitro investigations have demonstrated that, like β-lactam antibiotics, vancomycin is a concentration-independent or time-dependent killer of gram-positive organisms and exhibits minimal concentration-dependent killing. In vitro studies, however, can be limiting for several reasons [47]:

1. One compartment models represent only concentrations that would exist in the central compartment and not necessarily those that would exist at the site of infection.
2. Typically only bacteria in log phase growth at standard inocula (10^5 or 10^6 CFU/mL) are used.
3. The effects of the immune system or protein binding are generally not considered.

Despite the limitations, in vitro studies appear to correlate well with animal and human studies and therefore provide useful information for optimal dosing strategies in clinical situations.

Several investigators demonstrated the concentration-independent killing of vancomycin by exposing various bacteria to increasing amounts of the drug. Vancomycin's killing effect against *Staphylococcus aureus* was investigated in vitro by Flandrois et al. [48]. The early portion of the time–kill curve was the focus of the study to characterize the bactericidal activity in the initial phases of the dosing interval. A decrease in CFU of only 1 log was obtained at the end of the 8 h study at concentrations of 1, 2.5, 5, and 10 times the MIC, indicating a concentration-independent, slow rate of kill. The killing phase occurred between hours 2 and 4, with the CFU/mL being held constant for the remainder of the curve. Ackerman et al. generated mono- and biexponential killing curves for vancomycin over a 2–50 μg/mL concentration range to evaluate the relationship between concentration and pharmacodynamic response against *Staphylococcus aureus* and coagulase-negative *Staphylococcus* species. For all organisms tested, killing rates did not change with increasing concentrations of vancomycin, and maximum killing appears to be achieved once concentrations of 4–5 times the MIC of the pathogen are obtained.

Because the pharmacokinetics of vancomycin involve, at minimum, biexponential decay, further studies attempting to simulate this elimination and any effects on bacterial killing were investigated. Utilizing an in vitro model simulating mono- or biexponential decay, Larrson et al. [9] found no statistically significant difference in either the rate or extent of bacterial killing of *Staphylococcus aureus*. Again, varying concentrations did not induce a change in bactericidal activity, thereby demonstrating that the high drug concentrations achieved during the distribution phase did not enhance the bactericidal activity attained during the elimination phase.

With the understanding that vancomycin killed staphylococci in a concentration-independent fashion, the need to select a pharmacodynamic index that best predicts efficacy was warranted. Duffull et al. [47] used four different vancomycin regimens against *S. aureus* in an in vitro dynamic model.[47] Three dosing schedules with different peak concentrations but the same AUC and a fourth dosing regimen with a smaller AUC were compared for efficacy. The authors found that killing was independent of both peak concentrations and total exposure to drug (AUC). In addition, maintaining a constant concentration above the MIC was equally effective, even with an AUC that was half of that obtained by the other three dosing regimens. This investigation thus supported $T >$ MIC as the optimal parameter for efficacy.

Greenberg and Benes [50] produced time-kill curves from experiments performed in a static environment with 50% bovine serum and constant antibiotic concentrations. They reported a significantly increased rate and extent of killing of *Staphylococcus aureus* when the concentration of vancomycin increased from 20 to 80 mg/L, even though free drug concentrations for all regimens exceeded the MIC by at least three fold. This experiment is one of a few that demonstrated significant concentration-dependent killing with vancomycin alone with concentrations beyond the MIC of the organism.

Vancomycin in combination with other antimicrobials has also been evaluated. Houlihan et al. [51] investigated the pharmacodynamics of vancomycin alone and in combination with gentamicin at various dosing intervals against *Staphylococcus aureus*–infected fibrin-clots in an in vitro dynamic model. Vancomycin monotherapy simulations included continuous infusion, 500 mg every 6 h, 1 g every 12 h, and 2 g every 24 h all of which produced varying peaks and troughs. While all regimens produced concentrations above the MIC for 100% of the dosing intervals, no difference in kill was seen with higher peak concentrations. The investigators also discovered that vancomycin killing was significantly enhanced by the addition of gentamicin whether it was given every 12 or 24 h and, in fact, it killed in a concentration-dependent fashion. The 2 g dosing scheme of vancomycin significantly reduced bacterial counts to a greater extent than any other combination regimen. Whether this finding is due to augmented penetration into the fibrin clots in the presence of gentamicin is unknown.

The vast majority of pharmacodynamic investigations with vancomycin include the use of *Staphylococcus aureus,* few studies involve other gram-positive or anaerobic organisms. Levett [52] demonstrated time-dependent killing of *Clostridium difficile* by vancomycin in vitro. Vancomycin was sub inhibitory at concentrations below the MIC of the organism. Once concentrations at the MIC were obtained, no difference in kill was seen whether 4 mg/L (at the MIC) or 1000 mg/L (250 × MIC) was utilized. Therefore, as for other organisms, vancomycin kills *C. difficile* in a concentration-dependent manner until the MIC is achieved, beyond which time-dependent killing is observed.

Odenholt-Tornqvist, Lowdin, and Cars have been the primary source of investigations on the SMEs and PA SMEs of vancomycin. In an initial study with *Streptococcus pyogenes* and *Streptococcus pneumoniae*, the investigators found that the PA SME with concentrations as low as 0.3 × the MIC prevented regrowth of both Steptococcus species for 24 h [53]. In a recent in vitro investigation of the pharmacodynamic properties of vancomycin against *Staphylococcus aureus* and *Staphylococcus epidermidis*, the same authors detected no concentration-dependent killing [46]. Low killing rates were demonstrated by time to 3 log kill (T3K) at 24 h with all strains, the exception being a methicillin-sensitive strain of *Staphylococcus epidermidis* (MSSE) that attained T3K at 9 h. Regrowth occurred between 12 and 24 h when drug concentration had declined to the MIC. PA SME, SME, and post-MIC effect (PME) were also evaluated in this study. Long PA-SMEs (2.3 to $\gg$20 h) were found with all strains while SMEs were shorter (0.0–15.8 h). Both PA-SMEs and SMEs increased with increasing multiples of the MIC. Interestingly, longer PMEs, "the difference in time for the numbers of CFU to increase 1 log/mL from the values obtained at the time when the antibiotic concentration has declined to the MIC compared with the corresponding time for a antibiotic-free growth control" [46], were found with shorter half-lives. Other investigations have suggested that the regrowth of bacteria can occur if insufficiently inhibited bacteria are allowed to synthesize new peptidoglycan to overcome the antimicrobial's bactericidal effect [54]. The authors assumed that the PAE, PA SME, and PME would emulate the time for which the amount of peptidoglycan is kept below a critical level needed for bacterial growth [46]. Subsequently, the investigators postulated that longer PMEs may occur with shorter half-lives due to the fact that the MIC is obtained faster, thereby not allowing adequate peptidoglycan production to initiate regrowth. Conversely, shorter PMEs were found with longer half-lives. With a slower decline to the MIC and a longer period of time at the MIC, sufficient peptidoglycan could be produced to allow regrowth. How PA-SMEs, SMEs, and PMEs will influence dosing schedules is unknown and further investigations are needed.

5.3 Animal Studies

Animal studies focusing on pharmacodynamic predictors of efficacy for vancomycin are quite limited. Peetermans et al. [10], with a granulocytopenic mouse thigh infection model, showed concentration-dependent killing of staphylococcus for concentrations at or below the MIC. Once concentrations exceeded that value, however, no further kill was seen with increasing doses.

The activity of vancomycin was again evaluated against penicillin-resistant pneumococci using a mouse peritonitis model [55]. In comparing various pharmacokinetic/pharmacodynamic parameters at the ED_{50}, values investigators concluded that both $T >$ MIC and Cmax were important predictors of efficacy in their model. These parameters were deemed best predictors because they varied the least. Also, of significance with this study was the discovery that vancomycin activity was not influenced by the penicillin susceptibility of the organism.

Cantoni et al. [56], in an attempt to compare the efficacy of amoxicillin–clavulanic acid against methicillin-sensitive and methicillin-resistant *Staphylococcus aureus* (MSSA and MRSA, respectively) versus vancomycin in a rat model of infection, found vancomycin activity to be dependent upon strain. Against the MSSA strain, vancomycin at 30 mg/kg given every 6 h was more effective than the same dose every 12 h. Against the MRSA strain, the four times daily regimen only marginally improved outcome compared to the twice-daily regimen. In that vancomycin concentrations were undetectable after 6 h of therapy, the four times daily regimen was the only therapy that allowed concentrations to remain above the MIC for a majority of the dosing interval. This finding further supports the dependence of vancomycin activity upon the $T >$ MIC.

5.4 Human Studies

In vivo, serum bactericidal titers (SBTs) have been evaluated to determine antimicrobial efficacy. An SBT of 1:8 with vancomycin has been associated with clinical cure in patients with staphylococcal infections [57–58]. This SBT was associated with serum concentrations greater than 12 mg/L. James et al. [59] conducted a prospective, randomized, crossover study to compare conventional dosing of vancomycin versus continuous infusions in patients with suspected or documented gram-positive infections. In that the most effective concentration of vancomycin against staphylococcus is not known, the investigators chose a target concentration of 15 μg/mL via continuous infusion and peak and trough concentrations of 25–35 and 5–10 μg/mL, respectively, with conventional dosing of 1 g every 12 h. Despite variability in actual concentrations obtained, continuous infusion produced SBTs of 1 : 16, whereas conventional dosing produced trough SBTs of 1 : 8, which was not found to be statistically insignificant. Concentrations remained above the MIC throughout the entire dosing intervals for all patients, whether they received conventional dosing or continuous infusion, and therefore the authors concluded that both methods of intravenous administration demonstrated equivalent pharmacodynamic activities. Although continuous infusion therapy was more likely than conventional dosing to produce SBTs of 1:8 or greater, this study did not attempt to evaluate clinical efficacy associated with such values. Therefore it is unknown, whether improved patient outcome was obtained.

Klepser et al. [60], in a preliminary report of a multicenter study of patients with gram-positive infections receiving vancomycin therapy, found increased rates of bactericidal activity with vancomycin trough concentrations greater than 10 mg/L [60]. Bacterial eradication was also correlated with trough SBTs of 1:8 or greater. Patients that failed therapy had pathogen MICs of >1 mg/L. Hyatt et al. [61] suggest that the area under the inhibitory serum concentration–time curve (AUIC) as well as the organism's MIC were associated with clinical outcome. By performing a retrospective analysis of 84 patients receiving vancomycin therapy for gram-positive infections, these authors found that therapy that produced AUIC <125 and pathogens with MICs >1 mg/L had a higher likelihood of failure. Therefore, these two studies propose that not only $T >$ MIC but also trough values may be important for maximum clinical efficacy.

In summary, vancomycin demonstrates concentration-independent killing of gram-positive bacteria, and peak concentrations do not appear to correlate with rate or extent of kill. Maximum killing is achieved at serum concentrations of 4–5 times the MIC of the infecting pathogen, and sustaining concentrations at or above these levels for the entire dosing interval will likely produce the best antimicrobial effect. Dosing strategies should therefore be aimed at maximizing the time in which concentration at the site of infection remains above the MIC of the pathogen. Whether the most efficient killing is obtained by continuous infusion of vancomycin or by intermittent bolus is controversial. Several studies revealed that no difference in killing is seen between the two methods of administration [51,59,62]; however, such benefits as predictable serum concentrations and ease of administration might be advantageous [62]. Conversely, due to vancomycin's long half-life and the perceived better tolerability associated with intermittent bolus injections, continuous infusion of this drug may not be needed and is often discouraged [62].

6 CLINICAL APPLICATION

6.1 Clinical Uses

Vancomycin is available as vancomycin hydrochloride (Vancocin, Lyphocin, Vancoled, and others) for intravenous use, as powder for oral solution, and as capsules for oral use (Vancocin Pulvules). The indications for vancomycin use are limited in relation to its strong gram-positive spectrum. Although vancomycin is bactericidal against most gram-positive cocci and bacilli, the intravenous preparation should be reserved for serious gram-positive infections not treatable with β-lactams or other traditional options. The use of vancomycin should not precede therapy with β-lactams for susceptible organisms. Clinical outcomes in both staphylococci and enterococci show vancomycin inferiority as compared to nafcillin and ampicillin regarding bactericidal rate and rapidity of blood sterility [63–67].

Vancomycin is the drug of choice for serious staphylococcal infections that cannot be treated with β-lactams due to bacterial resistance [methicillin-resistant *Staphylococcus aureus* (MRSA), and methicillin-resistant *Staphylococcus epidermidis* (MRSE)] or to the patient's inability to receive these medications [68–70]. Staphylococcal infections include bacteremia, endocarditis, skin and soft tissue infections, pneumonia, and septic arthritis. Dialysis peritonitis due to staphylococci may also be treated with IV vancomycin. Although vancomycin is indicated for *S. aureus* osteomyelitis, bone penetrations are extremely variable, especially between published studies, and treatment with other options could prove more effective [71–75]. Vancomycin is also indicated for infections due to coagulase-negative staphylococci including catheter-associated bacteremia, prosthetic valve endocarditis, vascular graft infections, prosthetic joint infections, central nervous system shunt infections, and other infections associated with indwelling medical devices [68–70]. Complete cure of most medical-device-related infections usually requires the removal of the device due to the biofilm secreted by the *S. epidermidis*. Staphylococcal treatment with vancomycin may require up to 1 week or longer for clinical response in serious infections such as MRSA [70]. Courses of vancomycin that fail to cure serious staphylococcal infections may require the addition of gentamicin, rifampin, or both [69,70,76].

Two significant clinical issues surround the use of vancomycin for the treatment of staphylococcal endocarditis. First, controversy exists as to whether the addition of rifampin is synergistic or antagonistic. Although certain studies have proven the combination to be more efficacious than single therapy with vancomycin [77–79], other more recent publications site the combination as antagonistic [65]. Additionally, clinical experience with the combination has been inconsistent [80].

The second issue that surrounds vancomycin use for staphylococcal endocarditis is the potentially better outcome with β-lactams. In addition to the in vitro data that suggest that vancomycin is less rapidly bactericidal than nafcillin, clinical data exist to support this conclusion [63–67]. Although no large-scale comparison studies exist to evaluate the efficacy of vancomycin versus β-lactams in staphylococcal endocarditis, assumptions can be formulated from published studies. In a study by Korzeniowski and Sande [67], the duration of bacteremia due to *S. aureus* endocarditis lasted a median of 3.4 days after treatment with nafcillin, whereas bacteremia lasted a median of 7 days for patients treated with vancomycin in a study conducted by Levine et al. [65]. The patients in the Levine study were infected with methicillin-resistant *S. aureus* in comparison to the methicillin-sensitive organisms from the Korzeniowski study, yet, in general, the morbidity and mortality of bacteremic infections due to MSSA and MRSA are comparable [66]. In a small study that compared vancomycin to nafcillin in *S. aureus* endocarditis, the investigators found that patients treated with nafcillin plus tobramycin had a cure rate of 94%, whereas only 33% of patients treated with vancomycin plus tobramycin were cured [64]. Worth mentioning, however, is the fact that while the nafcillin plus tobramycin group consisted of 50 patients, only three patients received vancomycin plus tobramycin due to β-lactam allergy. Small and Chambers [63] performed another study that evaluated the use of vancomycin in 13 patients with staphylococcal endocarditis, five of whom failed therapy. The reason for vancomycin ineffectiveness in these cases may be the need for prolonged high levels of a bactericidal antibiotic, however, with longer durations of bacteremia and poorer clinical outcomes, serious consideration needs to be given to whether vancomycin should be considered at all in patients with MSSA endocarditis who can tolerate β-lactam therapy.

Streptococcal infections not treatable with β-lactams or other traditional options are also proper indications for vancomycin [68–70]. Endocarditis due to β-lactam-resistant *S. viridans* or *S. bovis* is a common use of vancomycin, although organisms with elevated MIC values may require that it be combined with an aminoglycoside. Vancomycin is the drug of choice for pneumococcal infections showing high-level resistance to penicillin [68–70]. Cefotaxime or ceftriaxone plus rifampin may be needed to adequately cover *S. pneumoniae* meningitis due to vancomycin's poor penetration in the central nervous system [81–82]. Although penetration is enhanced while meninges are inflamed, as in meningitis and shunt infections, certain cases may require intrathecal or intraventricular administration to obtain therapeutic levels.

As for enterococcal infections, vancomycin represents the treatment of choice for ampicillin-resistant enterococcus [68–70]. Enterococcus endocarditis and other infections may require the addition of an aminoglycoside, such as gentamicin. Vancomycin is also the treatment of choice for corynebacterial infections [68–70].

Empirically, vancomycin should be used only in limited situations. Vancomycin can be considered for febrile neutropenic patients presenting with clinical signs and symptoms of gram-positive infections in areas of high MRSA prevalence [39]. Other indications for empirical use of vancomycin in neutropenic patients with fever include the presence of severe mucositis, colonization with MRSA or penicillin-resistant *Streptococcus pneumoniae*, prophylaxis with quinolone antibiotics, or obvious catheter-related infection [83]. Vancomycin should be discontinued after 4–5 days if no infection is identified or if initial cultures for gram-positive organisms are negative after 24–48 h. For prophylaxis, vancomycin may be used perioperatively with prosthesis implantation only in severely β-lactam allergic patients [39]. Vancomycin is also used for endocarditis prophylaxis for β-lactam allergic patients.

Orally, vancomycin is indicated for metronidazole-refractory antibiotic-associated colitis caused by *Clostridium difficile* [39,68–70]. Intravenous administration of vancomycin typically does not achieve adequate levels in the colon lumen to successfully treat antibiotic-associated colitis; however, there are rare reports of success with this route cited in the literature.[84] Administration via nasogastric tube, enema, ileostomy, colostomy, or rectal catheter may be needed if the patient presents with severe ileus. Oral vancomycin has also been used prophylactically to prevent endogenous infections in cancer and leukemia patients. This regimen seems to decrease the *C. difficile* associated with the chemotherapy [85–87].

6.2 Inappropriate Uses

Although vancomycin is an effective option for most gram-positive infections, the drug needs to be judiciously used to prevent the emergence and spread of resistance. Vancomycin should not be used when other drug options such as β-lactams are viable. Microbial susceptibilities need to be treated to determine the appropriateness of vancomycin therapy, and the antibiotic should be changed if the organism is susceptible to a different agent.

The CDC has published guidelines for the appropriate use of vancomycin (Tables 1 and Table 2) [39]; however, vancomycin misuse around the nation is widespread. A retrospective study from May 1993 to April 1994 identified 61% of vancomycin usage as inappropriate according to the CDC criteria [88]. A similar evaluation published in 1997 found that only 47% of vancomycin orders prescribed for 7147 patients were appropriate [89]. According to this study, inade-

Table 1 Appropriate Use of Vancomycin

Treatment of serious infections due to β-lactam-resistant gram-positive pathogens
Treatment of gram-positive infections in patients with serious β-lactam allergies
Antibiotic-associated colitis failure to metronidazole
Endocarditis prophylaxis per American Heart Association recommendations
Antibiotic prophylaxis for implantation of prosthetic devices at institutions with a high rate of infections due to methicillin-resistant staphylococci

Source: Ref. 37.

Table 2 Inappropriate Use of Vancomycin

Routine surgical prophylaxis
Empirical treatment for febrile neutropenic patients without strong evidence of gram-positive infection and high prevalence of β-lactam resistant organisms in the institution
Treatment in response to a single positive blood culture for coagulase-negative staphylococci when other blood cultures taken appropriately in the same time frame are negative
Continued empirical use without positive culture for β-lactam-resistant gram-positive pathogen
Systemic or local prophylaxis for central or peripheral catheter
Selective gut decontamination
Eradication of methicillin-resistant *Staphylococcus aureus* colonization
Primary treatment of antibiotic-associated colitis
Routing prophylaxis for patients on chronic ambulatory peritoneal dialysis
Routine prophylaxis for very low birthweight infants
Topical application or irrigation

Source: Ref. 37.

quate use and inappropriate control patterns were similar whether large teaching centers or small rural hospitals were evaluated. As such, alternative methods of vancomycin control need to be implemented to ensure adequate use and limit resistance.

6.3 Toxicity and Adverse Drug Reactions

A variety of adverse reactions have been associated with vancomycin, including fever, rash, phlebitis, neutropenia, nephrotoxicity, auditory toxicity, interstitial nephritis, and infusion-related reactions. Many of the infusion-related reactions were likely due to impurities in the initial formulations and have been significantly reduced with the newer formulations. The red man or red neck syndrome is an anaphylactoid reaction related to rapid infusion of large doses, typically >12 mg/(kg · h) [13,69–70]. The reaction begins 10 min after infusion and generally resolves within 15–20 min after stopping the dose. Patients may experience tachycardia, chest pain, dyspnea, urticaria, and swelling of the face, lips, and eyelids. Additionally, patients may experience a hypotensive episode with a 25–50% reduction in systolic blood pressure. Interestingly, volunteers receiving vancomycin infusions have a higher propensity toward the reaction than patients [62]. The reason is unknown. Symptoms of red nan syndrome appear to be histamine-mediated; however, investigations are inconclusive. Extending the administration of vancomycin to 1 h or a maximum of 15 mg/min should prevent most infusion-related reactions.

Vancomycin toxicity was retrospectively studied by Farber and Moellering [90] in 98 patients. They noted a 13% incidence of phlebitis, a 3% incidence of fever and rash, and a 2% incidence of neutropenia. However, this report may overestimate true adverse reactions because of the inclusion of many potentially high-risk patients. Interestingly, whereas other studies have shown that concomitant aminoglycosides are not a risk factor for nephrotoxicity [91], patients receiving both vancomycin and an aminoglycoside experienced a 35% incidence of reversible nephrotoxicity, which is more than expected from either antibiotic alone. Only 5% of patients receiving vancomycin alone experienced nephrotoxicity. The authors also found that patients with nephrotoxicity had trough concentrations of 20–30 mg/L.

Vancomycin ototoxicity has been reported with peak serum concentrations of 80–100 mg/L [92]. Geraci [92] identified two patients with vancomycin-induced ototoxicity, one of whom had a history of renal disease, an elevated blood urea nitrogen on admission, and a recorded diastolic blood pressure of zero. Serum concentrations determined 3–6 h after the dose was administered ranged from 80 to 95 mg/L. Due to the biexponential nature of the vancomycin serum concentration–time curve, the true vancomycin peak was likely near 200–300 mg/L. Farber and Moellering [90] also reported the occurrence of ototoxicity in a patient who, at 1 h postinfusion, had serum concentrations of <50 mg/L; however, the true peak was likely in the toxic range as defined by Geraci [92].

In summary, the incidence of adverse reactions associated with vancomycin are relatively infrequent. Only approximately 40 cases of oto- and nephrotoxicity were reported in the medical literature in the years 1956–1984 despite incessant use. Most of these cases were complicated by concomitant aminoglycoside therapy and pre-existing renal problems, as well as investigator discrepancies in interpreting serum levels.

6.4 Dosing and Therapeutic Monitoring

Medical literature abounds that questions the need to therapeutically monitor vancomycin concentrations. Cantu et al. [93] suggest that monitoring vancomycin concentrations is unnecessary in that no correlation has been demonstrated between drug levels, toxicity, and clinical response. Opponents propose that vancomycin can be dosed using published nomograms based on the the patient's age, weight, and estimated creatinine clearance. Conversely, Moellering et al. [94] argue that therapeutic vancomycin monitoring would in fact be prudent for optimal clinical response and restriction of toxicity in such situations as patients on hemodialysis, patients with rapidly changing renal function, and patients receiving high dose vancomycin or concomitant aminoglycoside therapy.

Numerous strategies do exist for empirically dosing vancomycin. Administering 500 mg every 6 h, 1 g every 12 h, or 20–40 mg/kg body weight/day are commonly employed. In addition, nomograms exist such as those established by Matzke et al. [95], Moellering et al. [94], Lake and Peterson [96], and Nielsen et al. [97]. Serious faults lie in the dependence of these nomograms on efficacious use of vancomycin, however, because the authors assume rather than prove that their method of pharmacokinetically modeling the data was appropriate. Most empirical regimens were designed to provide peak concentrations of 20–40 mg/L and trough concentrations of 5–10 mg/L (or approximately 5 times the MIC of the infecting pathogen), however, such practices place only 3–23% of patients in this therapeutic range, according to one published study [98]. Unfortunately, although such goals in serum levels are set, no solid data are available to support this therapeutic range and accordingly, serum peak and trough concentrations have been selected somewhat arbitrarily, based on speculations from retrospective studies, case reports, and personal opinions. Peak concentrations appear to play little to no role in the efficacy of the drug and appear to have limited involvement in toxicity unless exceedingly large peak values are obtained. On the other hand, trough concentrations may be useful monitoring parameters. Because vancomycin is a concentration-independent killer, the goal of therapy should be to maintain the unbound concentration above the microbial MIC for a significant portion of the dosing interval because regrowth of most organisms will begin shortly after drug concentrations fall below the MIC. A depiction of predicted vancomycin pharmacodynamic indices obtained from a typical intravenous dose using various pathogen MICs is presented in Table 3.

The role of vancomycin degradation products also needs to be considered when interpreting levels in patients with renal failure where half-lives are significantly extended [99–100]. In vitro and in vivo, vancomycin breaks down over time to form crystalline degradation products. Antibodies in commercial assays, such as TDx fluorescence polarization immunoassay, cross react with major and

TABLE 3 Estimated Vancomycin Pharmacodynamic Ratios for Various MIC Values[a]

MIC (mg/L)	$C_{P_{max}}$/MIC	$T >$ MIC (h)	AUC_{24}/MIC
0.25	140	12	784
0.5	70	12	392
1.0	35	12	196
2.0	17.5	12	98
4.0	8.75	12	49
8.0	4.38	11	24.5

[a] Calculations based on a 1 g dose given every 12 h to a 70 kg patient with normal renal function.

minor degradation products thereby overstating factor B (active drug) content in the level. This can result in an overstated vancomycin concentration of 20–50%.

In summary, trough concentrations of 5–10 mg/L appear to be reasonable goals for vancomycin therapy in that MICs of most gram-positive pathogens are ≤1 mg/L. Such concentrations would allow the unbound concentrations to remain above the MIC of the organism for the entire dosing interval. Administering 10–15 mg/kg per dose and adjusting the dosing interval per renal function based upon numerous published nomograms is not likely to produce ''toxic'' peak concentrations and should allow ''therapeutic'' concentrations throughout the dosing interval in the majority of patients with normal renal function. Loading doses are not typically needed, because transiently high distribution phase concentrations are unlikely to enhance bacterial killing. However, loading doses may be reasonable in patients in whom the site of infection is distal to the central compartment or poorly accessible. Until a relationship among clinical efficacy, toxicity, and vancomycin concentration is established, vancomycin therapy will inevitably continue to be monitored in an attempt to improve patient outcome. Whether therapeutic monitoring of vancomycin should be a standard of practice or is necessary only in patients receiving high dose therapy, patients on concomitant aminoglycoside therapy, or patients with renal insufficiency or failure on dialysis is likely to remain a personal preference until further studies establish guidelines. However, if the CDC guidelines for appropriate vancomycin usage were stringently followed, at least half of vancomycin use could be eliminated, leaving the remaining patients to be monitored.

7. OTHER GLYCOPEPTIDES

7.1 Teicoplanin

Teicoplanin, like vancomycin, binds to the terminal D-alanyl-D-alanine portion of the peptidoglycan cell wall of actively growing gram-positive bacteria to exert its bactericidal activity [101]. Currently available only in Europe, teicoplanin can be used to treat infections caused by both methicillin-sensitive and -resistant strains of *Staphylococcus aureus, S. epidermidis*, streptococci, and enterococci. Clinical trials have demonstrated teicoplanin to be a safe, well tolerated agent, with reports of side effects occurring in 6–13% of recipients [101]. The most prevalent adverse reactions reported are pain at the injection site and skin rash. Nephro- and ototoxicity are uncommon even when the drug is used concomitantly with other nephro- and ototoxic drugs. Pharmacokinetically, teicoplanin differs from vancomycin. The half-life is considerably longer (~47 h) and the percent protein-bound nears 90% [101]. Also, teicoplanin can be administered by either the intravenous or intramuscular route as opposed to vancomycin, which is limited parenterally to the intravenous route. Pharmacodynamic evaluations virtually duplicate those of vancomycin once the heightened protein binding of teicoplanin and subsequent lower active free concentrations are accounted for [102]. Further reviews of teicoplanin can be found elsewhere [101,103].

7.2 LY333328

LY333328 (Eli Lilly and Company) is a synthetic glycopeptide that is currently being developed to treat gram-positive bacterial infections, including those resistant to vancomycin. Because it is still in the early stages of development, little is known about the antibiotic. The drug acts on the same molecular target as vancomycin and other glycopeptide antibiotics [104]; however, LY333328 appears to display concentration-dependent bactericidal activity against gram-positive pathogens [102–106]. The half-life is long, approaching 10.5 days, which may allow for infrequent dosing [107]. Pharmacodynamic investigations and clinical efficacy trials are needed prior to drug approval and utilization.

8. CONCLUSION

With years of clinical experience, vancomycin has proven to be a safe and efficacious agent against gram-positive pathogens, including many multidrug-resistant strains. Despite this history, to date the therapeutic range has not been rigorously defined, however, going beyond the currently suggested therapeutic range is not likely to improve antibiotic performance. The accumulation of in vitro and in vivo studies suggests that vancomycin is a concentration-independent killer of gram-positive organisms with maximum killing occurring at serum concentrations of 4–5 times the MIC of the infecting organism. High peak concentrations are not associated with an improved rate or extent of kill, and therefore therapy should be targeted toward sustaining serum concentrations above the MIC for a large portion of the dosing interval. With the high level of vancomycin use, the development and spread of vancomycin-resistant organisms is a formidable and predictable occurrence. At a time when we are attempting to be more prudent and judicious in the use of vancomycin, we also find ourselves more dependent on the drug. Unfortunately, this combination of factors may drive bacterial resistance and ultimately nullify a drug that has been a gold standard product for a half a century.

REFERENCES

1. KB Crossley, JC Rotschafer, MM Chern, KE Mead, DE Zaske. Comparison of a radioimmunoassay and a microbiological assay for measurement of serum vancomycin concentrations. Antimicrob Agents Chemother 1980;17:654–657.
2. GL Cooper, DB Given. The development of vancomycin. In: GL Cooper and DB

Given, eds. Vancomycin: A Comprehensive Review of 30 Years of Clinical Research. Park Row Publ, 1986:1–6.

3. HA Kirst, DG Thompson, TI Nicas. Historical yearly usage of vancomycin. Antimicrob Agents Chemother 1998;42:1303–1304.
4. National Committee for Clinical Laboratory Standards. Performance standards for antimicrobial susceptibility testing. 9th Informational Supplement, M100-S9, 1999, Vol 19(1). National Committee for Clinical Laboratory Standards, Wayne, PA.
5. RN Jones, CH Ballow, DJ Biedenbach, JA Deinhart, JJ Schentag. Antimicrobial activity of quinupristin/dalfopristin (RP 59500, Synercid®) tested against over 28,000 recent clinical isolates from 200 medical centers in the United States and Canada. Diagn Microbiol Infect Dis 1998;31:437–451.
6. Nature 1999;399:524–526,590–593.
7. PE Reynolds. Structure, biochemistry and mechanism of action of glycopeptide antibiotics. Eur J Clin Microbiol Infect Dis 1989;8:943–950.
8. PE Reynolds, EA Somner. Comparison of the target sites and mechanisms of glycopeptide and lipoglycodepsipeptide antibiotics. Drugs Under Exp Clin Res 1990;16: 385–389.
9. AJ Larsson, KJ Walker, JK Raddatz, JC Rotschafer. The concentration-independent effect of monoexponential and biexponential decay in vancomycin concentration on the killing of *Staphylococcus aureus* under aerobic and anaerobic conditions. J Antimicrob Chemother 1996;38:589–597.
10. WE Peetermans, JJ Hoogeterp, AM Hazekamp-VanDokkum, P Van Den Broek, H Mattie. Antistaphylococcal activities of teicoplanin and vancomycin in vitro and in an experimental infection. Antimicrob Agents Chemother 1990;34:1869–1874.
11. KC Lamp, MJ Rybak, EM Bailey, GW Kaatz. In vitro pharmacodynamic effects of concentration, pH, and growth phase on serum bactericidal activities of daptomycin and vancomycin. Antimicrob Agents Chemother 1992;36:2709–2714.
12. E Svensson, H Hanberger, LE Nilsson. Pharmacodynamic effects of antibiotics and antibiotic combinations on growing and nongrowing *Staphylococcus epidermidis* cells. Antimicrob Agents Chemother 1997;41:107–111.
13. TS Lundstrom, JD Sobel. Vancomycin, trimethoprim-sulfamethoxazole, and rifampin. Infect Dis Clin N Am 1995;9:747–767.
14. GD Morse, MA Apicella, JJ Walshe. Absorption of intraperitoneal antibiotics. Drug Intell Clin Pharm 1998;22:58–61.
15. RC Moellering. Pharmacokinetics of vancomycin. J Antimicrob Chemother 1984; 14(suppl D):43–52.
16. JC Rotschafer, K Crossley, DE Zaske, K Mead, RJ Sawchuk, LD Solem. Pharmacokinetics of vancomycin: Observation in 28 patients and dosage recommendations. Antimicrob Agents Chemother 1982;22:391–394.
17. H Sun, EG Maderazo, AR Krusell. Serum protein-binding characteristics of vancomycin. Antimicrob Agents Chemother 1993;37:1132–1136.
18. GR Matzke, RF Frye. Drug therapy individualization for patients with renal insufficiency. In: JT DiPiro, RL Talbert, GC Yee, GR Matzke, BG Wells, LM Posey, eds. Pharmacotherapy: A Physiologic Approach. 3rd ed. Stamford, CT: Appleton & Lange, 1997:1083–1103.

19. N Woodford, AP Johnson, D Morrison, DCE Speller. Current perspectives on glycopeptide resistance. Clin Microbiol Rev 1995;8:585–615.
20. RC Moellering. Vancomycin-resistant enterococci. Clin Infect Dis 1998;26:1196–1199.
21. J Ena, RW Dick, R Jones, RP Wenzel. The epidemiology of intravenous vancomycin usage in a university hospital. J Am Med Assoc 1993;269:598–602.
22. M Arthur, PE Reynolds, F Depardieu, et al. Mechanisms of glycopeptide resistance in enterococci. J Infect Dis 1996;32:11–16.
23. HS Gold, RC Moellering Jr. Drug therapy: Antimicrobial-drug resistance. N Engl J Med 1996;335:1445–1454.
24. WC Noble, Z Virani, RGA Cree. Co-transfer of vancomycin and other resistance genes from *Enterococcus faecalis* NCTC 12201 to *Staphylococcus aureus*. FEMS Microbiol Lett 1992;93:195–198.
25. R Quintiliani, S Evers, P Courvalin. The vanB gene confers various levels of self-transferable resistance to vancomycin in enterococci. J Infect Dis 1993;16:1220–1223.
26. B Perichon, PE Reynolds, P Courvalin. VanD-type glycopeptide-resistant *Enterococcus faecium* (abst LB12). In: Program and Abstracts of the 36th Interscience Conference on Antimicrobial Agents and Chemotherapy (New Orleans). Washington DC: Am Soc Microbiol, 1996:5.
27. Centers for Disease Control and Prevention. Nosocomial enterococci resistant to vancomycin—United States, 1989–1993. MMWR Morb Mortal Wkly Rep 1993; 42:597–599.
28. NC Clark, RC Cooksey, BC Hill, JM Swenson, FC Tenover. Characterization of glycopeptide-resistant enterococci from US hospitals. Antimicrob Agents Chemother 1993;42:597–599.
29. LG Rubin, V Tucci, E Cercenado, GM Eliopoulos, HD Isenberg. Vancomycin resistant *Enterococcus faecium* in hospitalized children. Infect Control Hosp Epidemiol 1992;13:700–705.
30. JF Boyle, SA Saumakis, A Rendo, et al. Epidemiologic analysis and genotypic characteristic of a nosocomial outbreak of vancomycin-resistant enterococci. J Clin Microbiol 1993;31:1280–1285.
31. S Handwerger, J Skoble, LF Discotto, MJ Pucci. Heterogeneity of the vanA gene cluster in clinical isolates of enterococci from the northeastern United States. Antimicrob Agents Chemother 1995;39:362–368.
32. F Biavasco, E Giovanetti, A Miele, C Vignaroli, B Facinelli, PE Varalso. In vitro conjugative transfer of vanA vancomycin resistance between enterococci and listeriae of different species. Eur J Clin Microbiol Infect Dis 1996;15:50–59.
33. C Poyart, C Pierre, G Quesne, et al. Emergence of vancomycin resistance in the genus *Streptococcus*: Characterization of a vanB transferable determinant in *Streptococcus bovis*. Antimicrob Agents Chemother 1997;41:24–29.
34. RS Schwalbe, JT Stapleton, PH Gilligan. Emergence of vancomycin resistance in coagulase-negative staphylococci. N Engl J Med 1987;316:927–931.
35. LA Veach, MA Pfaller, M Barrett, FP Koontz, RP Wenzel. Vancomycin resistance in *Staphylococcus haemolyticus* causing colonization and bloodstream infection. J Clin Microbiol 1990;28:2064–2068.

36. D Sanyal, AP Johnson, RC George, BD Cookson, AJ Williams. Peritonitis due to vancomycin-resistant *Staphylococcus epidermidis*. Lancet 1991;337:54.
37. RS Schwalbe, WJ Ritz, PR Verma, EA Barranco, PH Gilligan. Selection for vancomcyin resistance in clinical isolates of Staphylococcus haemolyticus. J Infect Dis 1990;161:45–51.
38. RS Daum, S Gupta, R Sabbagh, WM Milewski. Characterization of Staphylococcus aureus isolates with decreases in susceptibility to vancomycin and teicoplanin: Isolation and purification of a constitutively produced protein associated with decreased susceptibility. J Infect Dis 1992;166:1066–1072.
39. Hospital Infection Control Practices Advisory Committee. Recommendations for preventing the spread of vancomycin resistance: Recommendations of the Hospital Infection Control Practices Advisory Committee (HICPAC). MMWR Morb Mortal Wkly Rep 1995;44(12).
40. K Hiramatsu, H Hanaki, T Ino, K Yabuta, T Oguri, FC Tenover. Methicillin-resistant *Staphylococcus aureus* clinical strain with reduced vancomycin susceptibility. J Antimicrob Chemother 1997;40:135–136.
41. Centers for Disease Control and Prevention. Reduced susceptibility of *Staphylococcus aureus* to vancomycin—Japan 1996. MMWR Morb Mortal Wkly Rep 1997; 46(27):624–628.
42. Centers for Disease Control and Prevention. *Staphylococcus aureus* with reduced susceptibility to vancomycin—United States, 1997. MMWR Morb Mortal Wkly Rep 1997;46(33):756–766.
43. Centers for Disease Control and Prevention. Update: *Staphylococcus aureus* with reduced susceptibility to vancomycin—United States, 1997. MMWR Morb Mortal Wkly Rep 1993;46(35):813–815.
44. WA Craig, B Vogelman. The post-antibiotic effect. Ann Intern Med 1987;106: 900–902.
45. MA Cooper, YF Jin, JP Ashby, JM Andrews, R Wise. In vitro comparison of the postantibiotic effect of vancomycin and teicoplanin. J Antimicrob Chemother 1990; 26:203–207.
46. E Lowdin, I Odenholt, O Cars. In vitro studies of pharmacodynamic properties of vancomycin against *Staphylococcus aureus* and *Staphylococcus epidermidis*. Antimicrob Agents Chemother 1998;42:2739–2744.
47. SB Duffull, EJ Begg, ST Chambers, ML Barclay. Efficacies of different vancomycin dosing regimens against *Staphylococcus aureus* determined with a dynamic in vitro model. Antimicrob Agents Chemother 1994;38:2480–2482.
48. JP Flandrois, G Fardel, G Carret. Early stages of in vitro killing curve of LY146032 and vancomycin for *Staphylococcus aureus*. Antimicrob Agents Chemother 1988; 32:454–457.
49. Ackerman, AM Vannier, E Eudy. Analysis of vancomycin time-kill studies with *Staphylococcus* species by using a curve stripping program to describe the relationship between concentration and pharmacodynamic response. Antimicrob Agents Chemother 1992;36:1766–1769.
50. RN Greenberg, CA Benes. Time-kill studies with oxacillin, vancomycin, and teicoplanin versus *Staphylococcus aureus*. J Infect Dis 161:1036–1037, 1990.
51. HH Houlihan, RC Mercier, MJ Rybak. Pharmacodynamics of vancomycin alone

and in combination with gentamicin at various dosing intervals against methicillin-resistant *Staphylococcus aureus*-infected fibrin-platelet clots in an in vitro infection model. Antimicrob Agents Chemother 1997;41:2497–2501.
52. PN Levett. Time-dependent killing of *Clostridium difficile* by metronidazole and vancomycin. J Antimicrob Chemother 1991;27:55–62.
53. I Odenholt-Tornqvist, E Lowdin, O Cars. Postantibiotic sub-MIC effects of vancomycin, roxithromycin, sparfloxacin, and amikacin. Antimicrob Agents Chemother 1992;36:1852–1858.
54. D Greenwood, K Bidgood, M Turner. A comparison of the responses of staphylococci to teicoplanin and vancomycin. J Antmicrob Chemother 1987;20:155–164.
55. JD Knudsen, K Fuursted, F Espersen, N Frimodt-Moller. Activities of vancomycin and teicoplanin against penicillin-resistant pneumococci in vitro and in vivo and correlation to pharmacokinetic parameters in the mouse peritonitis model. Antimicrob Agents Chemother 1997;41:1910–1915.
56. L Cantoni, A Wenger, MP Glauser, J Bille. Comparative efficacy of amoxicillin-clavulanate, cloxacillin, and vancomycin against methicillin-sensitive and methicillin-resistant *Staphylococcus aureus* endocarditis in rats. J Infect Dis 1989;159:989–993.
57. UB Schadd, GH McCracken, JD Nelson. Clinical pharmacology and efficacy of vancomycin in pediatric patients. J Pediatr 1980;96:119–126.
58. DB Louria, T Kaminski, J Buchman. Vancomycin in severe staphylococcal infections. Arch Intern Med 1961;107:225–240.
59. JK James, SM Palmer, DP Levine, MJ Rybak. Comparison of conventional dosing versus continuous-infusion vancomycin therapy for patients with suspected or documented gram-positive infections. Antimicrob Agents Chemother 1996;40:696–700.
60. ME Klepser, SL Kang, BJ McGrath, et al. Influence of vancomycin serum concentration on the outcome of gram-positive infections. Presented at The American College of Clinical Pharmacy Annual Winter Meeting; Feb 6–9; 1994, San Diego.
61. JM Hyatt, PS McKinnon, GS Zimmer, JJ Schentag. The importance of pharmacokinetic/pharmacodynamic surrogate markers to outcome. Clin Pharm Concepts 1995;28:143–160.
62. ME Klepser, KB Patel, DP Nicolau, R Quintiliani, CH Nightingale. Comparison of bactericidal activities of intermittent and continuous infusion dosing of vancomycin against methicillin-resistant *Staphylococcus aureus* and *Enterococcus faecalis*. Pharmacotherapy 1998;18:1069–1074.
63. PM Small, HF Chambers. Vancomycin for *Staphylococcus aureus* endocarditis in intravenous drug users. Antimicrob Agents Chemother 1990;34:1227–1231.
64. HF Chambers, RT Miller, MD Newman. Right sided *Staphylococcus aureus* endocarditis in intravenous drug abusers: Two-week combination therapy. Ann Intern Med 1998;109:619–624.
65. DP Levine, BS Fromm, BR Reddy. Slow response to vancomycin or vancomycin plus rifampin in methicillin-resistant *Staphylococcus aureus* endocarditis. Ann Intern Med 1991;115:674–680.
66. AW Karchmer. *Staphylococcus aureus* and vancomycin: The sequel. Ann Intern Med 1991;115:739–741.

67. O Korzeniowski, MA Sande, National Collaborative Endocarditis Study Group. Combination antimicrobial therapy for *Staphylococcus aureus* endocarditis in patients addicted to parenteral drugs and in nonaddicts. Ann Intern Med 1982;97: 496–503.
68. Anonymous. The choice of antibacterial drugs. Med Lett Drugs Ther 1998;40:33–42.
69. RH Glew, MA Keroack. Vancomycin and teicoplanin. In: SL Grobach, JG Bartlett, NR Blacklow, eds. Infectious Diseases. WB Saunders, Philadelphia; 1998:260–269.
70. R Fekety. Vancomycin and teicoplanin. In: GL Mandell, JE Bennett, R Dolin. Principles and Practice of Infectious Diseases. 4th ed. Churchill Livingstone, New York; 1995:346–353.
71. CW Norden, K Niederreiter, EM Shinners. Treatment of experimental chronic osteomyelitis due to *staphylococcus aureus* with vancomycin and rifampin. J Infect Dis 1983;147:352–357.
72. C Martin, M Alaya, MN Mallet, X Viviand, K Ennabli, R Said, PD Micco. Penetration of vancomycin into mediastinal and cardiac tissues in humans. Antimicrob Agents Chemother 1994;38:396–399.
73. L Massias, C Dubois, P de Lentdecker, O Brodaty, M Fischler, R Farinotti. Penetration of vancomycin in uninfected sternal bone. Antimicrob Agents Chemother 1993;36:2539–2541.
74. AL Graziani, LA Lawson, GA Gibson, MA Steinberg, RR MacGregor. Vancomycin concentrations in infected and noninfected human bone. Antimicrob Agents Chemother 1998;32:1320–1322.
75. JR Torres, CV Sanders, AC Lewis. Vancomycin concentrations in human tissue: Preliminary report. J Antimicrob Chemother 1979;5:475.
76. V Gopal, AL Bisno, FJ Silverblatt. Failure of vancomycin treatment in *Staphylococcus aureus* endocarditis; In vivo and in vitro observations. J Am Med Assoc 1976; 236:1604–1606.
77. AS Bayer, K Lam. Efficacy of vancomycin plus rifampin in experimental aortic-valve endocarditis due to methicillin-resistant *Staphylococcus aureus*: In vitro-in vivo correlations. J Infect Dis 1985;151:157–165.
78. RM Massanari, ST Donta. The efficacy of rifampin as adjunctive therapy in selected cases of staphylococcal endocarditis. Chest 1978;73:371–375.
79. RJ Faville, DE Zaske, EL Kaplan, K Crossley, LD Sabath, PG Quie. *Staphylococcus aureus* endocarditis. Combined therapy with vancomycin and rifampin. J Am Med Assoc 1978;240:1963–1965.
80. DP Levine, RD Cushing, J Ji, WJ Brown. Community-acquired methicillin-resistant *Staphylococcus aureus* endocarditis in the Detroit Medical Center. Ann Intern Med 1982;97:330.
81. PF Viladrich, F Gudiol, J Linares, R Pallares, I Sabate, G Rufi, J Ariza. Evaluation of vancomycin for therapy of adult pneumoccocal meningitis. Antimicrob Agents Chemother 1991;35:2467–2472.
82. JS Bradley, WM Scheld. The challenge of penicillin-resistant *Streptococcus pneumoniae* meningitis: current antibiotic therapy in the 1990s. Clin Infect Dis 1997; 24(suppl 2):S213–S221.

83. WT Hughes, D Armstrong, GP Bodey, AE Brown, JE Edwards, R Feld, P Pizzo, KVI Rolston, JL Shenep, LS Young. 1997 guidelines for the use of antimicrobial agents in neutropenic patients with unexplained fever. Clin Infect Dis 1997;25: 551–573.
84. ST Donta, GM Lamps, RW Summers, TD Wilkins. Cephalosporin-associated colitis and *Clostridium difficile*. Arch Intern Med 1980;140:574–576.
85. JG Bartlett. Antibiotic-associated colitis. Disease-A-Month 1984;30:1–54.
86. SD Miller, HJ Koornhof. *Clostridium difficile* colitis associated with the use of antineoplastic agents. Eur J Clin Microbiol 1984;3:10–13.
87. MA Cudamore, J Silva, R Fekety, MK Liepman, KH Kim. *Clostridium difficile* colitis associated with cancer chemotherapy. Arch Intern Med 1982;142:333–335.
88. SV Johnson, LL Hoey, K Vance-Bryan. Inappropriate vancomycin prescribing based on criteria from the Centers for Disease Control and Prevention. Pharmacotherapy 1995;15:579–585.
89. C Gentry. Wide overuse of antibiotic cited in study. Wall St J 1997;4:B-1.
90. BF Farber, RC Moellering. Retrospective study of the toxicity of preparations of vancomycin from 1974 to 1981. Antimicrob Agents Chemother 1983;23:138.
91. K Vance-Bryan, JC Rotschafer, SS Gilliland, KA Rodvold, CM Fitzgerald, DR Guay. A comparative assessment of vancomycin-associated nephrotoxicity in the young versus the elderly hospitalized patient. J Antimicrob Chemother 1994;33: 811–821.
92. JE Geraci. Vancomycin. Mayo Clin Proc 1977;52:631.
93. TG Cantu, NA Yamanaka-Yuen, PS Lietman. Serum vancomycin concentrations: Reappraisal of their clinical value. Clin Infect Dis 1994;18:533–543.
94. RC Moellering, DJ Krogstad, DJ Greenblatt. Vancomycin therapy in patients with impaired renal function: A nomogram for dosage. Ann Intern Med 1981;94:343–346.
95. GR Matzke, JM Kovarik, MJ Rybak, SC Boike. Evaluation of the vancomycin-clearance: Creatinine-clearance relationship for predicting vancomycin dosage. Clin Pharm 1985;4:311–315.
96. KD Lake, CD Peterson. A simplified dosing method for initiating vancomycin therapy. Pharmacotherapy 1985;5:340–344.
97. HE Nielsen, HE Hansen, B Korsager, PE Skov. Renal excretion of vancomycin in kidney disease. Acta Med Scand 1975;197:261–264.
98. HZ Zokufa, HA Rodvold, RA Blum, LJ Riff, JH Fischer, KB Crossley, JC Rotschafer. Simulation of vancomycin peak and trough concentrations using five dosing methods in 37 patients. Pharmacotherapy 1989;9:10–16.
99. NJ Saunders, SV Want, DJ Adams. Vancomycin monitoring in renal failure: Variation between assays. In: Program and Abstracts of the 34th Interscience Conference of Antimicrobial Agents and Chemotherapy, 1994. Orlando, FL. Am Soc Microbiology, Washington, DC, A-31.
100. AL Somerville, DH Wright, JC Rotschafer. Implications of vancomycin degradation products on therapeutic drug monitoring in patients with end-stage renal disease. Pharmacotherapy 1999;19:702–707.
101. KW Shea, BA Cunha. Teicoplanin. Med Clin N Am 1995;79:833– 844.
102. H Lagast, P Dodion, J Klastersky. Comparison of pharmacokinetics and bacteri-

cidal activity of teicoplanin and vancomycin. J Antimicrob Chemother 1986;18: 513–520.

103. AP MacGowan. Pharmacodynamics, pharmacokinetics, and therapeutic drug monitoring of glycopeptides. Therap Drug Monit 1998;20:473–477.
104. NE Allen, DL LeTourneau, JN Hobbs. Molecular interactions of a semisynthetic glycopeptide antibiotic with D-alanyl-D-alanine and D-alanyl-D-lactate residues. Antimicrob Agents Chemother 1997;41:66–71.
105. TI Nicas, JE Flokowitsch, DA Preston, DL Mullen, J Grissom-Arnold, NJ Snyder et al. Semisynthetic glycopeptides active against vancomycin-resistant enterococci: Activity against staphylococci and streptococci in vitro and in vivo. In Abstracts of the 35th Interscience Conference on Antimicrobial Agents and Chemotherapy. 1995:F-248.
106. M Robbins, D Felmingham. Cidal activity of LY 333328, a new glycopeptide, against Enterococcus spp. In: Program and Abstracts of the 20th International Conference of Chemotherapy, Syndey, Australia. 1997:4292.
107. J Chien, S Allerheiligen, D Phillips, B Cerimele, HR Thomasson. Safety and pharmacokinetics of single intravenous doses of LY333328 diphosphate (glycopeptide) in healthy men. In: Programs and Abstracts of the 38th Interscience Conference on Antimicrobial Agents and Chemotherapy, San Diego, CA, 1999:A-55.

9

Macrolide, Azalide, and Ketolide Pharmacodynamics

Charles H. Nightingale
Hartford Hospital, Hartford, Connecticut

Holly M. Mattoes
DesignWrite Incorporated, Princeton, New Jersey

1 INTRODUCTION

The macrolides and azalides have activity against gram-positive bacteria and are relatively weakly active against many gram-negative bacteria. These agents also penetrate well into mammalian tissue and achieve high concentrations in mammalian cells and are therefore very useful in the treatment of infections caused by intracellular pathogens. Their spectrum of activity makes them a good choice for the treatment of community acquired respiratory tract infections, because the organisms associated with such diseases usually involve *Streptococcus pneumoniae, Haemophilus influenzae,* and *Moraxella cattarhalis* and frequently involve intracellular organisms (Table 1) [1–3]. The macrolides and azalides (either as the parent compound or in combination with a microbiologically active metabolite) have adequate activity against these pathogens and have emerged as useful and popular agents for the treatment of milder forms of these diseases.

TABLE 1 MIC_{90} Values of Organisms Commonly Associated with Community Acquired Respiratory Tract Infections

Organism	Erythromycin	Clarithromycin	Azithromycin
S. pneumoniae	0.03	0.015	0.12
S. pyogenes	0.03	0.015	0.12
H. influenzae	4	1(w/14-OH)	0.5
M. catarrhalis	0.25	0.25	0.06
M. pneumoniae	0.01	0.03	0.001
C. pneumoniae	0.06	0.015	0.5
Legionella sp.	1	≤0.125	≤0.125

The macrolides and azalides bind to the 50S ribosome in the bacterial cell and therefore interfere with the production of bacterial protein [4,5]. The protein is essential for the bacterial life cycle, and because of the presence of the antibiotic the bacteria cannot make the needed protein and eventually die or stop reproducing. Although it is essential for bacterial life, apparently existing stores of the protein must be depleted before effects of the antibiotic are noticeable. As a result, many studies that use concentrations in the therapeutic range classify these compounds as bacteriostatic, and pharmacodynamic studies have shown them to be concentration independent (time-dependent) bacterial killers [6].

The first commercially available antibacterial agent in popular worldwide use was erythromycin. It is used as a single agent for the treatment of a variety of community associated respiratory tract infections and as a second agent (due to its effectiveness against intracellular pathogens) as part of a combination regimen for hospitalized patients. Although still popular as a less costly macrolide option, it does cause gastrointestinal side effects that many patients cannot tolerate for a complete course of therapy. This has implications for the selection of macrolide resistant organisms, which is the topic of another chapter in this book. Additionally its half-life is shorter than those of the newer agents, requiring daily frequent multi-dosing. The drug is also, owing to its metabolic pathway of elimination, involved in a number of drug interactions [7,8]. The popularity of erythromycin is decreasing, and it is being replaced in clinical use with the newer macrolide and azalide drugs (clarithromycin, roxithromycin, and azithromycin). As a result less attention will be devoted to erythromycin in this chapter and the pharmacodynamics of the macrolides/azalides will be discussed with a focus on the newer drugs.

Information on the new ketolide class of antibiotics, semisynthetic macrolide characterized by the replacement of the clandinose moiety with a ketone group, will also be discussed [9]. The ketolides are effective in treating gram positive pathogens, especially those exhibiting resistance to macrolides, by utilizing the same mechanism of action as the macrolide and azalide compounds [10]. Due to the high achievable drug concentrations in white blood cells and bronchopulmonary tissues, the ketolides are especially effective against common respiratory pathogens and intracellular organisms [11].

Because the purpose of this chapter is to discuss the pharmacodynamics of these agents, issues such as utility in clinical use, side effect profiles, and drug interactions will not be discussed. The reader is referred to standard textbooks and primary literature references on these topics. Additionally, no attempt will be made to provide every detail on pharmacodynamic properties of each drug. Rather there are certain principles that are important for this class of agents from a pharmacodynamic perspective, and these principles will be discussed and illustrated using some (but not all) of the newer agents.

2 OVERVIEW OF MACROLIDE AND AZALIDE PHARMACODYNAMICS

As discussed in an earlier chapter, antibiotics can be classified as either bacteriostatic or bactericidal drugs and further subcategorized as concentration dependent or time dependent bacterial killers. In reality, every antibiotic has all of these properties; however, the property that emerges, and upon which the classification is dependent, is a function of the concentrations achieved after clinical dosing relative to its activity against the pathogen. For the macrolides, the currently available data indicate that when the serum plasma concentrations are high enough the pharmacodynamic parameter that correlates best with bacterial eradication is the time for which the organism is exposed to adequate concentrations of these agents (clarithromycin, roxithromycin) [12]. Obviously, if the concentration of the drug is not high enough, one cannot make the simplifying assumption that the concentration part of the AUC ($C_p \times$ time) contributes little to the bacterial eradication process and can be ignored. In such a case bacterial eradication is related not just to the time of exposure of the bacteria to the drug ($T >$ MIC) but also to the concentration of drug to which the bacteria are exposed (AUC). Bacteria that have relatively high MICs may correlate clinical cure rates better to the pharmacodynamic parameter AUC/MIC. This may become an issue as the MICs of pathogens increase owing to the emergence of resistant strains. At the present time, however, most bacteria worldwide for which the macrolides have been useful agents still have MICs low enough such that the pharmacodynamic parameter of $T >$ MIC is appropriate. This will probably change as resistance increases and may already have changed in some countries. Although the exact duration of exposure that is adequate to cure or manage an infection in the clinical setting is not known, animal experiments and in vitro data [12] suggest that a good working number is a time above the MIC of approximately 50% of the dosing interval for patients with a functioning host defense system [12–15]. Animal studies in which neutropenia was induced indicate that superior animal survival was associated with drug concentrations of 4–5 times the MIC [12,13]. This suggests that more appropriate pharmacodynamic criteria for neutropenic patients might be a $T >$ MIC of 100% of the dosing interval.

It has been reported that azithromycin has a prolonged post antibiotic effect (PAE) [12,13]. It is controversial whether this PAE is sufficiently long to significantly affect clinical outcome. The usual regulatory agency approved doses of drugs are based on clinical studies that are derived after treatment with a particular dose and dosing regimen. This incorporates the total properties of the drugs and is then correlated to clinical outcome. To state this in another way, good clinical outcomes are due to the dose and dosing regimen of the drug used. This takes into account concentration issues and drug exposure issues, which include issues of protein binding and PAE. It has been stated, however, that because of the long PAE of azithromycin, the proper pharmacodynamic parameter would not be the $T >$ MIC but rather the AUC/MIC ratio. Unfortunately, there are insufficient data to substantiate this assumption in humans. Another assumption, also unsubstantiated, is that azithromycin, like the macrolides, eradicates bacteria by having an adequate exposure time ($T >$ MIC). For the macrolides we suggested a $T >$ MIC of approximately 50% of the dosing interval. Because of the PAE of azithromycin, an appropriate number might be somewhat less than 50%, i.e., 35% or 40%. This hypothesis is also possible; however, further investigation is needed to clarify this issue.

3 TISSUE DISTRIBUTION

The macrolides and azalides share the common property of extensive distribution into mammalian tissues. Other drug classes such as the quinolones also have this property, but not to the extent exhibited by the macrolides and azalides. One consequence of this, as noted above, is that the latter particularly useful in the treatment of infections caused by intracellular pathogens. Another consequence of this property is that it is responsible for the drugs' longer serum half-life compared to erythromycin (Table 2) [16,17]. Examination of Table 2 reveals that all of the newer agents have a longer half-life than erythromycin. The azithromycin half-life is particularly long (actually this is a working half-life, the true half life is even longer than shown in this table) [4,16,18–20]. The reason for the long azithromycin half-life is not the fact that the normal excretory routes of the body have difficulty in eliminating this drug. Rather the body can only eliminate what is available to it. The rate of appearance to excretory organs is a function of its release from tissue storage sites. Kinetically we can calculate only the slowest step in the elimination process, which in the case of azithromycin is release from tissue. The long half-life of azithromycin, therefore, is really an estimate of the half-life of tissue elimination.

TABLE 2 Important Parameters of the Pharmacokinetics of Macrolides

Parameter	Erythromycin (250 mg)	Clarithromycin (500 mg)	Azithromycin (250 mg)	Roxithromycin (150 mg)
Half-life	2–4	3–4	68	8–15
$C_{p_{max}}$/(μg/mL)	0.25–0.5	2	0.24	6.6–7.9
% Absorption	3.5–40%	50–55%	37%	—
AUC (μg/mL)	—	12.14	2.1	72.6–81

Distribution into tissue sites has ramifications related to the clinical use of these agents. This can be illustrated by referring to two studies of a similar nature [12,13]. In these studies human volunteers were dosed to steady state with clarithromycin and azithromycin. Plasma samples were obtained and bronchial lavage was performed, allowing the calculation of epithelial lining fluid (ELF) drug concentrations and determination of alveolar macrophage (AM) concentrations of both drugs. The results of both experiments demonstrate the same relationships between drug concentrations in these sites as they relate to the microbiological activity of target pathogens.

It is interesting to examine three figures that emanate from these studies. Figure 1 shows the plasma concentrations of both agents at steady state, and in

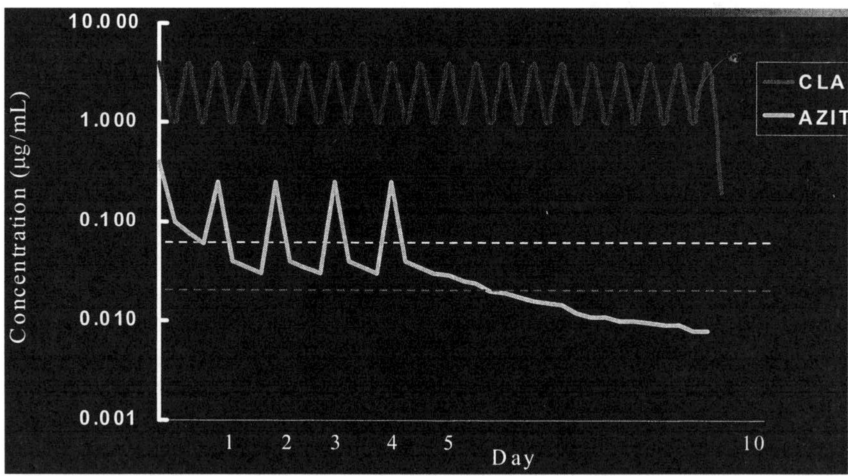

FIGURE 1 Plasma concentrations of clarithromycin and azithromycin with *S. pneumoniae* MIC_{90}.

this figure the typical MIC for *S. pneumoniae* is superimposed upon the kinetic curves. One can see that for clarithromycin, concentrations in plasma at steady state yield a $T >$ MIC of 100% of the dosing interval. The azithromycin curve indicates that this drug stays above the MIC of this pathogen (when a 250 mg once per day dose is used) for somewhat less than 50% of its dosing interval. Of course, if all the pathogens are eradicated or if the remaining pathogens can be eliminated by the patient's host defense mechanisms, then this drug would be expected to be clinically useful against this organism. However, if any bacteria survive such a dose and dosing regimen, they are exposed to subtherapeutic concentrations of active azithromycin for long periods of time. Theoretically this is a condition that can select for resistant organisms and exists because of the extensive tissue distribution properties of azithromycin [12]. Resistance issues are discussed more completely in another chapter of this book.

As described in an earlier chapter, the drug and bacteria need to be in the same place at the same time in order for the antibiotic to function by interfering with the bacterial life cycle. The question of where the bacteria reside in relationship to the drug is an important and yet unresolved issue. This affects the application of pharmacodynamics to any agent that has extensive tissue distribution and is a topic of discussion in the next section. Assuming, however, that in a lung infection the extracellular bacteria reside in some interstitial fluid such as the ELF, it is the concentration in the ELF that might be of clinical importance. Figure 2 shows the calculated ELF concentrations for each agent, and again the MIC for *S. pneumoniae* is superimposed on the kinetic curves. In this case both drugs clearly show that the $T >$ MIC is 100% of the dosing interval. This analysis

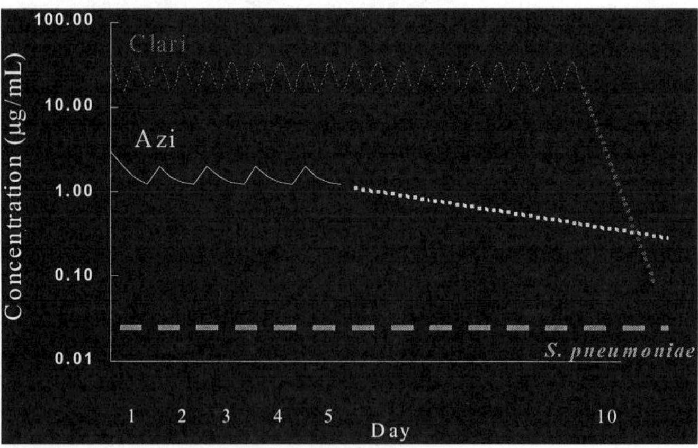

FIGURE 2 Epithelial lining fluid concentrations of clarithromycin and azithromycin with *S. pneumoniae* MIC_{90}.

needs to be determined with each target pathogen to predict clinical differences in the treatment of respiratory infections between these drugs.

Finally, as mentioned previously, the macrolides and azalides have utility in the treatment of respiratory tract infections caused by intercellular organisms. Examination of Fig. 3 allows one to understand the relationship between penetration into mammalian tissue and the MIC of these target organisms. Figure 3 shows the penetration of these drugs into the alveolar macrophage, which is used as a marker for mammalian tissue uptake. It can be seen that the AM concentrations for both drugs are well above the MIC for some typical intracellular pathogens ($T >$ MIC for 100% of the dosing interval). One would predict that the two agents would be equally effective in eradicating intracellular bacteria in a clinical setting.

Pharmacodynamically, the ketolide telithromycin demonstrates a concentration dependent kill, rather than a time dependent kill. *In vitro* studies also have supported the theory that telithromycin exhibits primarily concentration dependent and inoculum dependent bacteriostatic activity [21]. Additionally, animal studies have determined the AUC/MIC ratio to be the best predictor of *in vivo* efficacy for telithromycin and, therefore, once daily dosing is an appropriate dosing regimen for this ketolide [22]. A study evaluating telithromycin's pharmacokinetics after an 800 mg oral dose demonstrated a Cmax of 1.90 mg/l, AUC of 8.96 mg*h/l, and Tmax of 1.0 h [23]. As a result of this favorable kinetic profile, effective AUC/MIC ratios are observed for respiratory pathogens. A summary of MICs of telithromycin for these organisms is listed in Table 3. *H. influenzae*

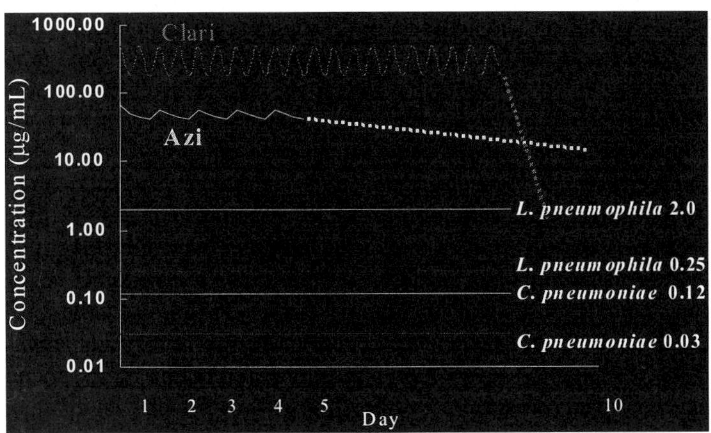

FIGURE 3 Alveolar macrophage concentrations of clarithromycin and azithromycin with *S. pneumoniae* MIC_{90}.

TABLE 3 Ketolide Pharmaacodynamics

	Telithromycin	ABT773
	MIC_{90}	MIC_{90}
Streptococcus pneumoniae	0.06 mg/L	0.03mg/L
Haemophilus influenzae	2 mg/L	4 mg/L
Moraxella cattarhalis	0.06 mg/L	0.12 mg/L
Mycoplasma pneumoniae	0.004 mg/L	NR
Chlamydia pneumoniae	0.25 mg/L	NR
Legionella spp.	0.03 mg/L	1 mg/L

NR = Not reported at this time.

has an increased MIC for telithromycin but still demonstrates similar *in vitro* activity to azithromycin and clarithromycin against this organism. Treatment success relies heavily on factors other than the interaction of the antibiotic with the bacteria. These were previously described and include the patient's immunocompetency. ABT 773 demonstrates time dependent kill, but unfortunately there are few pharmacokinetic data published and, therefore, the T>MIC cannot be accurately determined at the present time. However, it is expected to demonstrate an adequate pharmacodynamic profile against its target organisms, i.e., those causing community-acquired respiratory infections.

For good clinical cure of respiratory intracellular organisms, the alveolar macrophage drug concentration is an important consideration, because this is where the organism is believed to reside. A study evaluating steady state pharmacodynamics of the ketolide telithromycin in healthy volunteers demonstrated good penetration into the bronchopulmonary tissues, surpassing the plasma concentration in these individuals. The mean concentrations of this ketolide in the alveolar macrophages, epithelial lining fluid and bronchial mucosa exceeds the MIC for most common respiratory pathogens [24]. High intracellular concentrations of this drug were also observed in the white blood cells of healthy volunteers, again exceeding the MIC for the typical intracellular organisms for 100% of the dosing interval [25].

It is unfortunate that one is exposed to the pseudo pharmacodynamic term *penetration ratio.* We call the term pseudo pharmacodynamic because the way it is used implies that it has pharmacodynamic meaning, but usually insufficient information is given to understand its meaning. To illustrate this point we refer you to Table 4, which came from the same datasets. Examination of this table reveals that the clarithromycin AM/plasma ratio goes from approximately 340 to 1300, whereas that of azithromycin goes from approximately 1300 to 15,000. Also note that these data were obtained after the last dose of the drug was given. Generally the ratio increases as a function of time after the last dose. This is

TABLE 4 Clarithromycin/Azithromycin Alveolar Macrophage/Plasma Ratio

Time after dosing (h)	AM cell ratio	
	Clarithromycin	Azithromycin
4	543	1,292
8	465	15,237
12	1041	12,807
24	1265	14,386

intuitively problematic, because one expects to see concentrations decrease after dosing. Upon reflection one must realize that the ratio has a numerator and denominator. To make the ratio larger, one can increase the numerator or decrease the denominator or both. Usually insufficient data are presented to determine which is occurring, and the meaning of the ratio is therefore unknown. It is indeed unfortunate that when one sees a high ratio, one assumes that the numerator is large. Examination of this table and the plasma and AM concentration data (Figs. 1 and 3) reveals that the ratio is increasing because the denominator (plasma concentrations) is decreasing much faster than the numerator (AM concentrations) after dosing is stopped. The high ratios, in this case, are not a function of superior tissue concentration (Fig. 3) but of differences between the drugs' AM and plasma concentrations (Fig. 3), i.e., the lower the plasma concentration, the higher the ratio. As a result one must evaluate "penetration" data carefully to fully understand that importance of delivering drug to the body site where the bacteria may reside.

4 APPROPRIATE PHARMACODYNAMIC MODEL

To understand the practical applicability of the current pharmacodynamic model to drugs such as the macrolides and azalides we must remember two important criteria. First, the pharmacodynamic models index microbiological activity to serum or plasma concentrations. The question is whether this is appropriate for a drug class that has a large degree of tissue distribution. The second factor is where the pathogen reside in the body. Figure 4 helps clarify this latter issue [16,17]. Bacteria that are not in intimate contact with mammalian cells, e.g., in a mucus layer of the respiratory tract, are not pathogens. They may be detected after laboratory tests, but they are colonizers. For bacteria to be pathogens they usually need to attach to a mammalian cell membrane (extracellular organisms) or penetrate into the mammalian cell (intracellular organisms). Let us consider extracellular organisms that act as pathogens and examine the existing pharmacodynamic model to see how it applies to this class of agents.

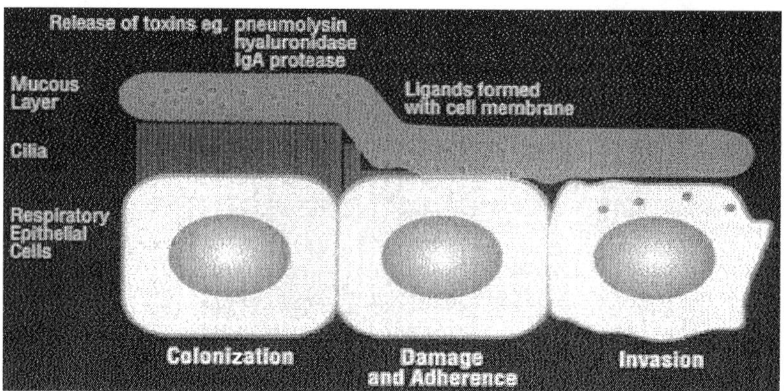

Figure 4 Proposed stages of infection of the bronchial mucosa. IgA, immunoglobulin A.

Figure 5 schematically shows the typical time dependent pharmacodynamic model as it applies to β-lactam antibiotics. These drugs do not penetrate into mammalian cells (the square boxes). The drug concentration, shown by the A's in the schematic, represent the *average* interstitial fluid concentration, which we assume is represented by the *average* serum or plasma concentration (which is what we usually measure). If this average concentration is high enough (2–4

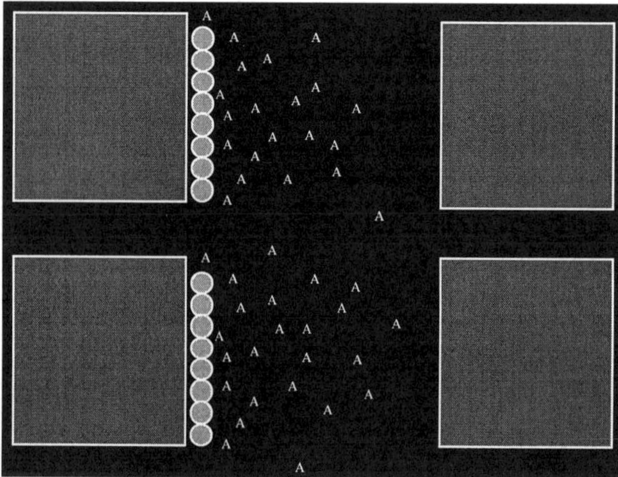

Figure 5 Time-dependent pharmacodynamic model.

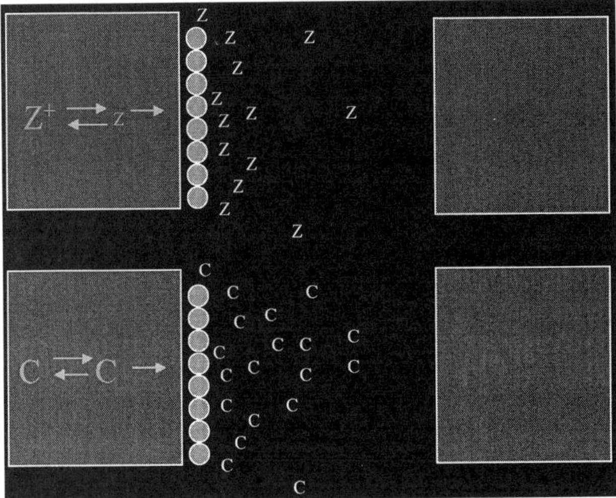

FIGURE 6 Macrolide pharmacodynamic model in mammalian cells.

times the MIC) and remains above the MIC for a long enough period of time ($T > \text{MIC}$ for >50% of the dosing interval), then the drug is expected to be clinically effective in eradicating the pathogens. A similar model is schematically shown in Fig. 6. In this figure the macrolides and azalides penetrate into the mammalian cells. If the *average* drug concentration is high enough (2–4 times the MIC) and is exposed to the bacteria for a long enough period of time ($T > \text{MIC}$ for >50% of the dosing interval), then the bacteria will be exposed to lethal concentrations of drug. This occurs when the MIC of the bacteria is very low, i.e., the bacteria is sensitive to the drug. In essence the model collapses to the β-lactam model. If the MIC of the bacteria were high relative to the *average* serum concentrations, then this model would predict that the bacterial would not be eradicated. This is illustrated in Table 5, which shows the pharmacodynamic prediction when the

TABLE 5 Macrolide Pharmacodynamic Analysis—*H. influenzae*

Macrolide	$T >$ MIC	C_{pk}/MIC	AUC/MIC
Erythromycin, 250 mg	0	0.13	—
Clarithromycin, 500 mg	3	0.25	12
Azithromycin, 250 mg	0	0.48	5

macrolides or azalides are targeted against an organism with a higher MIC such as *H. influenzae*. Whether one prefers the pharmacodynamic parameter of AUC/MIC, $T >$ MIC, or C_p/MIC, the result is the same. The pharmacodynamic parameters are too low to predict clinical success of these drugs against this pathogen. Clinical studies indicate that macrolides/azalides are effective in respiratory tract infections when *H. influenzae* is involved. Obviously there is a mismatch between what nature is telling us and what the existing model is predicting. It is our belief that this model does not fully apply when the pathogen has a relatively high MIC. Simply put, if the model indexes microbiological data to average serum or plasma concentrations and the organism resides elsewhere (attached to the outer membrane of the bacteria), indexing microbiological activity to serum concentration may not be correct if the MIC is high. To explain this further, one must recognize that although these drugs tend to easily move into tissues, they do not remain there forever. They slowly (azithromycin) or not so slowly (clarithromycin) come out of these tissue sites. A concentration gradient probably exists, with the highest concentrations just outside the mammalian cell membrane, the place where pathogens are believed to reside. These pathogens could be exposed to high concentrations of active antibiotic and be killed as a result. This could explain the apparent paradox between clinical results and pharmacodynamic predictions for bacteria with higher MICs. As time goes by and resistance continues to develop, the MICs will continue to increase. At some point the concentrations will be too high to

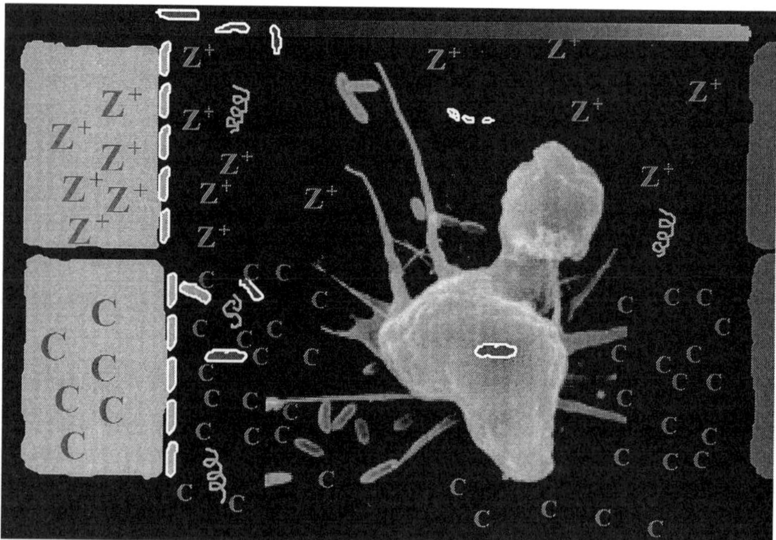

FIGURE 7 Macrolide pharmacodynamic model in the presence of white blood cells.

even evoke this expanded model, and we will clinically observe patient failures upon therapy. Of course, the entire situation is further complicated by the host's immune system (Fig. 7). White blood cells are attracted to the site of infection because the bacteria secrete chemotactic factors. They are also capable of engulfing bacteria and killing them, and it is believed that they actually bring active drug to the "battlefield." None of this has been adequately studied and represents hypothesis to some extent. It is necessary, however, to evoke an explanation like the one presented above to explain the discrepancy between the existing pharmacodynamic models and human clinical empirical data. The point is that the macrolide and azalide pharmacodynamic situation is rather complex and a simple pharmacodynamic model that indexes microbiological activity to serum concentrations cannot fully explain such a complex situation.

5 FUTURE CONSIDERATIONS

The macrolides, azalides, and ketolides are a useful class of drugs for the treatment of respiratory tract infections. For these agents, however, owing to their ability to easily penetrate into mammalian tissue, serum concentrations appear to be predictive of clinical outcome for only very sensitive organisms. For organisms with higher MICs the drug concentrations at the site in the body where the bacteria reside may be of more clinical relevance; however, these data are difficult or even impossible to obtain in humans. It is indeed unfortunate that the reporting of resistant organisms is not strongly base on the pharmacodynamic characteristics of these drugs. They are determined by the setting of so-called breakpoints, which are an interpretation of mostly in vitro and some clinical and pharmacodynamic data. These breakpoints can be somewhat arbitrarily set in spite of the good intentions and hard work of the officials setting them. It is possible, as in the case of macrolides, to report many isolates as resistant, but the reporting system does not provide any information about the magnitude of the resistance. Ketolides, which in a sense are macrolides with activity against macrolide resistant agents, are an exception to this phenomenon at the present time. Whether the drug (macrolide or azalide) can eradicate the organism depends on the serum and tissue concentrations achieved in relationship to the MIC. If drug concentrations are high enough for a long enough time after the usual clinical doses, then the organism will be adversely affected (die) regardless of whether one classifies it as resistant or sensitive. Clarithromycin has been developed in an extended release form in an attempt to increase drug concentrations over a longer period of time. These tablets are taken once daily and have a steady state AUC equivalent to conventional immediate release clarithromycin, which is taken twice daily [26].

Unfortunately the reporting of in vitro resistance data has a strong impact on the drug selection process, because for the most part macrolide and azalide therapy is empirical. This issue is not easy to address, because the existing pharmacodynamic data use serum or plasma as their index to microbiological efficacy, which may not be appropriate for the macrolides when they are targeted against organisms with higher MICs that reside in bodily fluids whose drug concentration profiles are not the same as that of serum. As time passes and more organisms become resistant and therefore have higher MICs, this situation will become more confused, and one can predict that the macrolide class of antibiotics will probably be replaced by the ''respiratory'' quinolones for the empirical therapy of respiratory tract infections. This may be an unfortunate occurrence that may relegate the macrolides to the role of adjunctive agent in the treatment or prophylaxis of infections believed to be caused by intracellular pathogens. This would be unfortunate if it is based upon erroneous resistance data and as a result deprives patients of an acceptable and somewhat unique (due to its high tissue penetration and immunological properties) class of agents.

REFERENCES

1. LA Mandell. Community-acquired pneumonia: Etiology, epidemiology, and treatment. Chest 1995;108(2):35S–41S.
2. D Lieberman, F Schlaeffer, I Boldur, D Lieberman, S Horowitz, MG Friedman, M Leiononen, O Horovitz , E Manor, A Porath. Multiple pathogens in adult patients admitted with community-acquired pneumonia: A one year prospective study of 346 consecutive patients. Thorax 1996;51:179–184.
3. HA Cassiere, MS Niederman. Community-acquired pneumonia. Disease of the Month 1998(Nov);622–675.
4. SC Piscitelli, LH Danziger, KA Roldvold. Clarithromycin and azithromycin: New macrolide antibiotics. Clin Pharm 1992;11:137–152.
5. MS Whitman, AR Tunket. Azithromycin and clarithromycin: overview and compariosn with erythromycin. Infection Control Hosp Epidemiol 1992;13:357–368.
6. A Bauernfeind, R Jungwirth, E Eberlein. Comparative pharmacodynamics of clarithromycin and azithromycin against respiratory pathogens. Infection 1995;23(5): 316–321.
7. TM Ludden. Pharmacokinetic interactions of the macrolide antibiotics. Clin Pharmacokinet 1985;10:63–79.
8. P Periti, T Mazzei, E Mini, A Novelli. Pharmacokinetic drug interactions of macrolides. Clin Pharmacokinet 1992;23:106–131.
9. C Agouridas, A Bonnefoy, JF Chanton. In vitro antibacterial activity of HMR 3647, a novel ketolide highly active against respiratory pathogens [abstract F-112]. In: Program and Abstracts of the 37th Interscience Conference on Antimicrobial Agents and Chemotherapy (Toronto, Ontario). Washington, DC: Am Soc Microbiol, 1997.
10. C Marie-Bigdot, D Decre, C Muller, E Salgado, E Bergogne-Berezin. In vitro activity of a novel ketolide antimicrobial agent HMR 3647 compared to erythromycin, roxithromycin, azithromycin and clarithromycin [abstract F-117]. In: Program and Abstracts of the 37th Interscience Conference on Antimicrobial Agents and Chemotherapy (Toronto, Ontario). Washington, DC: Am Soc Microbiol, 1997.

11. RP Smith, AL Baltch, W Ritz, M. Franke, P. Michelson. Antibacterial effect of ketolides HMR 3004 and HMR 3647 against intracellular Legionella pneumophilia [abstract F-249]. In: Program and Abstracts of the 37th Interscience Conference on Antimicrobial Agents and Chemotherapy (Toronto, Ontario). Washington, DC: Am Soc Microbiol, 1997.
12. RC Owens, DP Nicolau, R Quintiliani, CH Nightingale, Bactericidal activity of clarithromycin, azithromycin,and cefuroxime against penicillin-susceptible, -intermediate, and -resistant pneumococci. 20th Int Congress of Chemotherapy (Sydney, Australia), June 29–July 3, 1997.
13. JG Den Hollander, JD Knudsen, JW Mouton, F Fuursted, N Frimodt-Moller, HA Verbrugh, F Espersen. Comparison of pharmacodynamics of azithromycin and erythromycin in vitro and in vivo. Antimicrob Agents Chemother 1998;42:377–382.
14. WA Craig. Interrelationship between pharmacokinetics and pharmacodynamics in determining dosage regimens for broad-spectrum cephalosporins. Diagn Microb Infect Dis 1995;22:89–96.
15. B Vogelman, S Gudmundson, J Leggett, J Turnidge, S Ebert, WA Craig. Correlation of antimicrobial pharmacokinetic parameters with therapeutic efficacy in animal model. J Infect Dis 1998;158:831–847.
16. F Kees, M Wallenhofer, H Grobecker. Serum and cellular pharmacokinetics of clarithromycin 500mg q.d. and 250mg b.i.d. in volunteers. Infection 1995;23:168–172.
17. G Foulds, RM Shepard, RB Johnson. The pharmacokinetics of azithromycin in human serum and tissues. J Antimicrob Chemother 1990;25(suppl A):73–82.
18. A Wildfeuer, H Laufen, T Zimmermann. Uptake of azithromycin by various cells and its intracellular activity under in vivo conditions. Antimicrob Agents Chemother 1996;40:75–79.
19. GW Amsden, AN Nafziger, G Foulds. Pharmacokinetics in serum and leukocyte exposure of oral azithromycin, 1,500 milligrams, given over a 3- or 5-day period in healthy subjects. Antimicrob Agents Chemother 1999;43:163–165.
20. G Panteix, B Guillaumond, R Harf, A Desbos, V Sapin, M Leclercq, M Perrin-Fayolle. In-vitro concentration of azithromycin in human phagocytic cells. J Antimicrob Chemother 1993;31(suppl E):1–4.
21. FJ Boswell, JM Andrews, R Wise. Pharmacodynamic properties of HMR 3647, a novel ketolide demonstrated by studies of time-kill kinetics and post antibiotic effect [abstract F-254]. In: Program and Abstracts of the 37th Interscience Conference on Antimicrobial Agents and Chemotherapy (Toronto, Ontario). Washington, DC: Am Soc Microbiol, 1997.
22. O Vesga, C Bonnat, WA Craig. In vivo pharmacodynamic activity of HMR 3647, a new ketolide [abstract F-255]. In: Program and Abstracts of the 37th Interscience Conference on Antimicrobial Agents and Chemotherapy (Toronto, Ontario). Washington, DC: Am Soc Microbiol, 1997.
23. F Namour, DH Wessels, MH Pascual, D Reynolds, E Sultan. Dose proportionality of the pharmacokinetics of HMR 3647, a new ketolide antimicrobial, in healthy adult males [abstract 79]. In: Program and Abstracts of the 37th Annual Meeting of the Infectious Diseases Society of America (Philadelphia, PA). Alexandria, VA: Infect Dis Soc America, 1999.

24. CM Serieys, C Cantalloube, P Soler, HP Gia, F Brunner. HMR 3647 achieves high and sustained concentrations in broncho-pulmonary tissues [abstract P78]. In: Abstracts of the 21st International Congress of Chemotherapy (Birmingham, UK). Oxford, UK: Br Soc Antimicrob Chemother, 1999.
25. HP Gia, V Roeder, F Namour, E Sultan, B Lenfant. HMR 3647 achieves high and sustained concentrations in white blood cells in man [abstract P79]. In: Abstracts of the 21st International Congress of Chemotherapy (Birmingham, UK). Oxford, UK: Br Soc Antimicrob Chemother, 1999.
26. LE Gustavson, GX Cao, SJ Semla, RN Palmer. Pharmacokinetics of a new extended-release clarithromycin tablet at doses of 500 and 1000 mg daily [abstract A-1191]. In: Program and Abstracts of the 39th Interscience Conference on Antimicrobial Agents and Chemotherapy (San Francisco, CA). Washington, DC: Am Soc Microbiol, 1999.

10

Metronidazole, Clindamycin, and Streptogramin Pharmacodynamics

Kenneth Lamp
Bristol-Myers Squibb
Plainsboro, New Jersey

Melinda K. Lacy
University of Kansas Medical Center
Kansas City, Kansas

Collin Freeman
Bayer Corporation, West Haven, Connecticut

1 METRONIDAZOLE

Metronidazole (Flagyl) is a nitroimidazole antibiotic that has been available for use in clinical practice for over 25 years. Its original indication was for treatment of infections caused by *Trichomonas vaginalis*, but over the years it has been discovered to be useful in treating a variety of infections caused by various organisms. Although the nitroimidazole class of antibiotics includes tinidazole, secnidazole, and ornidazole, the wealth of information about the pharmacokinetics and pharmacodynamics of these agents comes from published data about metronidazole. However, even with the vast amount of information about metronidazole, there is very little information regarding its pharmacodynamic properties compared to other antimicrobial agents such as the β-lactams, aminoglycosides, and fluoroquinolones. The only distinguishing features of tinidazole, ornidazole, or secnidazole are prolonged $T_{1/2}$ values compared to metronidazole.

1.1 Chemistry and Mechanism of Action

Metronidazole is a nitroimidazole (chemical name 1-[β-hydroxyethyl]-2-methyl-5-nitromidazole) that belongs to the same chemical class as tinidazole and ornidazole (structure shown in Fig. 1). The compound was discovered in the late 1950s when researchers at Rhône–Poulenc Research Laboratories in France were trying to create a synthetic product from a *Streptomyces* spp.–derived compound called azomycin that would have appreciable activity against *Trichomonas vaginalis* [1].

From the research of different investigators, metronidazole's mechanism of action is believed to involve four phases: (1) entry into the bacterium cell, (2) reduction of the nitro group, cytotoxic effect of the reduced product, and (4) liberation of end products that are inactive [2]. It is the redox intermediate intracellular metabolites that are believed to be the key components of microorganism killing for metronidazole. The intracellular targets for these intermediates could be organisms' RNA, DNA, or cellular proteins.

1.2 Antimicrobial Activity

Following their work in 1959, Cosar and Julou and other researchers over the next several years found a variety of potential human uses for metronidazole that went beyond treatment for *T. vaginalis* infection. The following is a summary of metronidazole's antimicrobial activity.

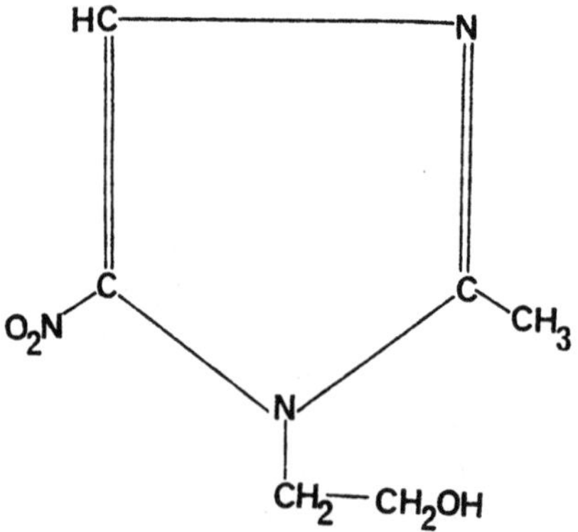

FIGURE 1 Metronidazole molecule.

1.2.1 Protozoa

In addition to *T. vaginalis*, metronidazole has exhibited activity against other protozoan organisms, including *Giardia lamblia* and *Entamoeba histolytica* [3–15].

1.2.2 Bacteria

Gram-Negative Bacteria. Shinn [8] and later Tally et al. [9] discovered the potential of using metronidazole for anaerobic infections. Metronidazole has since been used and studied extensively for treatment of various anaerobic infections [10–12]. Even today metronidazole is considered the gold standard by which other antimicrobials with perceived antianaerobic activity are compared. This is due primarily to metronidazole's rapid killing of *Bacteroides* species and the very low rate of resistance acquired by these bacteria [13–15]. Other *Bacteroides* species and *Fusobacterium* spp. have been reported as being at least as susceptible to metronidazole as *Bacteroides* as well as *Helicobacter* (formerly *Campylobacter*) *pylori*, *Actinobacillus*, and *Prevotella*, although resistance to metronidazole may be common in various regions of the world [9,13,14,16–20]. Minimum bactericidal concentrations (MBCs) of metronidazole when reported in these studies are the same or within one dilution of the reported MICs.

Gram-Positive Bacteria. As for gram-positive anaerobes, the peptostreptococci have usually been reported to exhibit MICs in the range of 0.25–4.0 mg/L [13,21,22].

Susceptibility of *Clostridium perfringens* to metronidazole is also in the MIC range of 1.0–4.0 mg/L, although not all clostridia are so susceptible [13,21,24,21]. Metronidazole is also considered to be one of the few drugs with activity against *Clostridium difficile* [21,25,26].

1.2.3 Other Organisms

Metronidazole has also been reported to have in vitro activity against *Campylobacter fetus*, *Gardnerella vaginalis*, *Leptotrichia buccalis*, and *Treponema pallidum* to varying degrees [27–32].

1.3 Pharmacokinetic and Pharmacodynamic Properties

The following is a brief summary of the many trials that have studied metronidazole's kinetics.

1.3.1 Absorption

The absorption of metronidazole has been studied for oral tablets, vaginal and rectal suppositories, and topical gel.

Oral Absorption. The oral absorption of metronidazole is excellent, with bioavailability often reported as ≥90% [37–39]. The oral C_{max} with a 500 mg dose is approximately 8.0–13.0 mg/L, with a corresponding T_{max} of 0.25–4.0 h [33–36].

Rectal Absorption. Rectal administration of metronidazole 500 mg has produced C_{max} values of approximately 4.0–5.5 mg/L at T_{max}'s of 0.5–1.0 for a retention enema to 4.0–12 h for suppositories [11,33,37,38]. Metronidazole absorption from the rectum has been reported as being approximately 67–82% based upon calculations with equivalent intravenous (IV) doses used as references [38].

Intravaginal Absorption. Intravaginal absorption of metronidazole has varied considerably depending on the vehicle used. The 0.75% metronidazole intravaginal gel at a dose of 5.0 g has produced C_{max} values of 0.2–0.3 mg/L with T_{max} values of 8.3–8.5 h [39]. For vaginal suppositories and inserts, the 500 mg dose C_{max} values have been approximately 1.9 mg/L with corresponding T_{max} values of 7.7–20 h [36,40]. The bioavailability of vaginal suppositories is 25% of an oral 500 mg dose, but the vaginal gel's bioavailability was 56% that of a 500 mg IV dose [36,39].

Topical Absorption. Systemic absorption of 1.0 g of 0.75% metronidazole gel is reportedly quite low. After 1.0 g of the gel was applied to the face of adults with rosacea, the resulting serum concentrations ranged from undetectable to 66 ng/mL in the following 24 h [41,42].

1.3.2 Distribution

Protein binding of metronidazole is <20% [35,43]. Metronidazole crosses cell membranes well in general and distributes well into a variety of tissues and fluids. The reported volumes of distribution (V_d) in studies for various age groups have ranged from 0.51 to 1.1 L/kg [43,44].

Single-dose studies using metronidazole 500 mg IV or oral doses have determined AUCs to be approximately 100–159 mg/(L · h) [36]. Oral or IV doses of 1.0 g have displayed AUCs of 214–257 mg/(L · h) [33,45]. The penetration of metronidazole into polymorphonuclear leukocytes has been described as equivalent to the concentration found in the extracellular fluid [46].

1.3.3 Metabolism

Metronidazole undergoes hepatic metabolism, forming five metabolites. The two major metabolites are an acid metabolite and a hydroxy metabolite. The acid metabolite's activity is considered to be clinically negligible, having only 5% of the activity of metronidazole [47].

Hydroxymetronidazole. The hydroxy metabolite of metronidazole is the most clinically important, because it also has antimicrobial activity but to a lesser extent than the parent compound. Hydroxymetronidazole has been reported as having 30–65% of the activity of the parent compound with respect to similar isolates [19,24,47].

1.3.4 Excretion

Metronidazole is primarily excreted in the bile as the parent drug and in the urine as its various metabolites. Only about 6–18% of metronidazole is excreted in the urine unchanged [35]. Hydroxymetronidazole is entirely excreted in the urine, being approximately 25% of the original dose [48].

The elimination half-life ($T_{1/2}$) has been reported to range from 6 to 10 h for metronidazole in volunteers and patients with normal hepatic and renal functions [37,44]. The hydroxy metabolite's $T_{1/2}$ reportedly ranges from 8 to 12 h [36]. Patients may have altered clearance values, such as $T_{1/2}$ values that are $\geq$10 h [49]. Metronidazole appears to exhibit dose-dependent clearance in doses ranging from 250 to 2000 mg [44,49].

1.4 Pharmacodynamics

1.4.1 Bactericidal Effect

Metronidazole appears to have an extremely rapid rate of killing against susceptible anaerobes [15,50].

Outcomes associated with the use of metronidazole in mixed aerobic–anaerobic infections, such as intra-abdominal infections, have yielded excellent results in terms of bacterial eradication when an antianaerobic agent such as metronidazole was included as part of the therapeutic regimen [51,52].

1.4.2 Concentration-Dependent Killing

Nix et al. [53] discovered that metronidazole had a concentration-dependent killing effect against *T. vaginalis* under anaerobic conditions at concentrations that ranged from 0.1 to >8.0 mg/L [53]. Time-kill kinetic studies of ciprofloxacin alone (concentration 0.5 mg/L; MIC 0.25 mg/L) compared to a combination of ciprofloxacin with metronidazole (10.0 and 40.0 mg/L) displayed more rapid killing with the combined antibiotics against *C. perfringens*. If this concentration-dependent effect truly exists for metronidazole, it would suggest that the general optimal dosing strategy for metronidazole against organisms like *T. vaginalis* and *B. fragilis* would be to give higher doses less frequently rather then smaller doses more frequently, similar to the use of aminoglycosides and fluoroquinolones against susceptible gram-negative aerobic bacteria.

1.4.3 Postantibiotic Effect

Like aminoglycosides and fluoroquinolones, metronidazole appears to exhibit a postantibiotic effect (PAE) extending over 3 h [54].

1.4.4 Serum Bactericidal Titers

Serum bactericidal titers (SBTs) have been used in studies as an ex vivo method of assessing metronidazole's effect on anaerobes, primarily *B. fragalis*. Rcsults from an SBT study reported a median metronidazole SBT of 1:2 against various *Bacteroides* species at 0.5, 1.0, and 6.0 h after administration of a single dose of metronidazole 500 mg IV [55]. Results with metronidazole against two strains of *B. fragilis* at the 6 h time point were <1:2, but titers related to *Fusobacterium*, *Peptostreptococcus*, and *Eubacterium lentum* were all >1:8 at all time points.

Fluoroquinolones have often been studied for use in combination with metronidazole for antibacterial activity against gram-negative aerobes and anaerobes. Boeckh et al. [56] studied the effect of fluoroquinolones (ofloxacin, ciprofloxacin, enoxacin, fleroxacin) in combination with antianaerobic antibiotics, including metronidazole, via SBTs. SBTs were performed from serum samples obtained at 1, 2, 6, and 8 h, depending upon the antibiotic combination, against various gram-positive and gram-negative aerobic pathogens as well as strains of *B. fragilis* and *B. thetaiotaomicron*. None of the combinations appeared to interfere with the individual antibiotics' antibacterial activities, and mean SBTs for the ciprofloxacin-metronidazole, ofloxacin-metronidazole, enoxacin-metronidazole, and fleroxacin-metronidazole combinations were all in the 1:2–1:4 dilution range for the various strains and species of *Bacteroides*. Similarly, Pefanis et al. [57] established greater effectiveness at eradicating mixed aerobic–anaerobic gram-negative pathogens from experimentally induced abscesses in a rat model based upon reduced CFU counts.

Serum bactericidal titer studies involving the combination of metronidazole 1.0 g with extended spectrum cephalosporins have also yielded results in the 1:4–1:8 range for *B. fragilis* at the end of 12 or 24 h for ceftizoxime or ceftriaxone, respectively [58–60].

1.5 Summary—Metronidazole

Although data are scarce, metronidazole's concentration-dependent bactericidal activity, prolonged $T_{1/2}$, and sustained bactericidal activity in plasma support the clinical evaluation of higher doses and longer dosing intervals. In vitro and ex vivo human studies have corroborated metronidazole's effectiveness as an antiprotozoal and antianaerobic agent.

The rapid concentration-dependent killing of anaerobes by metronidazole; its active metabolite, which helps to extend its effective duration of action; the penetrability of metronidazole into various tissues; the near lack of resistance of anaerobes like *B. fragilis* to metronidazole; and its low cost make metronidazole the preferred agent for antianaerobic therapy in many cases.

The other nitroimidazoles doubtless have identical pharmacodynamic properties, although their respective pharmacokinetics may be somewhat different from those of metronidazole. As newer nitroimidazoles are brought to market and are used with greater frequency, metronidazole's use may continue to gradually decline. However, the value of metronidazole is still readily apparent, and it still has an important role in today's antimicrobial armamentarium.

2 CLINDAMYCIN

Clindamycin (Cleocin, Pharmacia & Upjohn Co.), a lincosamide antibiotic, has been used in clinical practice for over 30 years. Compared to its parent compound lincomycin, clindamycin has improved oral absorption and a wider antibacterial spectrum of activity, making it the most popular agent in this classification of antibiotics. It is commercially available as an intravenous formulation, oral capsules, and suspension as well as in several topical preparations (solution, gel, lotion, individual pledgets, and vaginal cream). Clinically, clindamycin is used in the treatment of gram-positive and anaerobic bacterial infections of the abdomen, bone, lung, skin and soft tissues, and pelvis and is often an alternative agent in those who are allergic to β-lactam antibiotics. Additionally, it is used in the treatment of opportunistic protozoal infections of the lung and central nervous system in patients infected with the human immunodeficiency virus.

Usual oral doses in adults range from 150 to 450 mg every 6 h, whereas parenteral doses are generally 600–900 mg every 8 h [61].

2.1 Chemistry and Mechanism of Action of Clindamycin

Clindamycin (7-chloro-7-deoxylincomycin) is a semisynthetic derivative of lincomycin and is therefore classified as a lincosamide antibiotic. Similar to macrolides, streptogramins, and chloramphenicol, clindamycin exerts its activity against susceptible pathogens by binding to the 50S ribosomal subunit, which inhibits microbial protein synthesis through its effects on peptide chain initiation.

2.2 Antimicrobial Activity

Clindamycin is active against a variety of gram-positive and anaerobic bacterial pathogens [62]. Most streptococci, including *Streptococcus pneumoniae* and *Streptococcus pyogenes*, are susceptible, as are most methicillin-susceptible strains of *Staphylococcus aureus*. However, it is not active against enterococci or aerobic gram-negative organisms. Clindamycin is active against a broad range of anaerobic gram-negative bacilli including *Bacteroides* species, *Fusobacterium* species; anaerobic gram-positive bacilli such as *Propionibacterium*, *Eubacte-*

rium, and *Actinomyces*; and anaerobic gram-positive cocci such as *Peptococcus*, *Peptostreptococcus*, microaerophilic streptococci, and most strains of *Clostridium perfringens*. It is also active against pathogens that cause bacterial vaginosis, which include *Bacteroides*, *Gardnerella vaginalis*, *Mobiluncus*, and *Mycoplasma hominus*.

Additionally, many protozoa, including *Toxoplasma gondii*, *Plasmodium falciparum*, *Babesia*, and *Pneumocystis carinii*, are susceptible to clindamycin [62,63].

Two recent surveillance studies in the United States demonstrated that greater than 95% of all pneumococcal strains were susceptible to clindamycin with reported MIC_{90} values of 0.12 mg/L [64,65]. In one of the studies 76% of 969 *S. aureus* isolates were susceptible, with reported MIC_{50} and MIC_{90} values of 0.25 and >8 mg/L [65]. The susceptibility breakpoint is 0.5 mg/L for *Staphylococcus* spp. and 0.25 mg/L for *Streptococcus* spp. and *S. pneumoniae* [66].

2.3 Pharmacokinetic Properties of Clindamycin

Clindamycin oral preparations are rapidly absorbed, and reported oral bioavailability is around 90%. Other notable pharmacokinetic properties include >90% protein binding, wide distribution in body fluids and tissues except for cerebral spinal fluid, extensive hepatic metabolism to active metabolites, and a half-life of around 2.0–2.4 h [61,62,67–69]. For severe liver dysfunction, clindamycin doses should be reduced.

For 600 mg intravenous doses, peak serum concentrations are around 10.9 g/mL, while trough concentrations are 2.0 and 1.1 mg/L at 6 and 8 h, respectively [61]. Peak concentrations after intramuscular doses of 600 mg are 9.0 mg/L, which is slightly lower than those reported after intravenous dosing. For 900 mg intravenous doses, reported peak and trough concentrations at 8 h are 14.1 and 1.7 mg/mL, respectively [61].

2.4 Pharmacodynamics of Clindamycin

Until recently, little was known about the pharmacodynamic characteristics of clindamycin. Recent studies have demonstrated that clindamycin displays time-dependent pharmacodynamics against *S. pneumoniae*, methicillin-susceptible *S. aureus*, and *B. fragilis* [68,70]. Furthermore, clindamycin has an extended post-antibiotic effect against *Staphylococcus* [54,71].

2.4.1 In Vitro Studies

Two time-kill studies have evaluated clindamycin's activity against *B. fragilis* [71,72]. Clindamycin was shown to display concentration-independent activity in a study conducted by Klepser et al. [70]. In this study clindamycin concentrations were evaluated over a range of 1–64 times the MIC. Five strains of *B.*

fragilis with clindamycin MICs of 0.03–8.0 mg/L were studied. Bactericidal activity (≥3 log decrease in the starting inoculum) was independent of clindamycin concentration for three of the five strains. A bacteristatic effect was noted for the isolate with an MIC of 8.0 mg/L for all tested concentrations. Against another strain with an MIC of 1.0 mg/L, regrowth was observed at the MIC concentration, and bactericidal activity was observed for all other concentrations.

Aldridge and Stratton [72] described concentration-dependent activity for clindamycin, ceftizoxime, and cefotetan against *B. fragilis*. However, these investigators studied only antibiotic concentrations over a range of 0.5–4 times the MIC. In this study metronidazole, chloramphenicol, and cefoxitin were also evaluated, and reported clindamycin MIC values against the study isolates were 0.5 and 1.0 mg/L. As described in the above study, clindamycin clearly displays concentration-independent pharmacodynamic activity at concentrations that exceed 4 times the MIC [70]. Furthermore, several in vitro and in vivo studies demonstrate that cephalosporins have time-dependent, and not concentration-dependent, pharmacodynamics, which differs from the results reported by Aldridge [54].

2.4.2 Serum Inhibitory and Bactericidal Titers

Klepser et al. [68] evaluated the duration of serum bactericidal activity for 300 mg oral and intravenous doses of clindamycin dosed every 8 h and every 12 h against two isolates each of *S. aureus*, *S. pneumoniae*, and *B. fragilis* at steady state in healthy volunteers. Median MICs for the study isolates were 0.125 and 0.25 mg/L for *S. aureus*, 0.125 mg/L for both *S. pneumoniae* isolates, and 0.5 mg/L for the *B. fragilis* isolates. For the every 8 h regimens, measurable activity was observed for 87.5–100% of the dosing interval against all study isolates. For the every 12 h regimen, bactericidal activity was observed for 50–77% of the dosing interval against *S. aureus*, 100% for *S. pneumoniae*, and 80–88% for *B. fragilis*. These investigators concluded that dosing intervals of every 8 or every 12 h for 300 mg oral or intravenous doses of clindamycin provided adequate coverage against *S. aureus*, *S. pneumoniae*, and *B. fragilis*, except that an every 8 h interval may be necessary for treatment of *S. aureus* infections.

Serum inhibitory titers were measured by Flaherty et al. [67] in six volunteers participating in a multiple dose intravenous clindamycin study against a reference strain of *B. fragilis* with an MIC of 0.25–0.5 mg/L. Clindamycin regimens assessed in this study were as follows: 600 mg every 6 h, 900 mg every 8 h, and 1200 mg every 12 h. When considering the doses used in this study it is not surprising that activity was observed throughout the entire dosing interval for all regimens and that reciprocal inhibitory titers at the trough ranged from 5 to 12.

The synergistic effects of clindamycin with fluoroquinolones have also been studied [73,74]. Increased serum bactericidal activity was observed when clindamycin was combined with ciprofloxacin, ofloxacin, and fleroxacin against *S. aureus* and *S. pneumoniae* [73]. This single-dose study evaluated 600 mg intravenous and 300 mg oral doses of clindamycin given in combination with the quinolone test agents against both gram-positive organisms and anaerobes. Enhanced activity was observed when clindamycin (600 mg IV) was given in combination with ciprofloxacin (200 mg IV) and ofloxacin (200 mg IV) for *S. aureus* and *S. pneumoniae*. Against *S. aureus*, reported reciprocal titers at 6 h were 5.4 for ciprofloxacin-clindamycin compared to 2.3 for ciprofloxacin alone. Similarly, ofloxacin-clindamycin reciprocal titers of 4.1 were observed compared to 2 for ofloxacin alone at 6 h. Against *S. pneumoniae* reciprocal titers at 6 h were 2 and 13.6 for ciprofloxacin alone and ciprofloxacin-clindamycin, respectively. For ofloxacin and ofloxacin-clindamycin, reciprocal titers of 2 and 13.5 were noted at 6 h. Less activity was observed when oral clindamycin (300 mg) was given in combination with oral enoxacin (400 mg) and fleroxacin (400 mg) than either quinolone alone at 8 h against *S. aureus*.

The serum bactericidal activity of an oral combination of ciprofloxacin (750 mg every 12 h × 3 doses) and clindamycin (300 mg every 6 h × 5 doses) was studied by Weinstein et al. [74] in healthy elderly volunteers. Unlike the results reported by Boeckh et al. [73], the bactericidal activity of ciprofloxacin against *S. aureus* was antagonized by clindamycin when clindamycin-susceptible strains were tested. However, the reported MBCs for clindamycin against the three test *S. aureus* strains were either 4.0 or 8.0 mg/L. This antagonistic effect was not observed for the combination against *S. pyogenes* and *S. pneumoniae* in this study.

2.4.3 Postantibiotic Effect

Several investigators have studied the postantibiotic effect (PAE) for clindamycin against *S. aureus* [75,76]. Xue et al. [76] reported that the duration of the PAE for clindamycin is dependent on both concentration and duration of exposure to clindamycin, with longer PAEs observed at higher concentrations. In this study, which used 21 clinical osteomyelitis isolates of *S. aureus*, observed PAEs ranged from 0.4 to 3.9 h. Reported PAE values were not influenced by multiple dosing. When considering clinically achievable concentrations and estimated PAE values of 2.4 h, these investigators concluded that oral clindamycin could be administered at 300 mg every 8 h for the treatment of *S. aureus*, whereas recommended intravenous dosing is 300 mg every 6 h.

2.5 Summary—Clindamycin

Similar to that observed for β-lactams, macrolides, vancomycin, and others, only recently have the time-dependent pharmacodynamics of clindamycin been discovered. Studies demonstrating serum bactericidal activity against susceptible bacteria for either the majority or the entire dosing interval has been demonstrated with lower doses than are currently recommended. The application of the pharmacodynamics of clindamycin needs to be more fully evaluated in actual clinical situations.

3 STREPTOGRAMIN

The streptogramin class of antibiotics are new introductions into the United States; however, they have been available in Europe for many years for mild to moderate staphylococcal infections. Recent modifications to the structure allow for formulation of water-soluble forms of the compounds and subsequent use in intravenous solutions [77]. These efforts have led to the combination drug quinupristin-dalfopristin (RP 59500, Synercid) and its evaluation for treatment of severe, antibiotic-resistant infections.

3.1 Chemistry and Mechanism of Action of Streptogramin

Streptomyces pristinaespiralis produces two clinically unrelated antibiotics (streptogramin A and B), which in combination exert their antibacterial action. The streptogramin A antibiotics are polyunsaturated cyclic macrolactones and include pristinamycin IIA, virginiamycin M, and dalfopristin. Streptogramin B antibiotics are cyclic depsipeptides and include pristinamycin IA, quinupristin, and virginiamycin S [78]. Quinupristin was produced by modifying pristinamycin IA to quinuclindinylthiomethyl pristinamycin IA. Dalfopristin is diethylaminoethyl-sulfonyl-pristinamycin IIA [79]. A mixture of quinupristin, a streptogramin B, and dalfopristin, a streptogramin A, in a 30:70 ratio is capable of synergistically inhibiting protein synthesis. Streptogramin A binds to the 50S and 70S subunits of the ribosome when they are not actively synthesizing protein. It has been suggested that they block the elongation phase of bacterial protein synthesis. Conversely, streptogramin B can bind to active ribosomes at the 50S subunit. The synergistic activity of the streptogramins is achieved through a conformational change in the 50S subunit after binding a type A streptogramin, which leads to a strengthening of the binding of the type B streptogramin. Ultimately, the streptogramin combination inhibits early- and late-stage protein synthesis [80].

3.2 Antimicrobial Activity of Streptogramin

3.2.1 Gram-Positive Bacteria

The quinupristin-dalfopristin combination inhibits growth of most gram-positive bacteria. It has useful activity against *Staphylococcus aureus*, *Staphylococcus epidermidis*, *Streptococcus pneumoniae*, *Streptococcus agalactiae*, *Streptococcus pyogenes*, viridans streptococci, and *Enterococcus faecium*. *Enterococcus faecalis* is resistant to the streptogramins [81].

3.2.1 Gram-Negative Bacteria

Quinupristin-dalfopristin has acceptable activity for many respiratory pathogens. Most *Moraxella* spp., *Legionella* spp., *Mycoplasma* spp., and *Neisseria* spp. have an MIC_{90} of <4.0 mg/L. Against *Haemophilus influenzae*, it has less activity with MIC_{90} values of 4.0–8.0 mg/L [79,81]. Quinupristin-dalfopristin has no activity against Enterobacteriaceae or *Pseudomonas aeruginosa* [81].

3.22 Other Bacteria

Quinupristin-dalfopristin maintains useful activity against both *Bacteroides fragilis*, (MIC_{90} 4.0 mg/L) and other *Bacteroides* species (MIC_{90} 4–8 mg/L) [82,83].

3.3 Pharmacokinetic Properties of Streptogramin

The pharmacokinetics of quinupristin-dalfopristin are reported in a very small number of studies. Further data is needed for complete dosing recommendations, especially in patients.

3.3.1 Absorption

Quinupristin-dalfopristin is available only as an injectable product, although oral derivatives are being developed.

Etienne et al. [84] studied the pharmacokinetics in doses ranging from 1.4 to 29.4 mg/kg administered as a 1 h intravenous infusion. Maximum concentrations at the end of the infusion rose linearly from 0.95 to 24.2 mg/L for the doses studied. As would be expected, the area under the time–concentration curve (AUC) also increased linearly from 15.9 to 37.7 mg·h/L for the 12.6 and 29.4 mg/kg doses. Antibacterial activity was present for up to 6 h after the doses µg·h/ml or mg·h/L is the most frequently used units for AUC despite plasma concentrations below the typical MIC for staphylococci and streptococci, probably indicating the importance of active metabolites [84].

A more extensive study by Bergeron and Montay [85] used single doses of 5, 10, and 15 mg/kg given intravenously over 1 h to 18 healthy volunteers. At the 3 doses, quinupristin C_{max} increased linearly (from 1.2 to 2.3 to 3.6 mg/L), and dalfopristin C_{max} values were 4.6, 6.4, and 8.5 mg/L. The dalfopristin metabolite RP 12536 appeared rapidly and increased disproportionally from 0.9 to 2.5 to 3.8 mg/L. However, a combined $AUC_{0-\infty}$ for both dalfopristin and its metabolite did increase linearly. Quinupristin AUC values increased from 1.4 to 3.0 to 4.7 mg·h/L [85].

3.3.2 Distribution

In the Etienne et al. study, the mean $T_{1/2}$ for quinupristin/dalfopristin ranged from 1.27 to 1.53 h. The RP 12536 metabolite of dalfopristin had a $T_{1/2}$ of 0.75–0.84 h

[84]. Bergeron and Montay [85] reported that following biphasic plasma elimination, the elimination $T_{1/2}$ values for quinupristin and dalfopristin were 0.93–0.96 h and 0.39–0.91 h, respectively. Variability was higher for dalfopristin, and $T_{1/2}$ increased with increasing doses.

Quinupristin and dalfopristin are highly protein bound in animal infection models. Quinupristin in plasma was bound approximately 80% in rats and 90% in monkeys. Dalfopristin binding appears to increase over time from 45% to 90% or greater in rats and monkeys [85]. Protein binding ranges from 23% to 32% for quinupristin and from 50% to 56% for dalfopristin in humans [86]. Volume of distribution (V_d) and V_d at steady state (V_{dss}) were 1.37–1.44 L/kg and 0.79–0.83 L/lg, respectively, for quinupristin and were unaffected by dose. Dalfopristin V_d and V_{dss} rose with each dose. For the 5, 10, and 15 mg/kg doses V_d was 0.54, 0.88, and 1.8 L/kg, while V_{dss} was 0.33, 0.43, and 0.70 L/kg, respectively [85].

Radiolabeled quinupristin and dalfopristin were injected into rats and monkeys and radioactivity was assessed for distribution. Either drug was rapidly and extensively distributed to tissues in both species. High concentrations were seen in the gall bladder and in bile, indicating biliary excretion. Both components reached high concentrations in gastrointestinal tissues, kidneys, and liver. The brain and spinal cord had very low concentrations of quinupristin or dalfopristin [85].

Bernard measured blister fluid penetration after a single 12 mg/kg IV dose in six healthy male volunteers. Although a microbiological assay method was employed that is incapable of differentiating between the two components or metabolites, the mean percent tissue penetration was 82.4%, indicating good tissue penetration. Six hours after the end of the infusion, the combination was detectable at a concentration of 0.92 mg/L, which should be sufficient for bacterial activity [87].

3.3.3 Metabolism

Bergeron and Montay [85] reported that clearance rates were high and approximated hepatic blood flow, 1.1 L/(h·kg) and 1.0 to 1.2 L/(h·kg) for quinupristin anddalfopristin, respectively. Bernard et al. [87] found similar values after a single 12 mg/kg IV infusion, reported as 74 L/h for quinupristin-dalfopristin.

A single intravenous infusion of 430 mg for over 1 h was administered to six healthy male volunteers. The radioactivity of quinupristin and dalfopristin was measured to determine their metabolic fate. The two drugs are both metabolized to active metabolites in humans. Quinupristin's cysteine derivative (RP 100391) accounts for 38% and 7.5% of total radioactivity in urine and feces, respectively. No unchanged dalfopristin was recovered in either urine or feces. In urine, dalfopristin was recovered as pristinamycin IIA (RP 12536), 70%, and cysteine derivatives, 30% [85,88].

3.3.4 Excretion

After IV administration, both quinupristin and dalfopristin are excreted primarily in the feces. Fecal excretion as measured by radioactivity of quinupristin and dalfopristin accounted for 74.7% and 77.5%, respectively. The remainder of quinupristin and dalfopristin was recovered in urine, 15% and 18.7%, respectively. Thirty-five percent of quinupristin in urine was recovered unchanged, with a corresponding value of 15% in feces [88].

Renal Dysfunction. The pharmacokinetics of quinupristin and dalfopristin are not altered by the presence of continuous ambulatory peritoneal dialysis. The concentrations of quinupristin and dalfopristin in dialysis effluent were very low and below the MIC of most pathogens [86]. Patients with severe renal failure may have impaired clearance of quinupristin metabolites, and C_{max} and AUC values for dalfopristin were elevated 30% over those in healthy volunteers [86].

3.4 Pharmacodynamic Properties of Streptogramin

3.4.1 Bactericidal Effect

The MBC for streptogramin can be up to 5 dilutions higher than the MIC for *E. faecium* and 3–6 dilutions higher against *S. aureus*. Against streptococci, the MIC and MBC were within one dilution for each other [89].

Quinupristin-dalfopristin has been evaluated in several studies using time-kill studies. It exerts a time-dependent, bacteriostatic, and what is sometimes referred to as slow bactericidal activity against *E. faecium* and *S. aureus* [89,90]. However, in several studies, quinupristin-dalfopristin has a good bactericidal effect on certain strains of both organisms [91,92]. Further studies with many strains of *E. faecium* have shown that quinupristin-dalfopristin at a concentration of 6.0 mg/L can have a concentration-dependent bactericidal effect for isolates with MBCs of 4.0 mg/L; however, most strains appear to possess higher MBCs [91]. The quinupristin-dalfopristin concentration/MBC ratio and quinupristin MICs were significantly correlated with the bactericidal rate [91]. Other investigators have found that bactericidal activity is more likely to be demonstrated for enterococci in the log growth phase and those with at least intermediate susceptibility to erythromycin [93]. Against *S. aureus*, quinupristin-dalfopristin also demonstrates a variable bactericidal rate, presumably as a result of differences in MBCs. Against methicillin-susceptible *S. aureus* (MSSA) and methicillin-resistant *S. aureus* (MRSA), quionupristin-dalfopristin decreased the inoculum 1–2 $\log_{10}$ over 24 h compared to 3–4 $\log_{10}$ for oxacillin, vancomycin, or gentamicin [89]. In other experiments, quinupristin-dalfopristin has shown the ability to reduce the inoculum by 2–3 $\log_{10}$ in only 6–12 h [92]. The presence of a constitutively erythromycin-resistant phenotype is predictive of bacteriostatic activity [94].

Quinupristin-dalfopristin in early studies showed a consistent rapid bactericidal activity against penicillin-susceptible *S. pneumoniae*. The inoculum was decreased by 2–3 $\log_{10}$ in only 10 min. This bactericidal rate was faster than that of all comparators, including penicillin G, erythromycin, ciprofloxacin, sparfloxacin, and vancomycin. However, three out of ten strains only a bacteriostatic effect was seen [95]. Later studies with larger numbers of *S. pneumoniae* isolates demonstrated its rapid bactericidal effect against all *S. pneumoniae* regardless of penicillin or erythromycin susceptibility at 2 times the MIC [96,97]. Against viridans streptococci, quinupristin-dalfopristin exerts a bactericidal effect over 12–24 h. The bactericidal rate against viridans streptococci is less when the isolates are erythromycin-resistant through loss of quinupristin activity [98].

3.4.2 Postantibiotic Effect

The influence of postantibiotic effect (PAE) on antibiotic dosing is controversial. With quinupristin/dalfopristin possessing short half-lives, long PAEs may influence the dosing schedule.

The PAE against *E. faecium* in in vitro experiments has produced variable results. Against *E. faecium*, the PAE after a 1 h exposure to 0.25 times the MIC was 8.5 and 2.6 h for vancomycin-susceptible and -resistant strains, respectively [99]. However, others have found the PAE 4 times the MIC to be as short as 0.2–3.0 h for vancomycin-resistant strains and inversely related to the MBC and quinupristin MIC [91]. The presence of multiple and unmeasured antibiotic resistance may affect the results of PAE determinations for enterococci.

Staphylococci are also reported to possess a long concentration-dependent PAE after exposure to quinupristin/dalfopristin. The in vitro PAE at 10 times the MIC was 4.6–7.0 h for MSSA and MRSA, either erythromycin-susceptible or inducibly resistant. For MRSA containing the constitutively erythromycin-resistant phenotype, the PAE was reduced to 2.4 h [29]. Other investigators have also found a longer PAE in MSSA compared to MRSA at 4 times the MIC, ≥ 7 h versus 5 h, respectively [100].

Pneumococci show concentration-dependent PAEs to quinupristin-dalfopristin. The rapid bactericidal rate complicates the determination of PAE; however, at 0.5 times the MIC the PAE ranges from 1.7 to 4.1 h [99].

In the mouse thigh infection model, the PAEs against *S. aureus* and *S. pneumoniae* were 10 and 9.1 h, respectively [101].

3.4.3 Experimental Infection Models

Few studies have been published with quinupristin-dalfopristin, and limited information is available from in vitro or in vivo models. These models are also limited through the use of only a few bacterial strains in primarily endocarditis and may not be completely predictive of results in humans for other types of infections.

In Vitro Models. Quinupristin/dalfopristin was evaluated in an in vitro infection model of simulated endocardial vegetations. The drug was dosed to simulate a human dose of 7.5 mg/kg every 8 h for 96 h, low-dose continuous infusion (C_{ss} = 1.5 mg/L), and high-dose continuous infusion (C_{ss} = 9.2 mg/L). Two vancomycin-resistant and constitutively erythromycin-resistant *E. faecium* strains were used, and one of the isolates possessed an elevated MBC. Against the isolate with a low MBC, all regimens were bacteriostatic with the exception of the high-dose continuous infusion regimen, which achieved bactericidal activity after 90 h. The addition of doxycycline to the every 8 h regimen resulted in increased killing, although it did not reach a value indicating synergy. The isolate with an elevated MBC was unaffected by quinupristin/dalfopristin as an every 8 h regimen or low-dose continuous infusion. Doxycycline possessed the greatest activity alone, and no increased killing was observed when it was administered with quinupristin-dalfopristin. The use of a high-dose continuous infusion regimen or the addition of doxycycline reduced or eliminated the appearance of resistant isolates during the model [102].

Quinupristin-dalfopristin activity against *S. aureus* in a fibrin clot model was compared to vancomycin over 72 h. A 7.5 mg/kg every 8 h dose was simulated. Quinupristin-dalfopristin was more active than vancomycin; however, neither reached bactericidal activity. This was despite both the MSSA and MRSA isolate possessing MBCs close to the MIC. The combination of quinupristin-dalfopristin and vancomycin led to greater decreases in $\log_{10}$ counts (not synergistic) and prevented the emergence of quinupristin-dalfopristin resistance [103].

This same model further evaluated quinupristin-dalfopristin in simulated doses of 7.5 mg/kg given every 6, 8, and 12 h and by continuous infusion (6.0 mg/L) against *S. aureus.* One strain was an MRSA with constitutive erythromycin resistance, and the other was an MSSA and erythromycin-susceptible. All regimens were bactericidal against the MSSA strain, but no regimens reached this level of activity against the MRSA isolate. The $AUC_{0\text{-}24}$ was significantly correlated with activity against the MRSA strain [104].

In Vivo Models. Two inducibly erythromycin-resistant and one sensitive *E. faecium* strain were studied in a rabbit endocarditis model for 4 days. Quinupristin-dalfopristin was given in a dose of 30 mg/kg IM evert 8 h and compared to thrice daily regimens of amoxicillin or gentamicin or combinations. Quinupristin-dalfopristin when given alone had equivalent activity to amoxicillin against the erythromycin-susceptible strain. For the erythromycin-resistant strains, quinupristin-dalfopristin was not effective. Additional experiments against one of the erythromycin-resistant strains showed that combinations of quinupristin-dalfopristin with gentamicin or amoxicillin were more active than either of the drugs alone. No information was presented on pharmacodynamic parameters [105].

Quinupristin-dalfopristin has been studied in a rabbit infected fibrin clot model against two strains each of *S. aureus* and *S. epidermidis*. A rapid bactericidal rate was observed after the single dose of 50 mg/kg for *S. aureus*; however, only bacteriostatic activity was seen against *S. epidermidis*. The elevated MBCs for *S. epidermidis* at the inoculum tested may explain the disparate results. Also, the C_{max} obtained with this dose is considerably higher than that observed in humans and may not be predictive of human experience [106].

An early rabbit endocarditis model administered quinupristin-dalfopristin in a dose of 20 mg/kg intramuscularly (IM) every 6 h versus vancomycin 25 mg/kg IV every 12 h for 4 days. Three susceptible *S. aureus* strains with increasing quinupristin-dalfopristin MICs (0.5–2.0 mg/L) and MBCs (4.0–8.0 mg/L) were used. The peak serum concentration of quinupristin-dalfopristin measured by bioassay was 1.9 mg/L with a $T_{1/2}$ of 1.3 h. Vancomycin was effective against all strains, whereas quinupristin-dalfopristin was effective against the strains with MICs of 0.5 and 1.0 mg/L although less effective at sterilizing vegetations at an MIC of 1.0 mg/L. It failed against the strain with an MIC of 2.0 mg/L. Higher doses of 40 mg/kg in this model resulted in animal toxicity and death [107]. Given the pharmacokinetic data, these regimens would be expected to produce a time above the MIC during the dosing interval ($T >$ MIC) of approximately 57%, 36%, and 0% for *S. aureus* with MICs of 0.5, 1.0, and 2.0 mg/L, respectively. Therefore, it appeared that quinupristin-dalfopristin required a $T >$ MIC of approximately 50% for equivalent bactericidal activity.

Quinupristin-dalfopristin was compared to vancomycin in another *S. aureus* rabbit endocarditis model. The isolate had an MIC and MBC of 0.5 mg/L to quinupristin-dalfopristin. Vancomycin and quinupristin-dalfopristin were dosed at 30 mg/kg IM every 12 h for 4 days. Quinupristin-dalfopristin was as effective as vancomycin, and no resistant isolates were recovered from vegetations. The $T >$ MIC for quinupristin-dalfopristin was 33%. Concentrations were also measured in the vegetations, and at 1 h after a single injection the ratio of vegetation to serum concentration was 4.1. These data along with a prolonged PAE may explain the efficacy of quinupristin-dalfopristin [108]. However, this *S. aureus* strain may not be representative of most clinical isolates due to its equivalent MIC and MBC.

A *S. aureus* rat endocarditis model demonstrated that quinupristin-dalfopristin in a regimen simulating a human dose of 7 mg/kg every 12 h was as effective as vancomycin only against *S. aureus* strains that were erythromycin-susceptible. For constitutively erythromycin-resistant strains that had quinupristin MICs of >64 mg/L, the shorter dalfopristin $T_{1/2}$ in rats did not allow for the $T >$ MIC (<20%) to be sufficient for efficacy. A regimen that prolonged the dalfopristin concentration did allow the regimen to be effective for these macrolide-resistant strains. The authors recommended that efficacy would be improved through use of an every 8 h regimen or continuous infusion [24]. Similar findings were found in a rabbit endocarditis model evaluating the efficacy of quinupristin-dalfopristin against *S. aureus* with variable erythromycin susceptibilities. Quinupristin-dalfopristin doses were 30 mg/kg IM every 8 or 12 h and 10 mg/kg IV every 12 h. These regimens were as effective as vancomycin against erythromycin-susceptible or inducibly resistant strains regardless of oxacillin susceptibility. Quinupristin-dalfopristin was less active in all doses against the two strains with constitutively erythromycin-resistant phenotypes. The AUC for quinupristin-dalfopristin in plasma divided by the quinupristin MIC was most predictive of activity. The determination of quinupristin MICs may be necessary prior to beginning therapy with quinupristin-dalfopristin for endocarditis [77].

A mouse *S. aureus* septicemia model compared quinupristin-dalfopristin to vancomycin. Only one *S. aureus* strain was used, and no MBC or other drug resistant data were reported. Quinupristin-dalfopristin regimens of a single dose of 120 mg/kg, 60 mg/kg every 12 h, 40 mg/kg every 8 h, and 30 mg/kg every 6 h were administered for 24 h. Quinupristin-dalfopristin in all doses demonstrated a faster bactericidal rate than vancomycin, with some dose-dependent bactericidal activity being noted. No data were presented on which parameter was more closely associated with activity, because all AUCs were similar [109].

In a mouse thigh infection model, the influence of dosing interval on the activity of quinupristin-dalfopristin was evaluated against *S. aureus* and *S. pneumoniae*. The dose ranged from 12.5 to 800 mg/kg and administered in one, two, or four doses over 24 h. A sigmoidal dose–response model indicated that the AUC was best correlated with efficacy [101].

3.4.4 Synergy

The importance of synergistic combinations is well documented for certain enterococcal and staphylococcal infections. Given quinupristin-dalfopristin's slow bactericidal activity against many of these strains, synergy testing has been evaluated.

As already mentioned, quinupristin and dalfopristin are synergistic when used in combination. The IV product contains a quinupristin-dalfopristin ratio of 30:70. The more variable $T_{1/2}$ of dalfopristin and information on decreased penetration of dalfopristin into cardiac vegetations underlies the importance of investigating the effect of different ratios on activity [104]. Studies of in vitro and in vivo activity show that the combination remains synergistic and effective in a range from 16:84 to 84:16, which should accommodate most clinical situations [110].

Quinupristin-dalfopristin has no effect on the MIC of ciprofloxacin, gentamicin, or cefotaxime against *E. coli*, *K. pneumoniae*, *C. freundii*, *E. cloacae*, *S. marcescens*, or *P. aeruginosa*. Quinupristin-dalfopristin increased the MIC for ciprofloxacin against *B. fragilis* in nine out of 20 strains but had no effect on other *Bacteroides* species or *S. aureus* [82]. The quinupristin-dalfopristin MIC for vancomycin-resistant *E. faecium* was decreased when the combination combined with ciprofloxacin, teicoplanin, and tetracycline [100].

Using time-kill methods, quinupristin-dalfopristin was not found to have synergy against *E. faecium* when combined with clinafloxacin, LY333328, or eperozolid. These isolates had quinupristin-dalfopristin MBCs of ≥8.0 mg/L [111]. No synergy was seen defined by an FIC index of 0.5 when quinupristin-dalfopristin was combined with vancomycin; however, time-kill studies indicated synergy against *S. aureus* at higher inocula (5×10^7 CFU/mL) [103]. An inducibly erythromycin-reistant, gentamicin-resistant, amoxicillin-sensitive *E. faecium* strain was exposed to quinupristin-dalfopristin with and without gentamicin or amoxicillin, but the combinations did not demonstrate faster killing rates [105].

3.5 Summary—Streptogramins

Quinupristin-dalfopristin has been shown effective against *E. faecium*, *S. aureus*, and *S. pneumoniae*. The pharmacodynamic parameter most associated with efficacy in animal models is the AUC. The presence of erythromycin resistance has a dramatic effect on the activity of the combination drug quinupristin-dalfopristin. This phenotype will lead to elevated quinupristin MICs and may need to be determined prior to beginning therapy. Further data are needed from patients to determine the most appropriate dosing requirements that maximize its bactericidal effect.

REFERENCES

1. C Cosar, L Joulou. Activité de l'(hydroxy-2-éthyl)-1-méthyl-2-nitro-5-imidazole (8823 R.P.) vis-à-vis des infections expérimentales à trichomonas vaginalis. Ann Inst Pasteur 1959;96;238–241.
2. M Müller. Mode of action of metronidazole on anaerobic bacteria and protozoa. Surgery 1983;93:165–171.
3. B Korner, HK Jensen. Sensitivity of Trichomonas vaginalis to metronidazole, tinidazole, and nifuratel in vitro. Br J Vener Dis 1976;52:404–408.
4. SD Sears, J O'Hare. In vitro susceptibility of Trochomonas vaginalis to 50 antimicrobial agents. Antimocrob Agents Chemother 1988;32:144–146.
5. L Jokipii, AMM Jokipii. In vitro susceptibility of Giardia lamblia trophozoites to metronidazole and tinidazole. J Infect Dis 1980;141:317–325.
6. VK Vinayak, RC Mahajan, NL Chitkara. In-vitro activity of metronidazole on the cysts of Entamoeba histolytica. Ind J Pathol Bacteriol 1975;18:61–64.
7. RC Mahajan, NL Chitkara, VK Vinayak, DV Dutta. In vitro comparative evaluation of tinidazole and metronidazole on strains of Entamoeba histolytica. Indian J Pathol Bacteriol 1974;17:226–228.
8. DLS Shinn. Metronidazole in acute ulcerative gingivitis. Lancet 1962;1:1191.
9. FP Tally, VL Sutter, SM Finegold. Metronidazole versus anaerobes: In vitro data and initial clinical observations. Calif Med 1972;117:22–26.
10. JP Rissing, WL Moore Jr, C Newman, JK Crockett, TB Buxton, HT Edmondson. Treatment of anaerobic infections with metronidazole. Curr Ther Res 1980;27:651–663.

11. Study Group. An evaluation of metronidazole in the prophylaxis and treatment of anaerobic infections in surgical patients. J Antimicrob Chemother 1975;1:393–401.
12. SJ Eykyn, I Phillips. Metronidazole and anaerobic sepsis. Br Med J 1976;2:1418–1421.
13. B Olsson-Liljequist, CE Nord. In vitro susceptibility of anaerobic bacteria to nitroimidazoles. Scand J Infect Dis 1981;26(suppl):42–45.
14. KE Aldridge, M Gelfand, LB Reller, LW Ayers, CL Pierson, F Schoenknect, F Tilton, J Wilkins, A Henderberg, DD Schiro, M Johnson, A Janney, CV Sanders. A five-year multicenter study of the susceptibility of the Bacteroides fragilis group isolates to cephalosporins, cephamycins, penicillins, clindamycin, and metronidazole in the United States. Diagn Microbiol Infect Dis 1994;18:235–241.
15. JB Selkon. The need for and choice of chemotherapy for anaerobic infections. Scand J Infect Dis 1981;26(suppl):19–23.
16. GA Pankuch, MR Jacobs, PC Appelbaum. Susceptibilities of 428 gram-positive and -negative anaerobic bacteria to Bay y3118 compared with their susceptibilities to ciprofloxacin, clindamycin, metronidazole, piperacillin, piperacillin-tazobactam, and cefoxitin. Antimicrob Agents Chemother 1993;37:1649–1654.
17. CAM McNulty, J Dent, R Wise. Susceptibility of clinical isolates of Campylobacter pyloridis to 11 antimicrobial agents. Antimicrob Agents Chemother 1985;28:837–838.
18. M Lopez-Brea, E Martin, C Lopez-Lavid, JC Sanz. Susceptibility of Helicobacter pylori to metronidazole. Eur J Clin Microbiol Infect Dis 1991;10:1082–1083.
19. MJAMP Pavicic, AJ van Winkelhoff, J de Graaff. Synergistic effects between amoxicillin, metronidazole, and the hydroxymetabolite of metronidazole against Actinobacillus actinomycetemcomitans. Antimicrob Agents Chemother 1991;35:961–966.
20. MJAMP Pavicic, AJ van Winkelhoff, J de Graaff. In vitro susceptibilities of Actinobacillus actinomycetemcomitans to a number of antimicrobial combinations. Antimicrob Agents Chemother 1992;36:2634–2638.
21. AW Chow, V Patten, LB Guze. Susceptibility of anaerobic bacteria to metronidazole: Relative resistance of non-spore-forming gram-positive bacilli. J Infect Dis 1975;131:182–185.
22. AMM Jokipii, L Jokipii. Comparative activity of metronidazole and tinidazole against Clostridium difficle and Peptostreptococcus anaerobius. Antimicrob Agents Chemother 1987;31:183–186.
23. K Dornbusch, CE Nord, B Olsson-Liljeqvist. Antibiotic susceptibility of anaerobic bacteria with special reference to Bacteroides fragilis. Scand J Infect Dis 1979; 19(suppl 19):17–25.
24. JP O'Keefe, KA Troc, KA Thompson. Activity of metronidazole and its hydroxy and acid metabolites against clinical isolates of anaerobic bacteria. Antimicrob Agents Chemother 1982;22:426–430.
25. JL Whiting, N Cheng, AW Chow. Interactions of ciprofloxacin with clindamycin, metronidazole, cefoxitin, cefotaxime, and mezlocillin against gram-positive and gram-negative anaerobic bacteria. Antimicrob Agents Chemother 1987;31:1379–1382.

26. HM Wexler, SM Finegold. In vitro activity of cefotetan compared with that of other antimicrobial agents against anaerobic bacteria. Antimicrob Agents Chemother 1988;32:601–604.
27. H Hof, V Sticht-Groh. Antibacterial effects of niridazole: Its effect on microaerophilic campylobacter. Infection 1984;12:36–39.
28. AM Freydiere, Y Gille, S Tigaud, P Vincent. In vitro susceptibilities of 40 Campylobacter fetus subsp. jejuni strains to niridazole and metronidazole. Antimicrob Agents Chemother 1984;25:145–146.
29. BM Jones, I Geary, AB Alawattegama, GR Kinghorn, BI Duerden. In-vitro and in-vivo activity of metronidazole against Gardnerella vaginalis, Bacteroides spp. and Mobiluncus spp. in bacterial vaginosis. J Antimicrob Chemother 1985;16:189–197.
30. ABM Kharsany, AA Hoosen, J van den Ende. Antimicrobial susceptibilities of Gardnerella vaginalis. Antimicrob Agents Chemother 1993;37:2733–2735.
31. M Weinberger, T Wu, M Rubin, VJ Gill, PA Pizzo. Leptotrichia buccalis bacteremia in patients with cancer: Report of four cases and review. Rev Infect Dis 1991; 13:201–206.
32. AH Davies. Metronidazole in human infections with syphilis. Br J Vener Dis 1967; 43:197–200.
33. T Bergan, E Arnold. Pharmacokinetics of metronidazole in healthy volunteers after tablets and suppositories. Chemotherapy 1980;26:231–241.
34. GW Houghton, J Smith, PS Thorne, R Templeton. The pharmacokinetics of oral and intravenous metronidazole in man. J Antimicrob Chemother 1979;5:621–623.
35. ED Ralph, JT Clarke, RD Libke, RP Luthy, WMM Kirby. Pharmacokinetics of metronidazole as determined by bioassay. Antimicrob Agents Chemother 1974;6: 691–696.
36. J Mattila, PT Männistö, R Mäntylä, S Nykänen, U Lamminsivu. Comparative pharmacokinetics of metronidazole and tinidazole as influenced by administration route. Antimicrob Agents Chemother 1983;23:721–725.
37. T Bergan, O Leinebø, T Blom-Hagen, B Salvesen. Pharmacokinetics and bioavailability of metronidazole after tablets, suppositories and intravenous administration. Scand J Gastroenterol 1984;19(suppl 91):45–60.
38. GW Houghton, PS Thorne, J Smith, R Templeton. Plasma metronidazole concentrations after suppository administration. In: Phillips and Collier, eds. Metronidazole. Proceedings of the Second International Symposium on Anaerobic Infections, Geneva, April 1979:41–44.
39. FE Cunningham, DM Kraus, L Brubaker, JH Fischer. Pharmacokinetics of intravaginal metronidazole gel. J Clin Pharmacol 1994;34:1060–1065.
40. MM Alper, N Barwin, WM McLean, IJ McGilveray, S Sved. Systemic absorption of metronidazole by the vaginal route. Obstet Gynecol 1985;65:781–784.
41. IK Aronson, JA Rumsfield, DP West, J Alexander, JH Fischer, FP Paloucek. Evaluation of topical metronidazole gel in acne rosacea. Drug Intell Clin Pharm 1987; 21:346–351.
42. LK Schmadel, GK McEvoy. Topical metronidazole: A new therapy for rosacea. Clin Pharm 1990;9:94–101.

43. DE Schwartz, F Jeunet. Comparative pharmacokinetic studies of ornidazole and metronidazole in man. Chemotherapy 1976;22:19–29.
44. AH Lau, K Emmons, R Seligsohn. Pharmacokinetics of intravenous metronidazole at different dosages in healthy subjects. Int J Clin Pharmacol Ther Toxicol 1991; 29:386–390.
45. I Amon, K Amon, H Hüller. Pharmacokinetics and therapeutic efficacy of metronidazole at different dosages. Int J Clin Pharmacol Ther Toxicol 1978;16:384–386.
46. WL Hand, N King-Thompson, JW Holman. Entry of roxithromycin (RU 965), imipenem, cefotaxime, trimethoprim, and metronidazole into human polymorphonuclear leukocytes. Antimicrob Agents Chemother 1987;31:1553–1557.
47. KE Andersson. Pharmacokinetics of nitroimidazoles: Spectrum of adverse reactions. Scand J Infect Dis 1981;26(suppl 26):60–67.
48. I Nilsson-Ehle, B Ursing, P Nilsson-Ehle. Liquid chromatographic assay for metronidazole and tinidazole: Pharmacokinetic and metabolic studies in human subjects. Antimicrob Agents Chemother 1981;19:754–760.
49. TY Ti, HS Lee, YM Khoo. Disposition of intravenous metronidazole in Asian surgical patients. Antimicrob Agents Chemother 1996;40:2248–2251.
50. SK Spangler, MR Jacobs, PC Appelbaum. Time-kill study of the activity of trovafloxacin compared with ciprofloxacin, sparfloxacin, metronidazole, cefoxitin, piperacillin, and piperacillin/tazobactam against six anaerobes. J Antimicrob Chemother 1997;39(suppl B):23–27.
51. H Mattie, AC Dijkmans, C van Gulpen. The pharmacokinetics of metronidazole and tinidazole in patients with mixed aerobic-anaerobic infections. J Antimicrob Chemother 1982;10(suppl A):59–64.
52. JG Bartlett, TJ Louie, SL Gorbach, AB Onderonk. Therapeutic efficacy of 29 antimicrobial regimens in experimental intraabdominal sepsis. Rev Infect Dis 1981;3: 535–542.
53. DE Nix, R Tyrrell, M Müller. Pharmacodynamics of metronidazole determined by a time-kill assay for Trichomonas vaginalis. Antimicrob Agents Chemother 1995; 39:1848–1852.
54. WA Craig, SC Ebert. Killing and regrowth of bacteria in vitro: A review. Scand J Infect Dis 1991;74(suppl 74):63–70.
55. P Van der Auwera, Y Van Laethem, N Defresne, M Husson, J Klastersky. Comparative serum bactericidal activity against test anaerobes in volunteers receiving imipenem, clindamycin, latamoxef, and metronidazole. J Antimicrob Chemother 1987; 19:205–210.
56. M Boeckh, H Lode, KM Deppermann, S Grineisen, F Shokry, R Held, K Wernicke, P Koeppe, J Wagner, C Krasemann, K Borner. Pharmacokinetics and serum bactericidal activities of quinolones in combination with clindamycin, metronidazole, and ornidazole. Antimicrob Agents Chemother 1990;34:2407–2414.
57. A Pefanis, C Thauvin-Elipoulos, J Holden, GM Eliopoulos, MJ Ferraro, RC Moellering Jr. Activity of fleroxacin alone and in combination with clindamycin or metronidazole in experimental intra-abdominal abscesses. Antimicrob Agents Chemother 1994;38:252–255.
58. SF Kowalsky, RM Echols, EM McCormick. Comparative serum bactericidal activ-

ity of ceftizoxime/metronidazole, ceftizoxime, clindamycin, and imipenem against obligate anaerobic bacteria. J Antimicrob Chemother 1990;25:767–775.
59. CD Freeman, CH Nightingale, DP Nicolau, PP Belliveau, PR Tessier, Q Fu, D Xuan, R Quintiliani. Bactericidal activity of low-dose ceftizoxime plus metronidazole compared with cefoxitin and ampicillin-sulbactam. Pharmacotherapy 1994;14: 185–190.
60. CD Freeman, CH Nightingale, DP Nicolau, PP Belliveau, R Quintiliani. Serum bactericidal activity of ceftriaxone plus metronidazole against common intra-abdominal pathogens. Am J Hosp Pharm 1994;51:1782–1787.
61. Pharmacia & Upjohn. Cleocin Phosphate manufacturer's package insert. Pharmacia & Upjohn, 1998.
62. ME Falagas, SL Gorbach. Clindamycin and metronidazole. Med Clin N Am 1995; 79:845–867.
63. PG Kremsner. Clindamycin in malaria treatment. J Antimicrob Chemother 1990; 25:9–14.
64. GV Doern, MA Pfaller, K Kugler, J Freeman, RN Jones. Prevalence of antimicrobial resistance among respiratory tract isolates of Streptococcus pneumoniae in North America: 1997 results from the SENTRY antimicrobial surveillance program. Clin Infect Dis 1998;27:764–770.
65. MA Pfaller, RN Jones, GV Doern, K Kugler, and the SENTRY Participants Group. Bacterial pathogens isolated from patients with bloodstream infection: Frequencies of occurrence and antimicrobial susceptibility patterns from the SENTRY antimicrobial surveillance program (United States and Canada, 1997). Antimicrob Agents Chemother 1998;42:1762–1770.
66. National Committee for Clinical and Laboratory Standards. Performance standards for antimicrobial susceptibility testing: Eighth informational supplement. NCCLS document M100-S8. Wayne, PA, 1998.
67. JF Flaherty, LC Rodondi, BJ Guglielmo, JC Fleishaker, RJ Townsend, JG Gambertoglio. Comparative pharmacokinetics and serum inhibitory activity of clindamycin different dosing regimens. Antimicrob Agents Chemother 1988;32:1825–1829.
68. ME Klepser, DP Nicolau, R Quintiliani, CH Nightingale. Bactericidal activity of low-dose clindamycin administered at 8- and 12-hour intervals against Staphylococcus aureus, Streptococcus pneumoniae, and Bacteroides fragilis. Antimicrob Agents Chemother 1997;41:630–635.
69. JD Smilack, WR Wilson, FR Cockerill III. Tetracyclines, chloramphenicol, erythromycin, clindamycin, and metronidazole. Mayo Clin Proc 1991;66:1270–1280.
70. ME Klepser, MA Banevicius, R Quintiliani, CH Nightingale. Characterization of bactericidal activity of clindamycin against Bacteroides fragilis via kill curve methods. Antimicrob Agents Chemother 1996;40:1941–1944.
71. WA Craig, S Gudmundsson. Postantibiotic effect. In: V Lorian, ed. Antibiotics in Laboratory Medicine. 4th ed. Williams and Wilkins, Baltimore, 1996;296–329.
72. KE Aldridge, CW Stratton. Bactericidal activity of ceftizoxime, cefotetan, and clindamycin against cefoxitan-resistant strains of the Bacteroides fragilis group. J Antimicrob Chemother 1991;28:701–705.
73. M Boeckh, H Lode, KM Deppermann, S Grineisen, F Shokry, R Held, K Wernicke, P Koeppe, J Wagner, C Krasemann et al. Pharmacokinetics and serum bactericidal

activities of quinolones in combination with clindamycin, metronidazole, and ornidazole. Antimicrob Agents Chemother 1990;34:2407–2414.

74. MP Weinstein, RG Deeter, KA Swanson, JS Gross. Crossover assessment of serum bactericidal activity and pharmacokinetics of ciprofloxacin alone and in combination in healthy elderly volunteers. Antimicrob Agents Chemother 1991;35:2352–2358.
75. PJ McDonald, WA Craig, CM Kunin. Persistent effect of antibiotics on Staphylococcus aureus after exposure for limited periods of time. J Infect Dis 1977;135:217–223.
76. IB Xue, PG Davey, G Phillips. Variations in postantibiotic effect of clindamycin against clinical isolates of Staphylococcus aureus and implications for dosing of patients with osteomyelitis. Antimicrob Agents Chemother 1996;40:1403–1407.
77. B Fantin, R Lequercq, Y Merlé, L Saint-Julien, C Veyrat, J Duval, C Carbon. Critical influence of resistance to streptogramin B-type antibiotics on activity of RP 59500 (quinupristin-dalfopristin) in experimental endocarditis due to Staphylococcus aureus. Antimicrob Agents Chemother 1995; 39:400–405.
78. R Rende-Fournier, R Leclercq, M Galimand, J Duval, P Courvalin. Identification of the satA gene encoding a streptogramin A acetyltransferase in Enterococcus faecium BM4145. Antimicrob Agents Chemother 1993;37:2119–2125.
79. JM Andrews, R Wise. The in-vitro activity of a new semi-synthetic streptogramin compound, RP 59500, against staphylococci and respiratory patohgens. J Antimicrob Chemother 1994;33:849–853.
80. C Cocito, M Di Giambattista, E Nyssen, P Vannuffel. Inhibition of protein synthesis by streptogramins and related antibiotics. J Antimicrob Chemother 1997;39(suppl A):7–13.
81. DH Bouanchaud. In-vitro and in-vivo antibacterial activity of quinupristin/dalfopristin. J Antimicrob Chemother 1997;39(suppl A):15–21.
82. HC Neu, NX Chin, JW Gu. The in-vitro activity of new streptogramins, RP 59500, RP 57669 and RP 54476, alone and in combination. J Antimicrob Chemother 1992; 30(suppl A):83–94.
83. PC Appelbaum, SK Spangler, MR Jacobs. Susceptibility of 539 gram-positive and gram-negative anaerobes to new agents, including RP59500, biapenem, trospectomycin and piperacillin/tazobactam. J Antimicrob Chemother 1993;32:223–231.
84. SD Etienne, G Montay, A Le Liboux, A Frydman, JJ Garaud. A phase I, double-blind, placebo-controlled study of the tolerance and pharmacokinetic behaviour of RP 59500. J Antimicrob Chemother 1992;30(suppl A):123–131.
85. M Bergeron, G Montay. The pharmacokinetics of quinupristin/dalfopristin in laboratory animals and in humans. J Antimicrob Chemother 1997;39(suppl A):129–138.
86. CA Johnson, CA Taulor, SW Zimmerman, WE Bridson, P Chevlaier, O Pasquier, RI Baybutt. Pharmacokinetics of quinupristin-dalfopristin in continuous ambulatory peritoneal dialysis patients. Antimicrob Agents Chemother 1999, 43:152–156.
87. E Bernard, M Bensoussan, F Bensoussan, S Etienne, I Cazenave, E Carsenti-Etesse, Y Le Roux, G Montay, P Dellamonica. Pharmacokinetics and suction blister fluid penetration of a semisynthetic injectable streptogramin RP 59500 (RP 57669/RP 54476). Eur J Clin Microbiol Infect Dis 1994;13:768–771.

88. C Gaillard, J Van Cantfort, G Montay, D Piffard, A Le Liboux, S Etienne, A Scheen, A Frydman. Disposition of the radiolabelled streptogramin RP 59500 in healthy male volunteers. In: Programs and Abstracts of the 32nd Interscience Conference on Antimicrobial Agents and Chemotherapy, Anaheim, 1992, Abstract 1317. Am Soc Microbiol, Washington, DC.
89. RJ Fass. In vitro activity of RP 59500, a semisynthetic injectable pristinamycin, against staphylococci, streptococci, and enterococci. Antimicrob Agents Chemother 1991;35:553–559.
90. RL Hill, CT Smith, M Seyed-Akhavani, MW Casewell. Bactericidal and inhibitory activity of quinupristin/dalfopristin against vancomycin- and gentamicin-resistant Enterococcus faecium. J Antimicrob Chemother 1997;39(suppl A):23–28.
91. JR Aeschlimann, MJ Rybak. Pharmacodynamic analysis of the activity of quinupristin-dalfopristin against voncomycin-resistant Enterococcus faecium with differing MBCs via time-kill-curve and postantibiotic effect method. Antimicrob Agents Chemother 1998;42:2188–2192.
92. DE Low, HL Nadler. A review of in-vitro antibacterial activity of quinupristin/dalfopristin against methicillin-susceptible and -resistant Staphylococcus aureus. J Antimicrob Chemother 1997;39(suppl A):53–58.
93. F Caron, HS Gold, CB Wennersten, MG Farris, RC Moellering Jr, GM Eliopoulos. Influence of erythromycin resistance, inoculum growth phase, and incubation time on assessment of the bactericidal activity of RP 59500 (quinupristin-dalfopristin) against vancomycin-resistant Enterococcus faecium. Antimicrob Agents Chemother 1997;41:2749–2753.
94. JM Entenza, H Drugeon, MP Glauser, P Moreillon. Treatment of experimental endocarditis due to erythromycin-susceptible or -resistant methicillin-resistant Staphylococcus aureus with RP 59500. Antimicrob Agents Chemother 1995;39:1419–1424.
95. GA Pankuch, MR Jacobs, PC Applebaum. Study of comparative antipneumococcal activities of penicillin G, RP 59500, erythromycin, sparfloxacin, ciprofloxacin, and vancomycin by using time-kill methodology. Antimicrob Agents Chemother 1994;38:2065–2072.
96. GA Pankuch, MR Jacobs, PC Applebaum. MIC and time-kill study of antipneumococcal activities of RPR 106972 (a new oral streptogramin), RP 59500 (quinupristin-dalfopristin), pyostacine (RP 7293), penicillin G, cefotaxime, erythromycin, and clarithromycin against 10 penicillin-susceptible and -resistant pneumococci. Antimicrob Agents Chemother 1996;40:2071–2074.
97. GA Pankuch, C Lichtenberger, MR Jacobs, PC Appelbaum. Antipneumococcal activities of RP 59500 (quinupristin-dalfopristin), penicillin G, erythromycin, and sparfloxacin determined by MIC and rapid time-kill methodologies. Antimicrob Agents Chemother 1996;40:1653–1656.
98. F L'Heriteau, JM Entenza, F Lacassin, C Leport, MP Glauser, P Moreillon. RP 59500 prophylaxis of experimental endocarditis due to erythromycin-susceptible and -resistant isogenic pairs of viridans group streptococci. Antimicrob Agents Chemother 1995;39:1425–1429.
99. GA Pankuch, MR Jacobs, PC Appelbaum. Postantibiotic effect and postantibiotic sub-MIC effect of quinupristin-dalfopristin against gram-positive and -negative organisms. Antimicrob Agents Chemother 1998;42:3028–3031.

100. A Nougayrede, N Berthaud, DH Bouanchaud. Post-antibiotic effects of RP 59500 with Staphylococcus aureus. J Antimicrob Chemother 1992;30(suppl A):101–106.
101. W Craig, S Ebert. Pharmacodynamic activities of RP 50500 in an animal infection model. In: Programs and Abstracts of the 33rd Interscience Conference on Antimicrobial Agents and Chemotherapy, New Orleans, 1993, Abstract 470. Am Soc Microbiol Washington, DC.
102. JR Aeschlimann, MJ Zervos, MJ Rybak. Treatment of vancomycin-resistant Enterococcus faecium with RP 59500 (quinupristin-dalfopristin) administered by intermittent or continuous infusion, alone or in combination with doxycycline, in an in vitro pharmacodynamic infection model with simulated endocardial vegetations. Antimicrob Agents Chemother 1998;42:2710–2717.
103. SL Kang, MJ Rybak. Pharmacodynamics of RP 59500 alone and in combination with vancomycin against Staphylococcus aureus in an in vitro-infected fibrin clot model. Antimicrob Agents Chemother 1995;39:1505–1511.
104. MJ Rybak, Houlihan, RC Mercier, GW Kaatz. Pharmacodynamics of RP 59500 (quinupristin-dalfopristin) administered by intermittent versus continuous infusion against Staphylococcus aureus-infected fibrin-platelet clots in an in vitro infection model. Antimicrob Agents Chemother 1997;41:1359–1363.
105. B Fantin, R Leclercq, L Garry, C Carbon. Influence of inducible cross-resistance to macrolides, lincosamides, and streptogramin B-type antibiotics in Enterococcus faecium on activity of quinupristin-dalfopristin in vitro and in rabbits with experimental endocarditis. Antimicrob Agents Chemother 1997;41:931- 935.
106. A Turcotte, MG Bergeron. Pharmacodynamic interaction between RP 59500 and gram-positive bacteria infecting fibrin clots. Antimicrob Agents Chemother 1992; 36:2211–2215.
107. HF Chambers. Studies of RP 59500 in vitro and in a rabbit model of aortic valve endocarditis caused by methicillin-resistant Staphylococcus aureus. J Antimicrob Chemother 1992;30(supp A):117–122.
108. B Fantin, R Leclercq, M Ottaviani, JM Vallois, B Maziere, J Duval, JJ Pocidalo, C Carbon. In vivo activities and penetration of the two components of the streptogramin RP 59500 in cardiac vegetations of experimental endocarditis. Antimicrob Agents Chemother 1994;38:432–437.
109. N Berthaud, G Montay, BJ Conard, JF Desnottes. Bactericidal activity and kinetics of RP 59500 in a mouse model of Staphylococcus aureus septicaemia. J Antimicrob Chemother 1995;36:365–373.
110. DH Bouanchaud. In-vitro and in-vivo synergic activity and fractional inhibitory concentration (FIC) of the components of a semisynthetic streptogramin, RP 59500. J Antimicrob Chemother 1992;30(suppl A):95–99.
111. RC Mercier, SR Penzak, MJ Rybak. In vitro activities of an investigational quinolone, glycylcycline, glycopeptide, streptogramin, and oxazolidinone tested alone and in combinations against vancomycin-resistant Enterococcus faecium. Antimicrob Agents Chemother 1997;41:2573–2575.

11

Tetracycline Pharmacodynamics

Burke A. Cunha
Winthrop-University Hospital, Mineola, and the
State University of New York School of Medicine, Stony Brook, New York

Holly M. Mattoes
DesignWrite Incorporated, Princeton, New Jersey

1 INTRODUCTION

The first tetracycline to be discovered, chlortetracycline, was isolated from *Streptomyces aureufaciens* in 1944. Since 1944, several tetracycline analogs have been developed including oxytetracycline, which was introduced in 1950, tetracycline hydrochloride (1953), and demethylchlortetracycline (demeclocycline). In the late 1950s it was discovered that the 6-hydroxyl group could be removed from the basic tetracycline group, which resulted in 6-deoxytetracyclines, with significantly different microbiological and pharmacokinetic properties. In the 1960s, the long-acting tetracyclines were introduced. Doxycycline was isolated in 1962, and minocycline was introduced in 1967. Although all tetracyclines inhibit bacterial protein synthesis, there are significant differences in inherent antibacterial activity between short-acting tetracyclines, e.g., tetracycline, and long-acting second generation tetracyclines, e.g., doxycycline and minocycline [1–3]. The "second generation" tetracyclines have better activity, excellent pharmacokinetics, better intestinal absorption, better tissue penetration, and decreased toxicity [4].

Recently, the glycylcyclines, minocycline derivatives, have demonstrated potent activity against a wide range of pathogens including vancomycin-resistant enterococcus (VRE) [5]. The glycylcyclines have enhanced activity against aerobic and anaerobic bacteria that are typically resistant to tetracycline antimicrobials [6]. This enhanced activity is due to the agents' ability to overcome both of the major resistant mechanisms, ribosomal protection and active efflux, which result in tetracycline resistance. As a result, the glycylcycline spectrum of activity includes penicillin-resistant *Streptococcus pneumoniae*, VRE, and anaerobes like doxycycline [1–3,5].

2 PHARMACOKINETICS OF TETRACYCLINES

2.1 Tetracycline

The tetracycline class of antibiotics are variably absorbed, and their pharmacokinetic properties are often due to the differing relative lipid solubilities and protein-binding capacities. Tetracycline has a shorter serum half-life (6 h) than that of the second-generation antimicrobials, doxycycline (22 h) and minocycline (11–33 h). As a result, the short half-life of tetracycline means it needs to be given as four divided doses daily. In patients with renal failure the half-life of tetracycline dramatically increases, and in patients with severe renal failure the half-life can be prolonged to 57–120 h. Doxycycline does not accumulate in renal failure, and the dose of doxycycline remains unchanged even in dialysis patients with renal failure. Among the class of tetracyclines, protein binding is the lowest with tetracycline, demonstrated to be 20–65% depending on the method of analysis [3]. Unlike doxcycline, the absorption of tetracycline is significantly affected by food and milk, decreasing by up to 50%. Additionally, tetracycline is chelated by cations and therefore should not be used concurrently with antacids.

Pharmacokinetic studies of tetracycline found that serum concentrations after a single 500 mg oral dose peaked at 3–4.3 μg/mL after 2–4 h, whereas in patients with normal renal function at steady state the same dose achieved a peak concentration of 2–5 μg/mL. A 250 mg oral dose had an average peak serum concentration of 2.4 μg at 3 h, and this dropped to 1 μg/mL at 12 h. An in vitro model determined that at therapeutic doses the tissue distribution in the lung achieved concentrations of 0.2–2 μg/mL. Tissue penetration into the lungs appears to be the same whether the lungs are healthy or diseased [7]. Tetracycline has the ability to penetrate into reticuloendothelial cells, which allows for its use against infections by intracellular pathogens such as *Rickettsia*, *Chlamydia*, and *Legionella* [8]. Gram-positive resistance to tetracycline has dramatically limited its use to treat common infections, however, doxycycline and minocycline have no resistance after decades of extensive use [2,10].

2.2 Minocycline

Minocycline and doxycycline are considered second generation tetracyclines, owing to their pharmacokinetic advantages over tetracycline, which result in enhanced tissue and fluid penetration and more convenient once or twice daily dosing regimens. Fewer data have been published regarding the pharmacokinetics of minocycline than that of doxycycline. Minocycline may be given PO or IV, and serum concentrations following a typical dosing regimen of an initial 200 mg dose followed by 100 mg every 12 h results in steady state of 2.3–3.5 μg/mL. The half-life is approximately 17 h after a single dose and 21 h after multiple dosing, and, unlike tetracycline, the half-life is not prolonged or substantially increased in renal failure [8]. The absorption of minocycline is decreased by approximately 20% following ingestion of food and/or milk, but is not clinically significant. Chelation occurs with minocycline; therefore, concomittant antacid use should be avoided. Similar to tetracycline, doxycycline, minocycline demonstrate high concentrations intracellularly, which is useful in treating *Chlamydia* and *Legionella* infections.

2.3 Doxycycline

Doxycycline is highly protein-bound (82%) and has the advantage of being 5 times as lipid-soluble as tetracycline. It is rapidly and almost completely (93%) absorbed from the upper portion of the gastrointestinal tract following oral administration; tetracycline is less efficiently (25–80%) absorbed. Food does not have an important effect on the absorption of orally administered doxycycline, and serum levels are not decreased in the presence of antacids, gluten, or metallic cations. The absorption half-life of doxycycline is approximately 50 min, and detectable serum levels are achieved within 30 min following oral administration. Peak levels occur 2 h after dosing, and the serum $t_{1/2}$ is ~22 h. Oral antacids, however, have been found to increase the total clearance of IV doxycycline, resulting in a decreased half-life [28].

Peak serum levels of doxycycline following a single 200 mg oral dose are ~2.7 μg/mL (range 2.1–4.4 μg/mL). A single 200 mg dose of doxycycline results in serum levels of ~1.6 μg/mL (range of 1.5–1.7 μg/mL). After a 400 mg oral dose, doxycycline serum concentrations are approximately 4.0 μg/mL. Serum levels of doxycycline are the same with either oral or intravenous administration after a steady state is achieved. Intravenous administration of doxycycline results in higher initial serum concentrations, 100 mg (IV) q12h = 4 μg/mL; 100 mg (IV) q8h = 7 μg/mL; 200 mg (IV) q12h = 15 μg/mL. Doxycycline is widely distributed throughout body tissues. Lung levels after 200 mg of doxycycline (IV) achieve concentrations of 6.8 μg/g. Average levels of doxycycline are ~5.9 μg/g. Doxycycline achieves therapeutic levels in the gallbladder, bile duct wall, and bile and readily penetrates respiratory secretions. In patients with acute maxillary sinusitis, doxycycline reaches concentrations of 2.1 μg/mL in sinus secretion. Mean prostatic concentration of doxycycline is ~1.63 μg/g, and doxycycline accumulates in prostatic tissue. In patients given 200 mg doxycycline orally followed by 100 mg/day, average ovarian levels ranged from 3.04 to 3.24 μg/g. Levels of doxycycline in fallopian tubes were 3.21 μg/g. Mean doxycycline levels in breast milk at 24 h after drug administration were about 40% of serum levels. Moderate doxycycline concentrations are also found in umbilical blood and amniotic fluid [1–3,9,10].

Based on doxycyclines pharmacokinetics, therapy should be initiated with a 72 h loading regimen because of its high lipid solubility for serious infections, e.g., Legionnaire's disease. A dose of 200 mg IV q12h provides rapid tissue saturation of doxycycline and is effective in achieving maximum serum concentrations rapidly because ~5 serum half-lives are required before steady-state kinetics are achieved. Doxycycline 100 mg (IV) q12h basis requires 4–5 days of therapy before a therapeutic effect can be achieved. Since the serum $t_{1/2}$ of doxycycline is ~22 h, an initial 72 h loading regimen is required if a rapid therapeutic effect is desired [9,27]. Doxycycline does not significantly accumulate in patients with renal insufficiency. Blood levels of doxycycline in patients with severely impaired renal function are the same as in patients with normal kidneys. Thus, doxycycline should be administered in the usual dosage to patients with renal impairment without risk of accumulation. Hemodialysis has a negligible effect on the serum half-life of doxycycline, and a dosage adjustment is not needed when doxycycline is administered in patients undergoing hemodialysis [1–3,9,10].

2.4 Glycylcyclines

The glycylcyclines are a derivative of minocycline and have good activity against gram-positive/gram-negative pathogens. GAR-936, a member of the glycylcycline class, has good penetration into tissues, with a high tissue/plasma ratio, and a large volume of distribution, 1.01 L/kg, in rats [11]. A study evaluating healthy subjects found that the maximal serum concentration (C_{max}) and area under the serum concentration versus time curve (AUC) values of this antimicrobial agent was of proportional following a 1 h IV infusion of 12.5 mg, resulting in a C_{max} of 0.11 μg/mL and an AUC of 0.9 μg·h/mL. Following a 300 mg dose the C_{max} and AUC increased to 2.8 and 17.9 μg·h/mL, respectively. When GAR-936 was dosed at 50 mg/kg subcutaneously in a murine model of *Pseudomonas aeruginosa*, AUC values reached 63.3 μg·h/mL, achieving better concentrations than a similarly dosed gentamicin, which demonstrated an AUC of 51.1 μg·h/mL [12]. Additionally, the half-life of GAR-936 was found to be long at 36 h [13]. Similarly to tetracycline and minocycline, GAR-936 chelates calcium [11].

3 PHARMACODYNAMICS OF TETRACYCLINES

The tetracyclines are believed to be bacteriostatic when used in vitro; however, in high concentrations are bacteriocidal [3]. Tetracyclines to have time-dependent kill, meaning that the parameter of the time above the minimum inhibitory concentration of the pathogen ($T >$ MIC) best describes the killing by these drugs. For time-dependent killing, the killing is dependent on the length of time the bacteria are exposed to the antibiotic. As the area under the concentration versus time curve for plasma (AUC) approaches 2–4 times the MIC value of the organism, the effect is maximized. Here the rate of killing plateau and additional serum drug concentration have a negligible effect, and it is the time above the MIC is the important parameter related to bacterial kill and antibacterial activity. Generally for these agents the $T >$ MIC should be at least 50% of the dosing interval for immunocompetent patients, whereas immunocompromised patients may require the $T >$ MIC 100% of the dosing interval.

Tetracycline was once useful for a variety of gram-positive and gram-negative pathogens. However, as a result of increased resistance, it is now typically reserved for uncommon infections. Additionally, plasma-mediated resistance is occurring as a result of overuse in animal feeds containing tetracycline, and it appears that most acquired resistance of gram-positive and -negative pathogens is a result of this plasma-mediated problem [3]. This makes it difficult to treat infections by common gram-positive organisms, which currently demonstrate a high level of resistance to tetracycline. Tetracycline resistance is usually a result of active drug efflux due to an exogenous metal–tetracycline/H^+ antiporter. Similarly, doxycycline and minocycline do not share this resistance problem, these second generation tetracyclines have excellent antimicrobial activity [14].

Doxycycline is useful against a broad range of pathogens. However, it was introduced prior to the appreciation of current pharmacodynamic concepts, and as a result it is only recently that the optimal dosing regimen for doxycycline was determined [15–20]. Time-kill kinetic studies demonstrated that at low concentrations, i.e., at 2–4 times the MIC, 100 mg (IV/PO) q12h of doxycycline kills the organisms tested in a time-dependent manner. At higher serum concentrations, 200 mg (IV/PO) q12h or 400 mg (IV/PO) q24h, i.e., 8–16 times the MIC of the organisms, doxycycline exhibits concentration-dependent killling [17–20] (Fig. 1). Additionally, the postantibiotic effect (PAE) of doxycycline influences the pharmacodynamics of this agent. PAE $= T - C$, where T is the time required for the counts of CFU/mL in the test culture to increase by 1 $\log_{10}$ above the count observed immediately after antibiotic removal and c is the time required for the count of CFU/mL in an untreated control culture to increase 1 $\log_{10}$ above the count observed immediately after completion of the same procedure used on the test culture for antibiotic removal. Doxycycline has a PAE for gram-positive and gram-negative aerobic organisms that was found to be concentration-dependent. Doxycycline has a PAE of 2.1–4.2 h with gram-positive and gram-negative organisms [20] (Fig. 2). This is similar to the PAE of tetracycline, which varies between 2 and 3 h.

Glycylcyclines demonstrate time-dependent (concentration-independent) kinetics. This was demonstrated in a thigh infection model, which found that $T >$ MIC was the best correlated pharmacodynamic model [21]. The study compared two glycylcyclines, GAR 936 and WAY 152,288, against a variety of common gram-positive and gram-negative pathogens. Whereas the glycylcycline GAR 936 only required the concentration of free drug to remain above the MIC for 50% of the dosing interval for effective eradication of *Streptococcus pneumoniae*, *Escherichia coli*, and *Klebsiella pneumoniae*, similar killing with WAY 152,288 required the MIC to be exceeded for at least 75% of the dosing interval using the same isolates. Because of the long half-lives and PAEs of these agents, the AUC also may play a predictive role in the killing of organisms [21].

It has been determined that for GAR 936 a single dose of 300 mg IV would provide a concentration of 2 μg/mL for 75% of the time [22]. The glycylcyclines would also have excellent activity against *Staphylococcus aureus* (MSSA), which for GAR 936 demonstrates MICs ranging from 0.06 to 1 μg/mL, and the MIC_{90} values for MSSA is 0.5 μg/mL [23]. An endocarditis model [24] found that when serum levels fell below the MIC before 50% of the dosing interval GAR 936 was as effective in eradicating VanA-resistant *Enterococcus faecium* as when serum levels were constantly above the MIC throughout the dosing interval. The authors concluded that this result may be due to the low clearance of the agent, GAR 936, from the endocarditis vegetations as well as the long PAE against enterococci [24].

Glycylcyclines has good activity against anaerobic bacteria, covering most common anerobic pathogens. Unlike doxycycline and minocycline, glycylcyines have litle activity against *Bacteroides fragilis* and possibly *Clostridium perfringens* [25]. For *Mycoplasma pneumoniae* the susceptibility of GAR 936 measured by the MIC_{50} was 0.2 μg/mL, twice that of doxycycline/minocycline and twofold less than that of tetracycline [26].

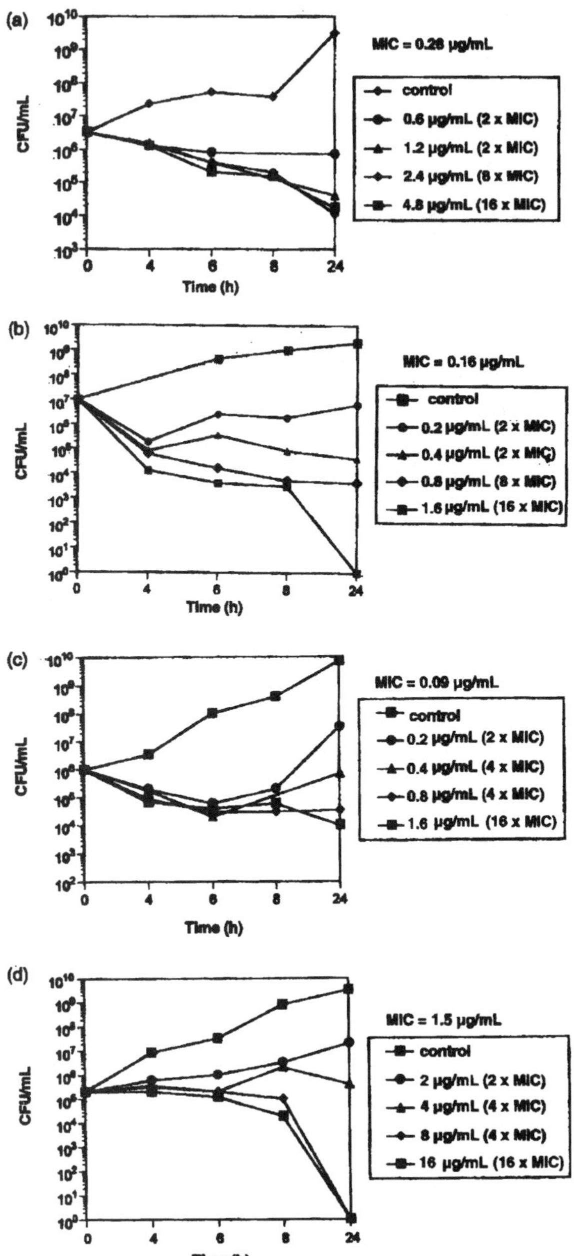

FIGURE 1 Doxycycline kill curves for (a) *Staphylococcus aureus*; (b) *Streptococcus pneumoniae*; (c) *Pasteurella multocida;* (d) *Escherichia coli*. (With permission from Ref. 20.)

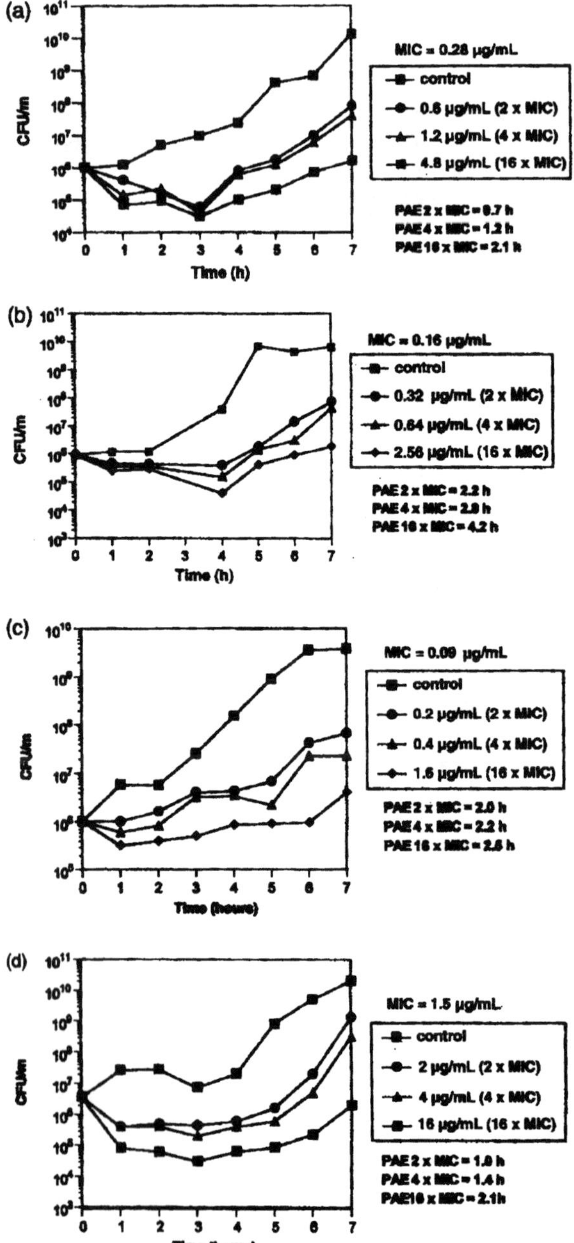

FIGURE 2 Doxycycline postantibiotic effects (PAEs) for (a) *Staphylococcus aureus*; (b) *Streptococcus pneumoniae*; (c) *Pasteurella maltophilia;* (d) *Escherichia coli*. (With permission from Ref. 20.)

DISCUSSION

Although tetracyclines have been useful in treating a wide variety of pathogens since the early 1900s, increased resistance has made tetracycline second-line therapy until recently with the advent of doxycycline and minocycline. Glycylcyclines appear to be effective in treating a wide range of gram-positive, gram-negative, and anaerobic bacteria. The second generation tetracyclines doxycycline and minocycline have increased pharmacokinetic and pharmacodynamic advantages over tetracycline, and other advantages in overall dosing, allowing for their potential once daily dosing as a result of their long PAEs and half-lives and increased activity against common pathogens which maintain their position in the antibiotic armamentarism as first line agents [27–30].

REFERENCES

1. BA Cunha. Clinical uses of tetracyclines. In: RK Blackwood, JJ Hlavka, JH Booth, eds. The Tetracyclines. Springer-Verlag, Berlin, 1985:393.
2. BA Cunha, JB Comer, M Jonas. The tetracyclines. Med Clin North Am 1982;66: 293.
3. NC Klein, BA Cunha. Tetracyclines. Med Clin North Am 1995;79:789–801.
4. N Joshi, DQ Miller. Doxycycline revisited. Arch Intern Med 1997;157:1421–1428.
5. PJ Petersen, NV Jacobus, WJ Weiss, PE Sum, RT Testa. In vitro and in vivo antibacterial activities of a novel glycylcycline, the 9-t-butylglycylamido derivative of minocycline (GAR-936). Antimicrob Agents Chemother 1999;43:738–744.
6. RT Testa, PJ Petersen, NV Jacobus, P Sum, VJ Lee, FP Tally. In vitro and in vivo antibacterial activities of the glycylcyclines, a new class of semisynthetic tetracyclines. Antimicrob Agents Chemother 1993;37:2270–2277.
7. MP Fournet, R Zini, L DeForges, F Lange, J Lange, JP Tillement. Tetracycline and erythromycin distribution in pathological lungs of humans and rat. J Pharm Sci 1989; 78:1015–1019.
8. GK McEvoy, ed. Tetracyclines. In: American Hospital Formularly Service Drug Information. American Society of Health System Pharmacists, Bethesda, MD, 1997: 368–386.
9. BA Cunha. The pharmacokinetics of doxycycline. Postgrad Med Commun 1979;1: 43–50.
10. BA Cunha. Doxycycline. Antibiotics Clin 1999;3:21–27.
11. NL Tombs. Tissue distribution of GAR-936, a broad spectrum antibiotic, in male rats. 39th Interscience Conference on Antimicrobial Agents and Chemotherapy, 1999, abstr P-413.
12. SM Mikels, AS Brown, L Breden, S Compton, S Mitelman, PJ Petersen, WJ Weiss. In vivo activities of GAR-936 (GAR), gentamicin (GEN), piperacillin (PIP), alone and in combination in a murine model of Pseudomonas aeruginosa pneumonia. 39th Interscience Conference on Antimicrobial Agents and Chemotherapy, 1999, abstr P-414.

13. G Muralidaharan, J Getsy, P Mayer, I Paty, M Micalizzi, J Speth, B Webster, P Mojaverian. Pharmacokinetics (PK), safety and tolerability of GAR-936, a novel glycylcycline antibiotic, in healthy subjects. 39th Interscience Conference on Antimicrobial Agents and Chemotherapy, 1999, abstr P-416.
14. Y Someya, A Yamaguchi, T Sawai. A novel glycylcycline, 9-(n,n-dimethylglycylamido)-6-demethyl-6-deoxytetracycline, is neither transported nor recognized by the transposon TN10-endoced metal-tetracycline/H^+ antiporter. Antimicrob Agents Chemother 1995;39:247–249.
15. WA Craig. Pharmacokinetic/pharmacodynamic parameters: Rationale for antibacterial dosing of mice and men. Clin Infect Dis 1998;26:1–12.
16. K Totsuka, K Shimizu. In vitro and in vivo post-antibiotic effects (PAE) of CL 331,928 (DMG-DMDOT), a new glycylcycline against Staphylococcus aureus. 34th Interscience Conference on Antimicrobial Agents and Chemotherapy, 1994:179, abstr F114.
17. WA Craig, SC Ebert. Killing and regrowth of bacteria in vitro: A review. Scand J Infect Dis Suppl 1991;74:63–70.
18. O Cars, I Odenholt-Tornquist. The post-antibiotic sub-MIC effect in vitro and in vivo. J Antimicrob Chemother 1993;31:159–166.
19. WA Craig, S Gudmundsson. Post-antibiotic effect. In: V Lorian, ed. Antibiotics in Laboratory Medicine. 4th ed. Williams and Wilkins, Baltimore, 1996:296–329.
20. BA Cunha, P Domenico, CB Cunha. Pharmacodynamics of doxycycline. Clin Microb Infect Dis 2000;6:270–273.
21. ML van Ogtrop, D Andes, TJ Stamstad, B Conklin, WJ Weiss, WA Craig, O Vesga. In vivo pharmacodynamic activities of two glycylcyclines (GAR-936 and WAY 152,288) against various gram-positive and gram-negative bacteria. Antimicrobial Agents Chemother 2000;44:943–949.
22. HW Boucher, CB Wennersten, RC Moellering, GM Eliopoulos. In vitro activity of GAR-936 against gram-positive bacteria. 39th Interscience Conference on Antimicrobial Agents and Chemotherapy, 1999, abstr. P-406.
23. E Mahalingam, L Trepeski, S Pongporter, J De Azavedo, DE Lo, BN Kreiswirth. In vitro activity of new glycylcycline, Gar 936 against methicillin-resistant and -susceptible Staphylococcus aureus isolated in North America. 39th Interscience Conference on Antimicrobial Agents and Chemotherapy, 1999, abstr. P-408.
24. A Lefort, L Massias, A Saleh-Mghir, M LaFaurie, L Garry, C Carbon, B Fantin. Pharmacodynamics of GAR-936 (GAR) in experimental endocarditis due to VAN A-type Enterococcus faecium. 40th Interscience Conference on Antimicrobial Agents and Chemotherapy, 2000, abstr P-2256.
25. M Hedberg, CE Nord. In vitro activity of anaerobic bacteria to GAR-936, a new glycylcycline. 39th Interscience Conference on Antimicrobial Agents and Chemotherapy, 1999, abstr P-411.
26. GE Kenny, FD Cartwright. The susceptibility of human mycoplasmas to a new glycylcycline, GAR 936. 39th Interscience Conference on Antimicrobial Agents and Chemotherapy, 1999, abstr P-412.
27. VX Nguyen, DE Nix, S Gillikin, JJ Schentag. Effect of oral antacid administration on the pharmacokinetics of intravenous doxycycline. Antimicrob Agents Chemother 1989;33:434–436.

28. HW Boucher, CB Wennersten, GM Eliopoulis. In vitro activities of the glycycline GAR-936 against gram positive bacteria. Antimicrob Agents Chemother 2000;44: 2225–2229.
29. KW Shea, Y Ueno, F Abumustafa, SMH Qadri, BA Cunha. Doxycycline activity against streptococcus pneumoniae. Chest 1995;107:1775–1776.
30. BA Cunha. Doxycycline revisited. Intern Med 1997;10:65–69.

12

Pharmacodynamics of Antivirals

George L. Drusano, Sandra L. Preston, and Peter J. Piliero
Albany Medical College, Albany, New York

1 INTRODUCTION

Although pharmacodynamic relationships for antibacterial agents have been sought and identified for a long period of time, it has been a general feeling that the treatment of viral and fungal infections was different in kind. A corollary to this is that delineation of pharmacodynamic relationships would be much more difficult.

In reality, the exact principles that govern the delineation of pharmacokinetic/pharmacodynamic (PK/PD) relationships for antibacterials also govern antifungals and, as will be shown here, antivirals.

The first issue, as always in the development of dynamics relationships, is to decide upon an endpoint. Most of the data for this chapter have been derived from studies of the human immunodeficiency virus (HIV), Type 1. Consequently, this chapter addresses the in vitro and in vivo data for this virus. Other viruses should behave in a similar fashion (as is seen with cytomegalovirus). An exception to the rule is hepatitis C virus (among others), because of our inability to obtain more than one round of viral replication in vitro.

With HIV-1, there are a number of endpoints that may be chosen. Some are

1. Survivorship
2. Change in CD_4 count consequent to therapy
3. Change in viral load consequent to therapy
4. Change in the hazard of emergence of resistance consequent to therapy
5. Durability of maintaining the viral load below detectable levels

Survivorship is, as always, the ultimate test of an intervention. With the advent of potent HIV chemotherapy, this disease process has been converted from a relatively rapid killer to one that will likely take its toll over a number of decades. Consequently, survivorship may not be the best endpoint to examine for clinical studies, because of the long lead times. In this chapter, we concentrate on endpoints 2–5 for clinical studies.

In anti-HIV chemotherapy, as in antibacterial chemotherapy, one can generate pharmacodynamic relationships from in vitro approaches as well as from clinical studies. One difference between these areas is the ease of employing animal systems for the generation of dynamic relationships. For antibacterials, there are many examples of the generation of dynamic relationships for different drug classes [1–3]. For HIV, the cost and ethical implications of using simian models has prevented much work in this area. The McCune model and its variants are attractive, but again, because of the cost of maintaining the system, little has been done to develop dynamic relationships for HIV in animal systems. Other retroviruses have been employed [4,5], but it is difficult to draw inferences for human chemotherapy of HIV from a different pathogen with different pathogenetic properties.

Consequently, in this chapter, in vitro but not animal model systems are also reviewed to add insight gleaned from these systems.

2 IN VITRO SYSTEMS

Although one might consider determination of viral EC_{50} or EC_{90} to be a pharmacodynamic system measurement, this chapter takes the view that this is simply a static measure of drug potency. It will play (see below) an important role in determining the final shape of the pharmacodynamic relationship when added to other measures. Alone, it is merely a measure of compound potency.

For in vitro systems to be true pharmacodynamic systems, there must be the possibility of changing drug concentrations over time to examine the effect for a pathogen of known susceptibility to the drug employed. The only system with peer-reviewed publication for HIV-1 is shown in Fig. 1. In addition, it is important to factor in the effect of protein binding, as only the free drug is virologically active.

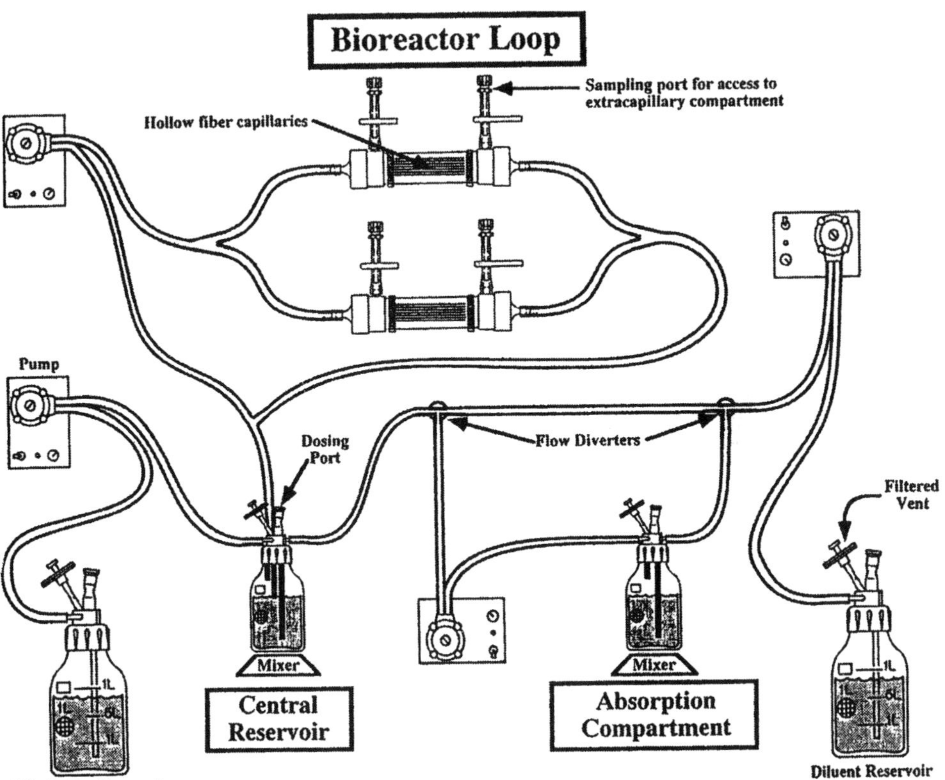

FIGURE 1 Schematic diagram of the in vitro pharmacodynamic model system. One of the two systems enclosed within a single incubator housed in a biological safety cabinet is shown. Cells are grown, and samples are removed from the extracapillary compartment of HF bioreactors. Constant infusion, oral, or intravenous bolus doses are introduced through the dosing ports in the diluent reservoir, absorption compartment, or central reservoir, respectively. Exposure of cells to fluctuating concentrations of D4T is affected by programmed dilution of drug within the central reservoir, while the volume of the central compartment is maintained constant by elimination. The mean pore diameter of the HF capillaries (10 kDa) would prevent HIV or HIV-infected cells from exiting the bioreactor and from circulating through the tubing. (Further information is available upon request.)

3 PROTEIN BINDING

The effect of protein binding has been examined in greatest detail for its effect on the anti-HIV potency of a drug by this laboratory. Bilello et al. [6] examined an HIV-1 protease inhibitor (A-80987) and determined the effect of protein binding on free-drug concentration, on drug uptake into infected cells, and, finally, on the virological effect of the drug. This set of experiments has a ''transitive logic'' organization.

In the first experiment (Fig. 2), increasing concentrations of the binding protein, α−1 acid glycoprotein, were introduced into the test system and the concentration of unbound drug was determined. As can be seen, increasing binding protein concentration leads to monotonically decreasing free-drug concentrations.

In Fig. 3, the amount of drug that penetrates infected CEM cells is shown as a function of the free fraction of the drug. Increased external free-drug concentration results in an increased amount of intracellular drug (stop oil experiments) in a linear function. Finally (Fig. 4), the amount of intracellular drug is related to the decrement of p24 output, as indexed through an inhibitory sigmoid-Emax model. It is clear through this series of experiments that only the free-drug concentration can induce a decrease in viral production.

These data make it clear that it is important to interpret drug concentrations in the hollow fiber system as representing the external free-drug concentrations necessary to induce the desired antiviral effect.

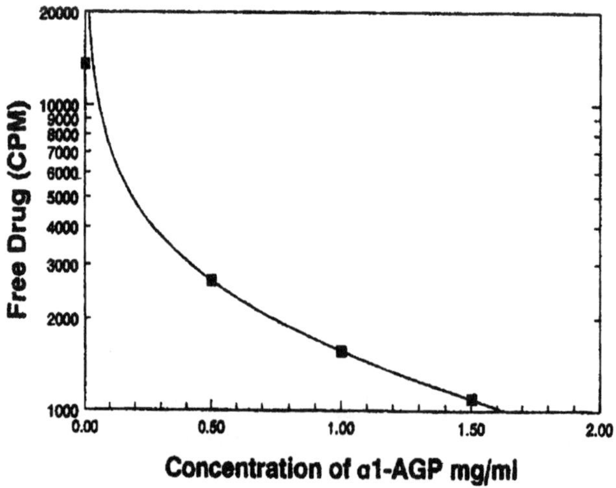

FIGURE 2 Relationship between increasing ″−1 acid glycoprotein concentration and A-80987 free drug concentration.

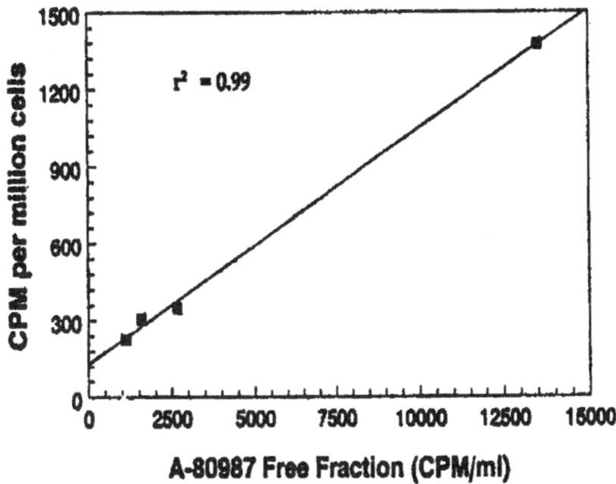

FIGURE 3 Relationship between increasing A-80987 free fraction and intracellular A-80987.

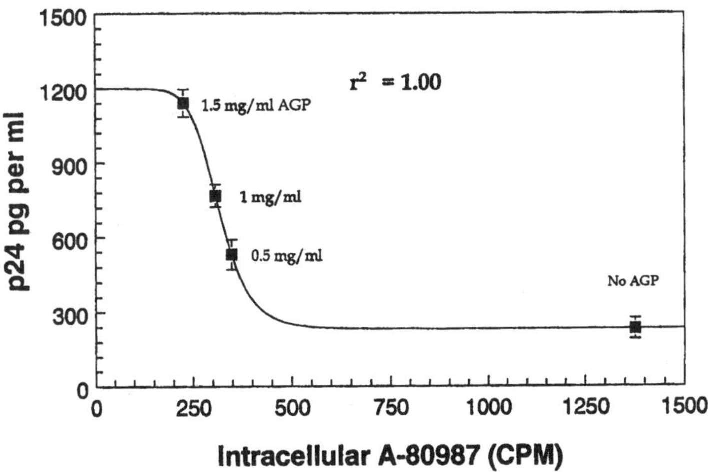

FIGURE 4 Relationship (inhibitory sigmoid E_{max}) between intracellular A-80987 and HIV viral output from infected PBMCs.

The most obvious place to initiate evaluation of anti-HIV agents is with the nucleoside analogs and with the HIV-1 protease inhibitors. The first published hollow fiber evaluation of an antiviral was the nucleoside analog stavudine (d4T). Bilello et al. [7] examined issues of dose finding and schedule dependency for this drug.

It is important to examine the development of stavudine in order to place its evaluation in the hollow fiber system in the proper perspective. The initial clinical evaluation of stavudine was initiated at a total daily dose of 2 mg/kg per day. The initial schedule chosen was every 8 h. Whereas the initial dose had an effect, dose escalation to 12 mg/kg per day produced no change in effect but much higher rates of drug-related neuropathy [8].

After this, the dose was de-escalated to 4 mg/kg per day and the schedule was lengthened to every 12 h. Further dose de-escalation was taken from this point on a 12 h schedule, and nine dosing cohorts were eventually examined. This process took approximately 2 years.

The hollow fiber evaluation took approximately 3 months. The identified dose was ultimately the dose chosen by the phase I/II trial and has stood the test of time and usage. It is, at least to our knowledge, the first prospective identification of a drug dose and schedule from an in vitro test system with clinical validation. The outcome of the experiments is illustrated in Fig. 5. This evaluation makes clear that for nucleoside analogs the pharmacodynamically linked variable is AUC/EC_{90}. With matching AUCs (Fig. 5), there was no difference in outcome between the exposure being given in a continuous infusion mode and half the exposure every 12 h (data not shown). The reason is likely the phosphorylation of the parent compound into the virologically active form of the molecule (the triphosphate for stavudine, or diphosphate for prephosphorylated compounds such as tenofovir). It is clear from Figs. 6 and 7 that there is full effect at 0.5 mg/kg every 12 h, irrespective of starting challenge. At half the exposure (0.25 mg/kg q12h), there is a hint of loss of control late in the experiment. Finally, at 0.125 mg/kg q12h, there is no discernible antiretroviral effect.

HIV-1 protease inhibitors have also been examined in this system. The first to be examined was the early Abbott inhibitor A-77003. This drug was a proof-of-principle agent and was administered intravenously as a continuous infusion. Consequently, the hollow fiber evaluation was performed as a continuous infusion. When protein binding was taken into account, the concentrations required for effect were above those tolerable clinically. Consequently, the drug was predicted to fail. Indeed, an extensive phase I/II evaluation came to this conclusion [9,10].

The next protease inhibitor evaluated was amprenavir (141W94). Here [11], time $> EC_{90}$ was demonstrated to be the pharmacodynamically linked variable. Dosing intervals of q12h and q8h with matching AUCs were compared to

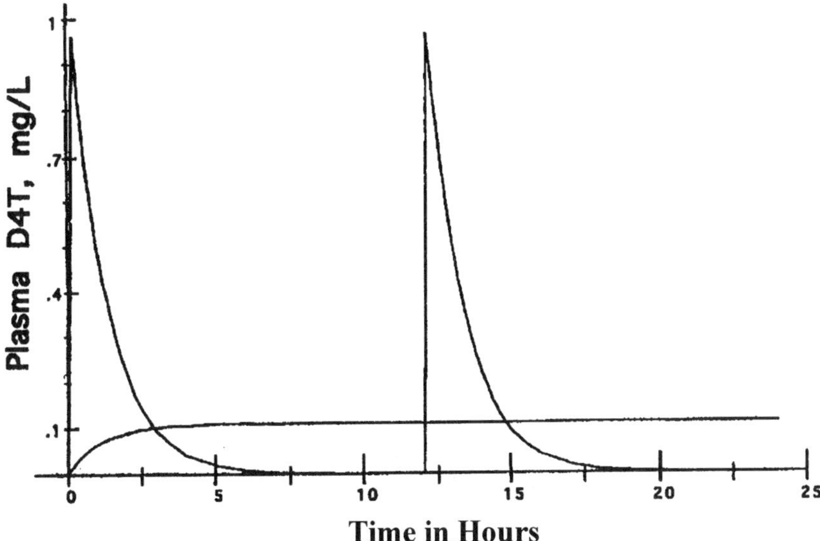

FIGURE 5 The concentration–time profile for stavudine in the hollow fiber unit is displayed for a 1 mg/(kg · day) dose administered either as a continuous infusion or as 0.5 mg/kg administered every 12 h. The AUCs developed are identical. The ability to suppress viral replication was identical for the regimens.

continuous infusion of the same AUC. Continuous infusion provided the most robust viral control, followed closely by q8h dosing. Every 12 h dosing lost a significant fraction of the control of viral turnover. This outcome was to be expected, as HIV-1 protease inhibitors are reversible inhibitors, freely cross cell membranes without the requirement for energy or a transporter, and do not require activation (phosphorylation) for effect as the nucleoside analogs do.

A third protease inhibitor was examined, the potent once-daily PI BMS 232632 [12]. In addition to the hollow fiber unit evaluation, the technique of Monte Carlo simulation was also brought to bear on the outcome of these experiments.

In Fig. 8, it is clear that time $> EC_{90}$ is the pharmacodynamically linked variable. In the one instance, complete control of viral replication in vitro is achieved with a continuous infusion regimen at $4 \times EC_{50}$ (about EC_{90-95}). This same daily AUC administered as a bolus allows breakthrough growth. Four times this daily AUC administered as a bolus regains control of the viral replication. Indeed, this latter part of the experiment demonstrates that free-drug concentraa

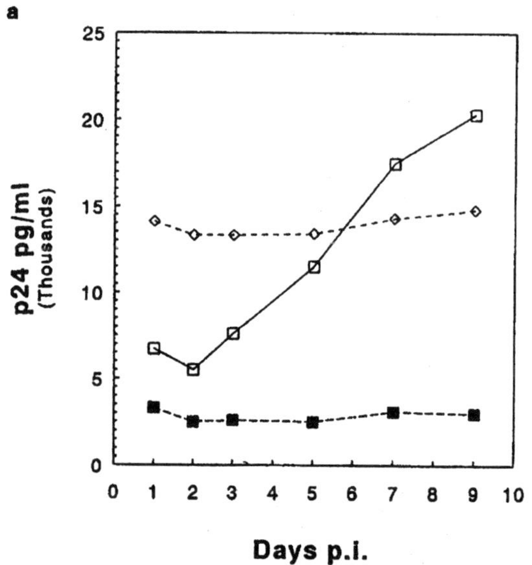

b

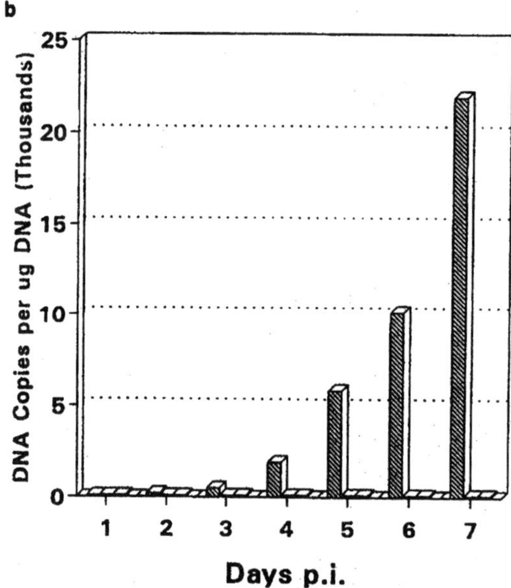

Figure 6 Panel a displays the increase in p24 output over time in a hollow fiber tube that was an untreated control (□), in a treated (0.5 mg/kg q12h) tube where 1/1000 cells were chronically HIV-infected at start (■) or where 1/100 cells were HIV-infected at start (◇). Panel b shows numbers of HIV DNA copies in treated and untreated hollow fiber units.

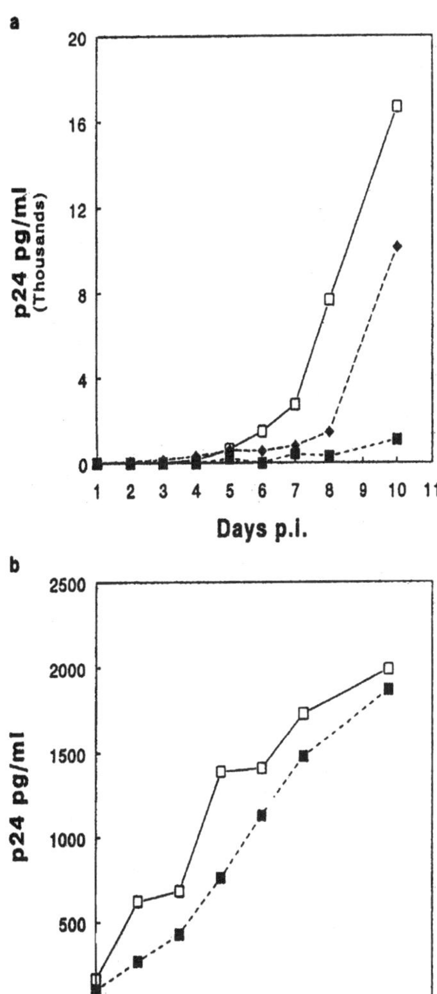

FIGURE 7 Panel a displays the increase in p24 output over time in a hollow fiber tube that was an untreated control (□), in a treated (0.25 mg/kg q12h) tube where 1/1000 cells were chronically HIV-infected at start (■) or where 1/100 cells were HIV-infected at start (◆). Panel b shows p24 output in a treated hollow fiber unit (0.125 mg/kg q12h [■]) and untreated control (□).

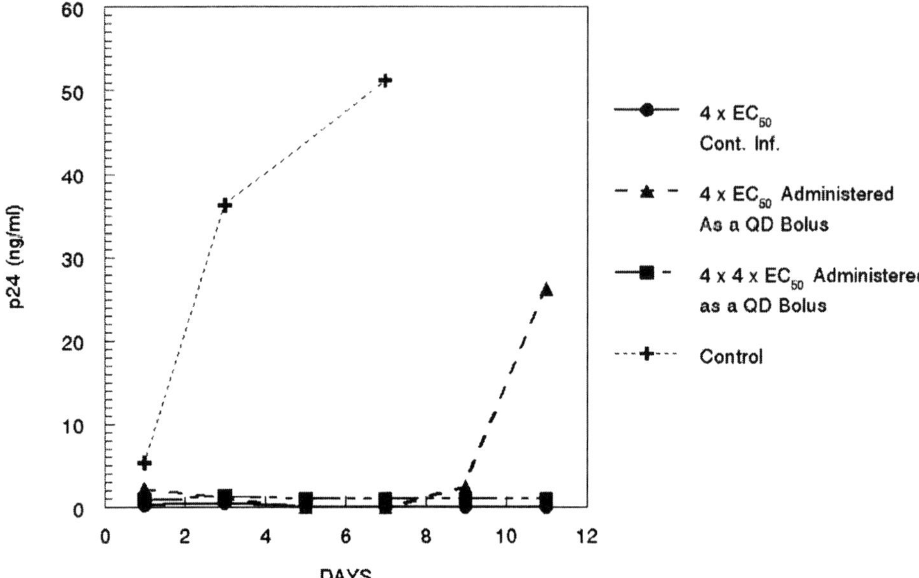

FIGURE 8 Effect of BMS 232632 on HIV replication. Three infected hollow fiber units were treated with BMS 232632. One tube was treated with a concentration of four times the EC_{50} as a continuous infusion. This produced a 24 h AUC of $4 \times 24 \times EC_{50}$. The second tube received the same 24 h AUC but was given in a peak-and-valley mode once daily. The third tube received an exposure calculated a priori to provide a time $> EC_{90}$ that would give essentially the same suppression as the continuous infusion of $4 \times EC_{50}$.

tions need to exceed the EC_{90} for approximately 80–85% of a dosing interval in order to maintain control of the HIV turnover. This served as the therapeutic target for further evaluation.

The sponsor provided pharmacokinetic data for BMS 232632 administered to normal volunteers at doses of 400 mg and 600 mg orally, once daily at steady state. Population pharmacokinetic analysis was performed, and the mean parameter vector and covariance matrix were employed to perform Monte Carlo simulation. The ability to attain the therapeutic target was assessed, accounting for the population variability in the handling of the drug. This is demonstrated in Fig. 9. The viral isolate susceptibilities to BMS 232632 are displayed as EC_{50} values. However, an internal calculation corrects for the difference between EC_{50} and EC_{90} as well as for the protein binding of the drug. The fractional target attainment is for free drug being greater than the nominal EC_{90} for 85% of the dosing interval

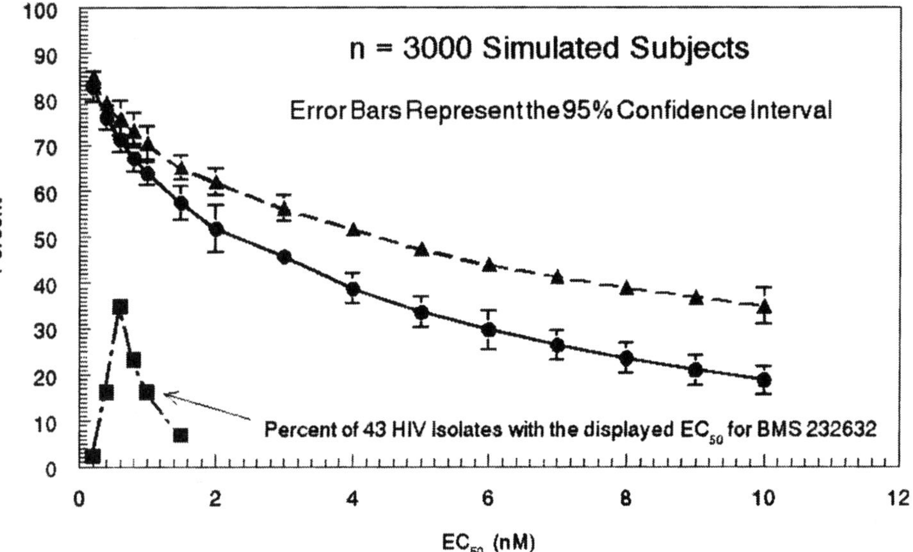

FIGURE 9 A Monte Carlo simulation of 1000 subjects performed three times was employed to estimate the fraction of these subjects whose concentration–time curve would produce maximal viral suppression on the basis of the data presented in Fig. 2. The evaluation was performed for doses of (●) 400 mg and (▲) 600 mg of BMS 232632, administered once daily by mouth. (■) Forty-three isolates from a clinical trial of BMS 232632 were tested by the Virologics Phenosense assay.

(the therapeutic target determined in Fig. 8). As can be seen, as the viral isolates become less and less susceptible to BMS 232632, the greater the difference between the 400 mg and 600 mg doses. The sponsors also determined the viral susceptibility to 43 clinical isolates from a phase I/II clinical trial of the drug in patients who were HIV-treatment naive. As can be seen, all had EC_{50} values below 2 nM. Consequently, this allows us to take an expectation over the distribution of measured EC_{50} values to determine the fraction of patients who will attain a maximal response to the drug, under the assumptions that the viral susceptibility distribution is correct for naive patients and that the kinetics in normal volunteers and its distribution are a fair representation of the kinetics of the drug in infected but treatment-naive patients. When this calculation is performed, approximately 69% of subjects taking the 400 mg dose will obtain a complete response, whereas slightly greater than 74% of patients taking 600 mg will obtain a complete response.

A clear lesson learned regarding the chemotherapy of HIV is that combination chemotherapy is more effective than monotherapy. However, little has been done to determine optimal combination dosing regimens. An initial effort to determine the interaction of antivirals in a fully parametric system was published by Drusano et al. [13]. The Greco model was fit to the data from an in vitro examination of 141W94 (amprenavir, an HIV-1 protease inhibitor) plus 1592U89 (abacavir, a nucleoside analog). This interaction is displayed in Figs. 10–12. Figure 10 displays the full effect surface from these two agents. The effects of protein binding are taken into account as the effects are developed in the presence of

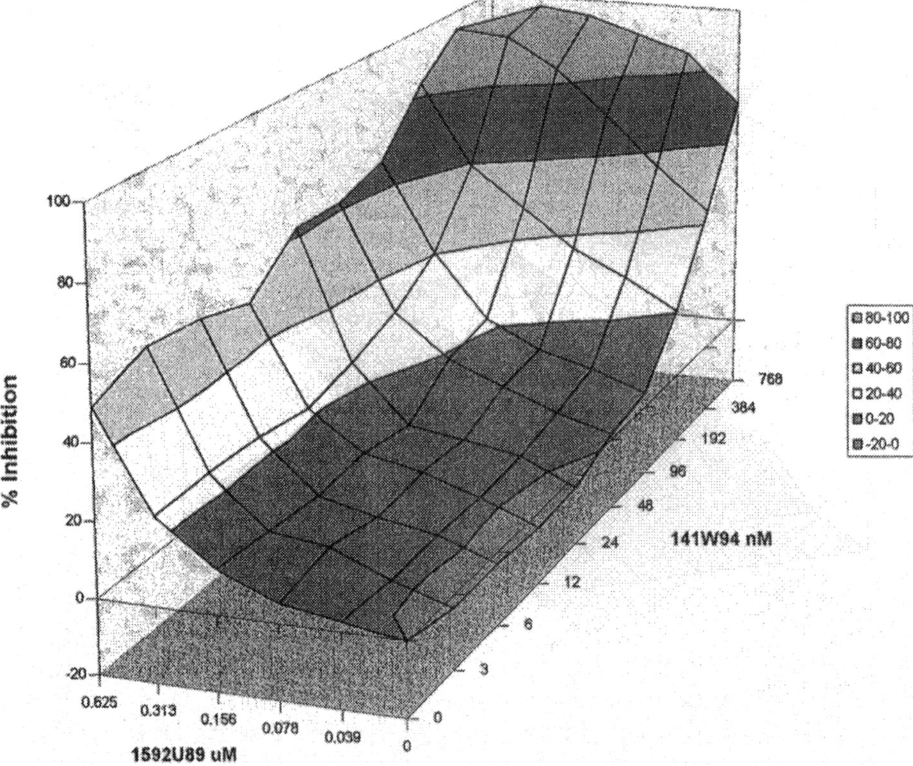

FIGURE 10 1592U89 and 141W94 combination study with albumin (40 mg/mL) and α−1 acid glycoprotein (1 mg/mL). A three-dimensional response surface representing the interaction from the in vitro matrix is displayed. Percent inhibition data from a 3-(4.5-dimethylthiazol-2-yl)-2,5-diphenyltetrazolium bromide assay with HIV-1_{IIIB} and MT-2 cells is displayed.

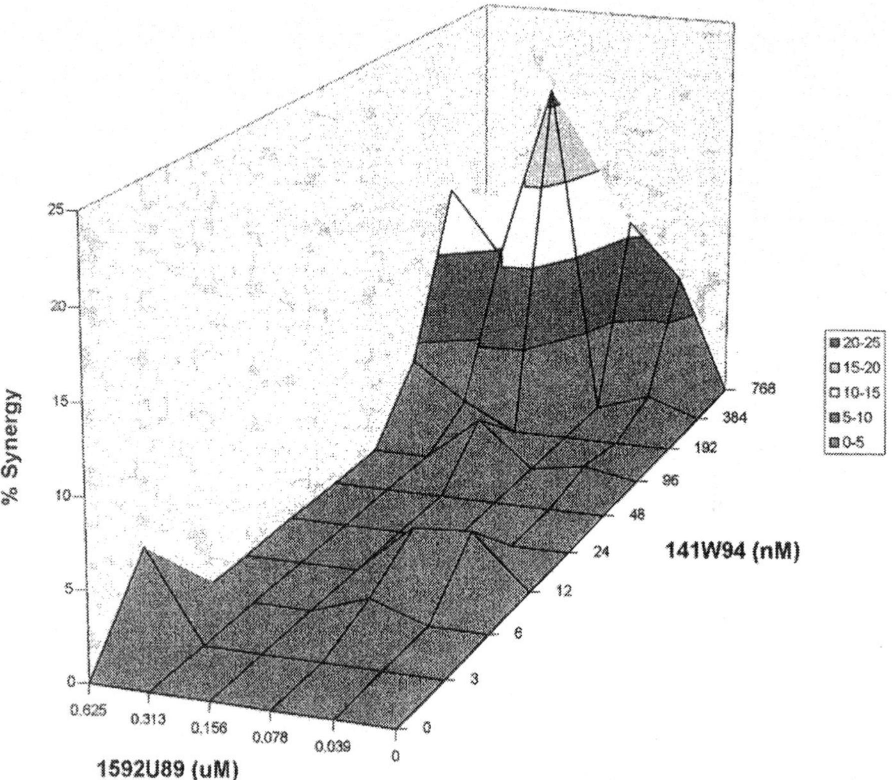

FIGURE 11 Synergy plot drawn from the data displayed in Figure 10. Plotted at the 95% confidence level.

physiological amounts of the binding proteins human albumin and human $\alpha-1$ acid glycoprotein. The drug interaction can be seen by subtracting the theoretical additive surface, and the synergy surface is seen in Fig. 11. It is important to note that there in synergy across all concentrations of the agents. As a model was fit to the data, the weighted residuals are displayed in Fig. 12 to demonstrate that the actual regression process was unbiased. The actual degree of interaction is given by estimation of the interaction parameter, α, which is 1.144. The 95% confidence bound about the interaction parameter is from 0.534 to 1.754. As this boundary does not cross zero, the synergy is significant at the 0.05 level.

This fully parametric analysis was employed in combination with Monte Carlo simulation to examine whether the drugs at the doses used clinically would

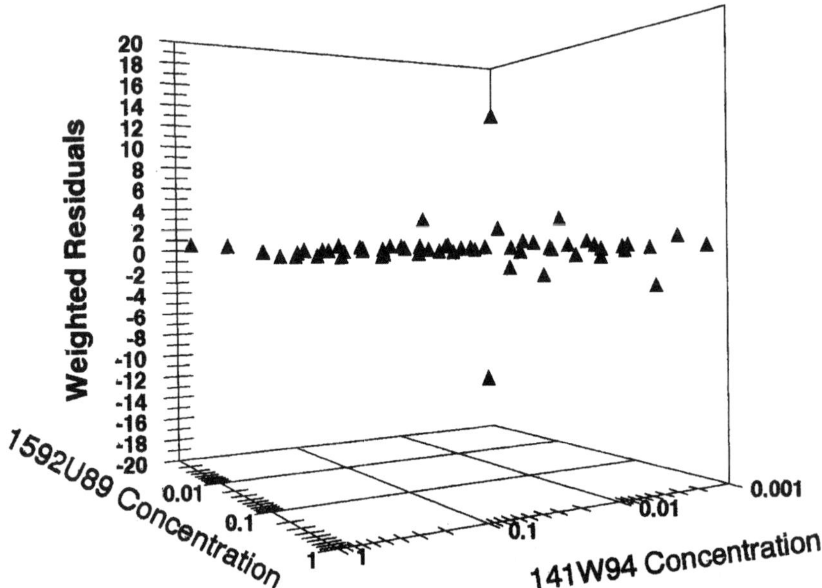

FIGURE 12 Weighted residual plot from the fully parametric analysis. The residuals are scattered about the zero line without bias.

be synergistic and whether the dosing interval affected the outcome [14]. The answer to both these questions was found to be yes. The data are displayed in Chapter 14.

4 CLINICAL STUDIES OF ANTIVIRAL PHARMACODYNAMICS

As noted previously, the first decision required for determining a pharmacodynamics relationship in the clinic is the choice of an endpoint. In this section, the change in CD_4 counts, the change from baseline viral load, prevention of resistance, and durability of maintenance of viral loads below detectability are the endpoints examined. Where possible, they are examined for both nucleoside analogs and HIV-1 protease inhibitors, both alone and in combination.

Use of nucleoside analogs as monotherapy occurred mostly at a time when viral copy number determinations were not freely available. Consequently, virtually all the available studies employed change in CD_4 cell count or p24 as the dynamic endpoint.

One of the first studies in this regard examined dideoxyinosine (ddI) use in a naive patient population [15]. No concentration–effect response was found for CD_4 cells, but a clear relationship was discerned between the number of CD_4 cells present at baseline and the number of cells that returned with the initiation of ddI therapy (Fig. 13). In addition, this study found a relationship between ddI exposure (as indexed to the area under the plasma concentration–time curve, AUC) and the fall in p24, both within patients and across the population (Fig. 14). The finding reported in the study just cited was also found for zidovudine [16].

More recently, Fletcher et al. [17] examined the relationship between ddI AUC and fall in viral load in children (Fig. 15). This study is flawed by the fact that the relationships were developed in patients receiving combination chemotherapy without any effort being made to account for the interaction between drugs.

With regard to emergence of resistance, there was one important study, largely ignored, that demonstrated the importance of viral susceptibility for effect. Kozal et al. [18] examined patients switching from zidovudine to didanosine (ddI). Over half of such patients developed a mutation at codon 74 by week 24 of ddI therapy that is known to confer ddI resistance. The effect on the number

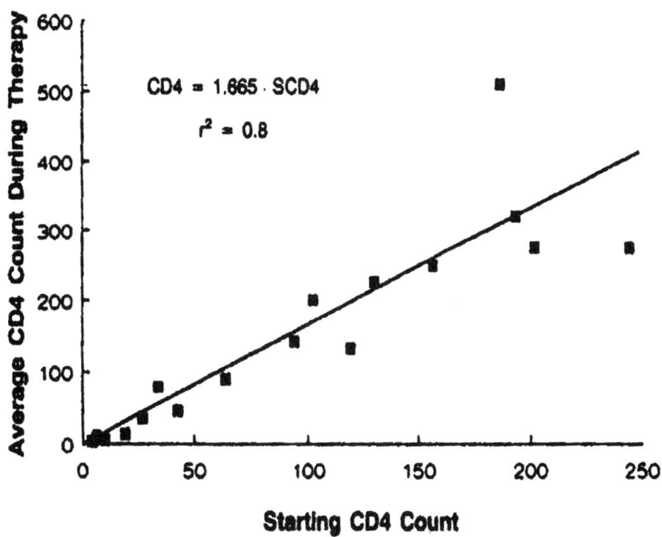

FIGURE 13 Linear regression between the number of CD_4-positive T-lymphocytes during therapy with dideoxyinosine and the baseline CD_4 count.

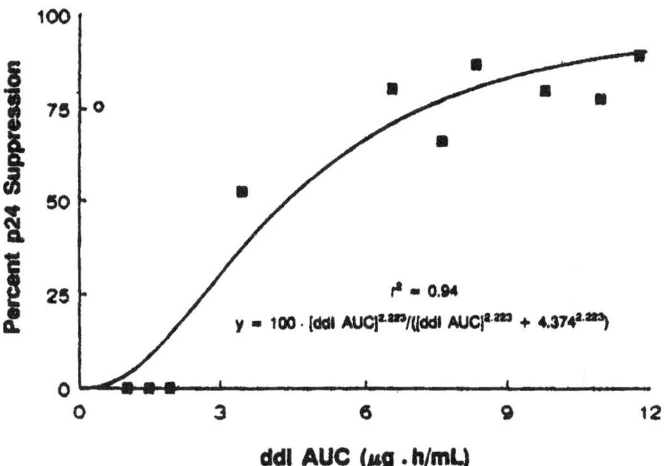

FIGURE 14 Relation between the suppression of p24 antigen and the steady-state area under the plasma concentration–time curve of dideoxyinosine.

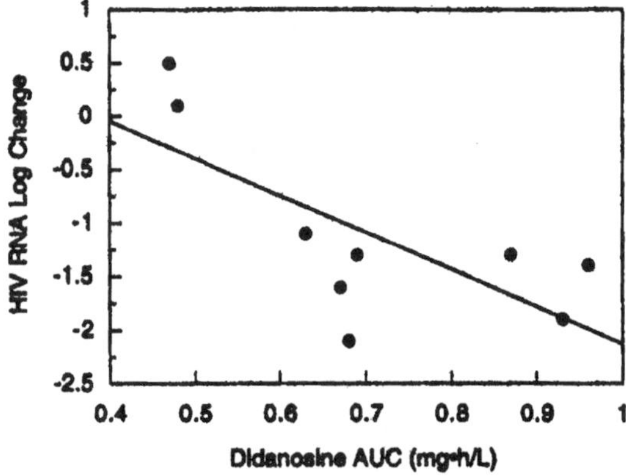

FIGURE 15 Didanosine AUC versus baseline to week 24 changes in plasma HIV RNA levels. The solid line represents the line of best fit as determined with linear regression; the equation for this line is $y = 1.337 - (3.47 \times \text{AUC})$; r^2 0.51; $p = 0.03$.

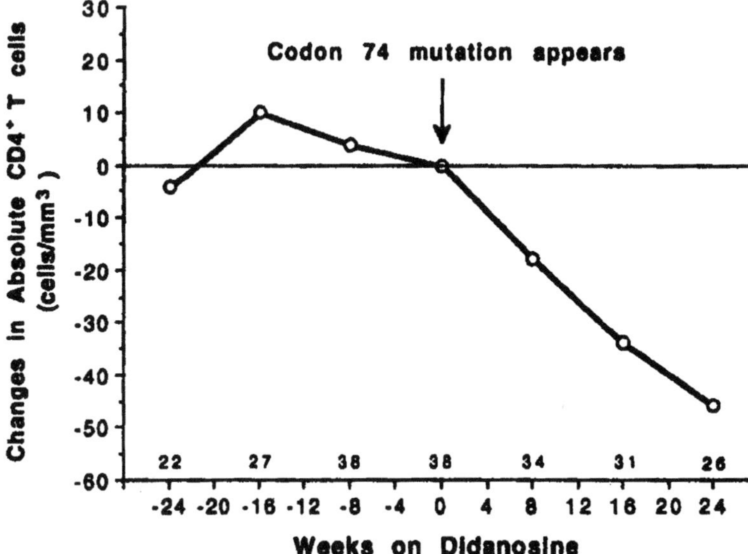

FIGURE 16 Mean CD_4^+ T-cell changes before the appearance of the HIV-1 reverse transcriptase mutation at codon 74 and CD_4^+ T-cell changes after the appearance of the mutation in 38 patients switched from zidovudine to didanosine.

of CD_4 cells is demonstrated in Fig. 16. At the time of appearance of the mutation, the CD_4 count dips below the baseline number of CD_4 cells, indicating that the increase in EC_{90} attendant to the mutation drives a loss of virological effect.

There is considerably more information relating exposure to effect for the HIV-1 protease inhibitors. Because of the time at which they were studied, virtually all of the data link some measure of exposure to the change from baseline in the viral load. Early publications examining the relationship between indinavir exposure and the CD_4 count were published by Stein and Drusano [19,20]. In the first of these publications, it was demonstrated that the return of CD_4 count was related to the baseline CD_4 count, as with nucleoside analogs. In the second, it was demonstrated that the return of CD_4 cells had another component attached to it. The model was expanded to include the decline in viral load. The return of CD_4 cell count was better explained by the larger model of baseline CD_4 count plus viral load change as the independent variables than either alone.

The first published paper examining the relationship between drug exposure and viral load decline studied high dose saquinavir. Schapiro et al. [21] demonstrated a relationship between the saquinavir AUC and the change in viral load.

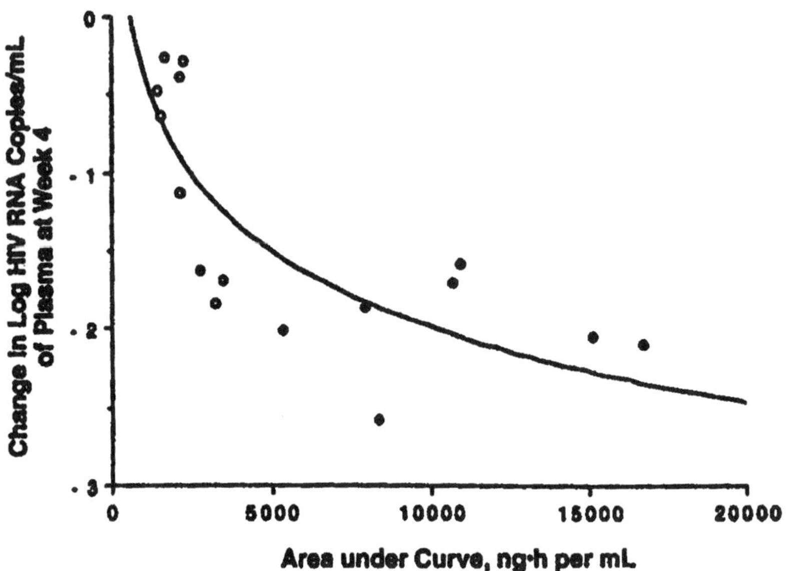

FIGURE 17 Drug levels at week 4 (AUC to 24 h) plotted against the decrease in plasma HIV RNA levels at week 4 for each patient in whom pharmacokinetics were studied. The line represents best fit and was determined using the least squares algorithm, $r = 0.801$, expressed as the Pearson correlation coefficient. (○) Patients receiving 3600 mg of saquinavir per day; (●) patients receiving 7200 mg of saquinavir per day.

A problem with this analysis is that the form of the function is not specified. Consequently, interpretation is difficult.

Shortly thereafter, Stein et al. published a small phase I/II study of indinavir [22]. This was the first ‘‘high dose’’ indinavir study (2400 mg/day) and was the first to demonstrate robust viral suppression with this drug. In addition, the authors examined the relationship between indinavir exposure and both CD_4 cell return and viral load decline. These relationships are shown in Fig. 18. One should

FIGURE 18 Modeling of data using a sigmoid E_{max} relationship and inhomogeneous differential equations. (a) The relationship of baseline CD_4 lymphocyte count to the average CD_4 lymphocyte count obtained over 24 weeks of therapy. (b) The relationship of the inhibition of HIV generation to total drug exposure (AUC). (c) The relationship of the inhibition of HIV generation to C_{min} serum concentration.

(a)

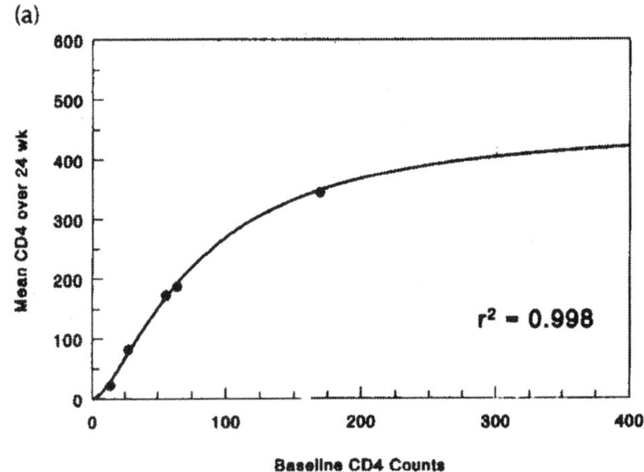
600
500
400
300
200
100
0
Mean CD4 over 24 wk
r² = 0.998
0
100
200
300
400
Baseline CD4 Counts

(b)

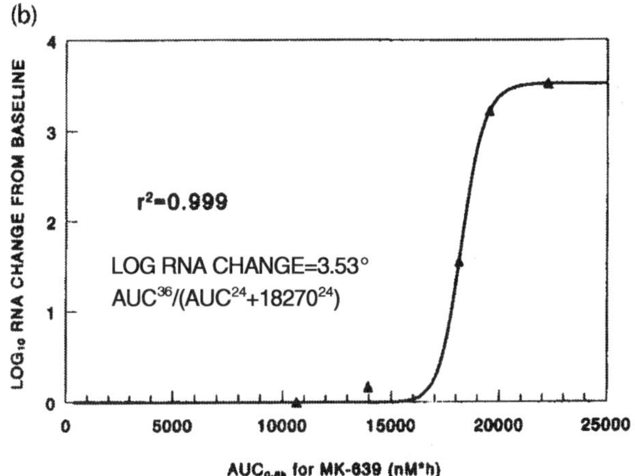
4
3
2
1
0
LOG₁₀ RNA CHANGE FROM BASELINE
r²=0.999
LOG RNA CHANGE=3.53°
AUC³⁶/(AUC²⁴+18270²⁴)
0
5000
10000
15000
20000
25000
AUC0-8h for MK-639 (nM*h)

(c)

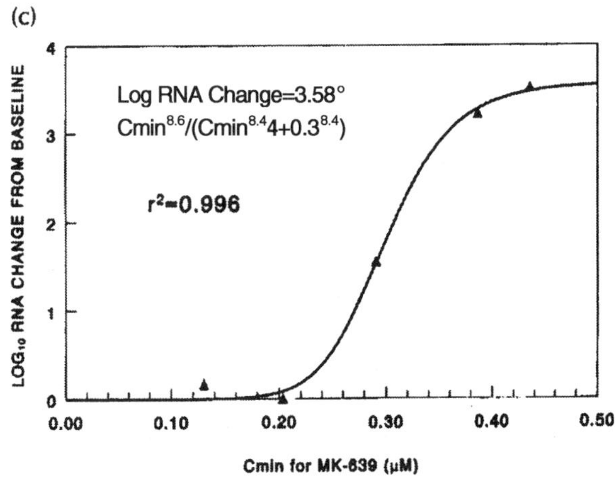
4
3
2
1
0
LOG₁₀ RNA CHANGE FROM BASELINE
Log RNA Change=3.58°
Cmin^8.6/(Cmin^8.4 4+0.3^8.4)
r²=0.996
0.00
0.10
0.20
0.30
0.40
0.50
Cmin for MK-639 (µM)

not draw the conclusion that HIV suppression is linked to AUC (as this has a slightly better r^2). In this study, the drug was administered on a fixed dose and schedule, maximizing the co-linearity (i.e., one could not make the AUC rise without also increasing the C_{min}). The in vitro studies simulated different doses and schedules, minimizing the co-linearity, and definitively showed that time > EC_{90} is the dynamically linked variable. This is correlated with C_{min}. The comparison of the in vitro and in vivo results also raises the issue of the importance of the EC_{90}.

Drusano et al. demonstrated for both indinavir [23] and amprenavir [24] that normalizing the measure of drug exposure to the EC_{50} (or EC_{90}) of a particular patient's isolate decreased the variance and increased the r^2. This makes sense, as the amount of exposure needed to suppress a sensitive isolate will, on first principles, be less than that needed to suppress a resistant isolate (see above for the case of ddI and CD_4 cells).

An issue that is not addressed by these studies is the duration of HIV suppression and the closely linked issue of suppression of emergence of resistance. The first study to examine this issue was that of Kempf et al. [25], who showed that obtaining a viral load below the detectability limit of the assay was important to the duration of control of the infection. Shortly, thereafter, Drusano et al. [26] examined this issue both for protease inhibitor monotherapy with indinavir and, for the first time, for combination therapy that included indinavir. The results for monotherapy are displayed in Fig. 19. It is clear that patients who attain viral loads that are below the detectability of the assay have the lowest hazard of losing control of the infection or emergence of resistance. The time to loss of control of infection is clearly related to the nadir viral load attained.

Of greater interest is the situation with combination chemotherapy, as this is the clinical norm. This study also examined the influence of different combination regimens on the hazard of loss of control of the viral infection. Combination regimens of zidovudine-indinavir, zidovudine-didanosine-indinavir and zidovudine-lamivudine-indinavir were examined and compared to their monotherapy arms in a stratified analysis. The results are displayed in Table 1. Only the regimen of zidovudine-lamivudine-indinavir remained significantly different from monotherapy after adjustment for the fall in viral copy number.

This result caused the in vitro investigation of this regimen [27]. A fully parametric analysis demonstrated that the interaction among all three drugs was key to the effect obtained in the clinical studies with this regimen. This is shown in Table 2, where the α's represent the interaction parameters. There are three two-drug interaction parameters and one for the interaction of all three compounds. Indinavir plus zidovudine interact in an additive manner as the value is close to zero and the 95% confidence interval overlaps zero. The same is true of indinavir plus lamivudine. Zidovudine plus lamivudine has a value that is positive and a 95% confidence interval that does not overlap zero, indicating a

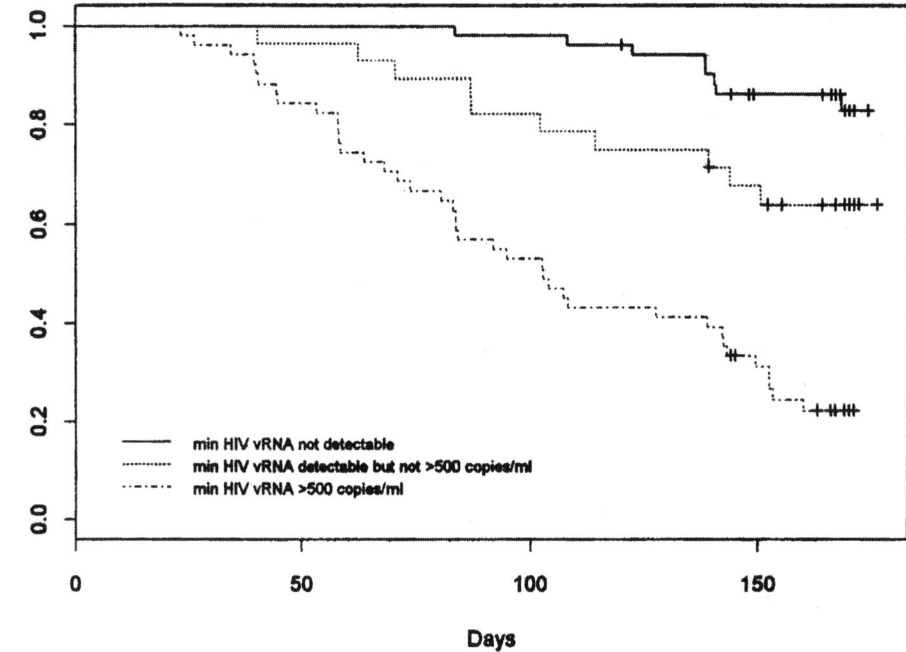

FIGURE 19 Kaplan–Meier estimate of probability that patient's isolate is not resistant to therapy (lack of sustained increase of ≥0.75 $\log_{10}$ copies/mL of HIV-1 RNA from patient's minimum level) at a given study day, stratified by minimum HIV-1 RNA achieved. Plot shows that probability of remaining susceptible is largest for patients who achieve undetectable level of HIV-1 RNA. Vertical slashes on plot indicate censoring events.

TABLE 1 Effect of Combination Therapy Versus Indinavir Monotherapy Before and After Adjusting for the Effect of the Minimum Level of HIV-1 RNA

Combination therapy	*P* before adjustment	Coefficient[a]	Hazard ratio[b] (95% CI)	*P*
IDV/AZT	.264	-0.35 ± 0.52	0.705 (0.254,1.957)	.497
IDV/AZT/ddI	.002	-1.36 ± 0.90	0.258 (0.044,1.514)	.105
IDV/AZT/3TC	<.001	-1.68 ± 0.80	0.186 (0.039,0.893)	.016

[a] Estimate + S.E. [b] Hazard ratio is vs. IDV monotherapy group in the same study.

TABLE 2 In Vitro Assessment of Drug Interaction of AZT-3TC-Indinavir

Parameter[a]	Estimate	95% Confidence interval
E_{con}	98.99	97.80–100.2
$IC_{50,IND}$	146.90	128.30–165.60
m_{IND}	1.711	1.393–2.030
$IC_{50,AZT}$	118.4	108.20–128.60
m_{AZT}	12.89	5.576–20.20
$IC_{50,3TC}$	1029.0	1018–1041
m_{3TC}	68.75	36.9–100.6
αIND,AZT	0.0001301	−0.6191–0.6194
αIND,3TC	0.6881	−0.05189–1.428
αAZT,3TC	0.9692	0.9417–0.9966
αIND,AZT,3TC	8.94	3.434–14.45

[a] E_{con}, effect seen in the absence of drug (percent); IC_{50}, concentration of drug necessary to reduce HIV-1 turnover by half when used alone (nM); *m*, slope parameter, corresponding to the rate of rise of effect with increasing drug concentration; ″, interaction parameter.

degree of synergistic interaction that is statistically significant. Finally, the magnitude of the synergistic interaction for the three-drug term is very large (and significant). It may be this exceptionally strong synergistic interaction that explains the superb results seen with this particular three-drug combination.

It is of interest that lamivudine not only plays a key role in the regimen but is also its Achilles' heel. Holder et al. [28] demonstrated that when the triple regimen fails, in about 70% of cases, the failure is due to an M184V mutation that produces high level resistance to lamivudine. So that although lamivudine appears to be a key part of this therapeutic regimen and its synergy, it also has the lowest genetic barrier to resistance. If there is some nonadherence to the regimen, enough rounds of viral replication may occur to allow the point mutant (M184V) to be amplified in the total population. When this clone becomes dominant in the population, lamivudine will lose most of its contribution to the regimen. Most of the synergy is also lost, and the result is viral rebound. As Holder and colleagues demonstrated, this occurs most of the time with mutation solely affecting the low genetic barrier drug.

It is obvious, then, that optimal chemotherapeutic regimens for HIV (and other viral pathogens) are likely to require explicit modeling of the interaction of the drugs in the regimens.

Burger et al. [29] also examined this combination. In a multivariate logistic regression with attaining a viral load below the limit of assay detectability as the endpoint, they demonstrated that baseline viral load, indinavir trough concentrations, and prior HIV-1 protease inhibitor use influenced the probability of attaining this endpoint.

All of the above has related to HIV. Other viruses can also have a pharmacodynamic evaluation elucidated. For CMV, there is a clear-cut dynamic relationship [30] that has been set forth in Chapter 14.

In summary, viruses follow the same laws of physics as bacterial pathogens (and fungal pathogens). It is important to delineate relationships both in vitro and in vivo between different measures of drug exposure and the endpoint that is deemed important. The in vitro investigations allow delineation of the true dynamically linked variable in a more straightforward manner. The in vivo investigations are important for validation. The future is in generating exposure–response relationships for combinations of agents. In this way, optimal therapy regimens can be generated to provide the greatest benefit for patients infected with viral pathogens.

REFERENCES

1. B Vogelman, S Gudmundsson, J Leggett, J Turnidge, S Ebert, WA Craig. Correlation of antimicrobial parameters with therapeutic efficacy in an animal model. J Infect Dis 1988; 158:831–847.
2. GL Drusano, DE Johnson, M Rosen, HC Standiford. Pharmacodynamics of a fluoroquinolone antimicrobial in a neutropenic rat model of Pseudomonas sepsis. Antimicrob Agents Chemother 1993; 37:483–490.
3. A Louie, P Kaw, W Liu, N Jumbe, MH Miller, GL Drusano. Pharmacodynamics of daptomycin in a murine thigh model of Staphylococcus aureus infection. Antimicrob Agents Chemother 2001; 45:845–851.
4. JA Bilello, JL Eiseman, HC Standiford, GL Drusano. Impact of dosing schedule upon suppression of a retrovirus in a murine model of AIDS encephalopathy. Antimicrob Agents Chemother 1994; 38:628–631.
5. JA Bilello, JJ Kort, C MacAuley, TN Fredrickson, RA Yetter, JL Eiseman. ZDV delays but does not prevent the transmission of MAIDS by LP-BM% MuLV-infected macrophage-monocytes. J Acquir Immune Defic Syndr 1992; 5:571–576.
6. JA Bilello, PA Bilello, K Stellrecht, J Leonard, D Norrbeck, DJ Kempf, T Robbins, GL Drusano. The uptake and anti-HIV activity of A 80987, an inhibitor of the HIV-1 protease, is reduced by human serum 1-acid glycoprotein. Antimicrob Agents Chemother 1996; 40:1491–1497.
7. JA Bilello, G Bauer, MN Dudley, GA Cole, GL Drusano. The effect of 2′,3′-dideoxy-2′,3′-didehydrothymidine (D4T) in an in vitro hollow fiber pharmacodynamic model system correlates with results of dose ranging clinical studies. Antimicrob Agents Chemother 1994; 38:1386–1391.
8. MJ Browne, KH Mayer, SB Chafee, MN Dudley, MR Posner, SM Steinberg, KK

Graham, SM Geletko, SH Zinner, SL Denman, et al. J Infect Dis 1993; 167:21–29.
9. JA Bilello, PA Bilello, JJ Kort, MN Dudley, J Leonard, GL Drusano. Efficacy of constant infusion of A 77003, an inhibitor of the HIV protease in limiting acute HIV-1 infection in vitro. Antimicrob Agents Chemother 1995; 39:2523–2527.
10. M Reedijk, CA Boucher, T van Bommel, DD Ho, TB Tzeng, D Sereni, P Veyssier, S Jurruaans, R Grannemann, A Hsu, et al. Safety, pharmacokinetics and antiviral activity of A77002, a C2 symmetry-based human immunodeficiency virus protease inhibitor. Antimicrob Agents Chemother 1995; 39:1559–1564.
11. GL Drusano. Antiviral therapy of HIV and cytomegalovirus. Abstracts of the 37th Interscience Conference on Antimicrobial Agents and Chemotherapy. Abstract S-121. Sept 28–Oct 1, 1997, Toronto, ON, Canada.
12. GL Drusano, JA Bilello, SL Preston, E O'Mara, S Kaul, S Schnittman, R Echols. Hollow fiber unit evaluation of a new human immunodeficiency virus (HIV)-1 protease inhibitor, BMS232632, for determination of the linked pharmacodynamic variable. J Infect Dis 2000; 183:1126–1129.
13. GL Drusano, DZ D'Argenio, W Symonds, PA Bilello, J McDowell, B Sadler, A Bye, JA Bilello. Nucleoside analog 1592U89 and human immunodeficiency virus protease inhibitor 141W94 are synergistic in vitro. Antimicrob Agents Chemother 1998; 42:2153–2159.
14. GL Drusano, DZ D'Argenio, SL Preston, C Barone, W Symonds, S LaFon, M Rogers, W Prince, A Bye, JA Bilello. Use of drug effect interaction modeling with Monte Carlo simulation to examine the impact of dosing interval on the projected antiviral activity of the combination of abacavir and amprenavir. Antimicrob Agents Chemother 2000; 44:1655–1659.
15. GL Drusano, GJ Yuen, JS Lambert, M Seidlin, R Dolin, FT Valentine. Quantitative relationships between dideoxyinosine exposure and surrogate markers of response in a phase I trial. Ann Intern Med 1992; 116:562–566.
16. GL Drusano, FM Balis, SR Gitterman, PA Pizzo. Quantitative relationships between zidovudine exposure and efficacy and toxicity. Antimicrob Agents Chemother 1994; 8:1726–1731.
17. CV Fletcher, RC Brundage, RP Remmel, LM Page, D Weller, NR Calles, C Simon, MW Kline. Pharmacologic characteristics of indinavir, didanosine and stavudine in human immunodeficiency virus-infected children receiving combination chemotherapy. Antimicrob Agents Chemother 2000; 44:1029–1034.
18. MJ Kozal, K Kroodsma, MA Winters, RW Shafer, B Efron, DA Katzenstein, TC Merigan. Didanosin resistance in HIV-infected patients switched from zidovudine to didanosine monotherapy. Ann Intern Med 1994; 121:263–268.
19. DS Stein, GL Drusano. Modeling of the change in CD_4 lymphocyte cell counts in patients before and after administration of the human immunodeficiency virus protease inhibitor indinavir. Antimicrob Agents Chemother 1997; 41:449–453.
20. GL Drusano, DS Stein. Mathematical modeling of the interrelationship of CD_4 lymphocyte count and viral load changes induced by the protease inhibitor indinavir. Antimicrob Agents Chemother 1998; 42:358–361.
21. JM Schapiro, MA Winters, F Stewart, B Efron, J Norris, MJ Kozal, TC Merigan.

The effect of high-dose saquinavir on viral load and CD4+ T-cell counts in HIV-infected patients. Ann Intern Med 1996; 124:1039–1050.

22. DS Stein, DG Fish, JA Bilello, J Chodakewitz, E Emini, C Hildebrand, SL Preston, GL Martineau, GL Drusano. A 24 week open label phase I evaluation of the HIV protease inhibitor MK-639. AIDS 1996; 10:485–492.
23. GL Drusano. This volume, Chapter 14.
24. GL Drusano, BM Sadler, J Millard, WT Symonds, M Tisdale, C Rawls, A Bye, and the 141W94 International Product Development Team. Pharmacodynamics of 141W94 as determined by short term change in HIV RNA: Influence of viral isolate baseline EC_{50}. Abstract A-16. 37th Interscience Conference on Antimicrobial Agents and Chemotherapy. Sept 28–Oct 1, 1997, Toronto, ON, Canada.
25. DJ Kempf, RA Rode, Y Xu, E Sun, ME Heath-Chiozzi, J Valdes, AJ Japour, S Danner, C Boucher, A Molla, JM Leonard. The duration of viral suppression during protease inhibitor therapy for HIV-1 infection is predicted by plasma HIV-1 RNA at the nadir. AIDS 1998; 12:F9–F14.
26. GL Drusano, JA Bilello, DS Stein, M Nessly, A Meibohm, EA Emini, P Deutsch, J Condra, J Chodakewitz, DJ Holder. Factors influencing the emergence of resistance to indinavir: Role of virologic, immunologic, and pharmacologic variables. J Infect Dis 1998; 178:360–367.
27. S Snyder, DZ D'Argenio, O Weislow, JA Bilello, GL Drusano. The triple combination indinavir-zidovundine-lamivudine is highly synergistic. Antimicrob Agents Chemother 2000; 44:1051–1058.
28. DJ Holder, JH Condra, WA Schleif, J Chodakewitz, EA Emini. Virologic failure during combination therapy with crixivan and RT inhibitors is often associated with expression of resistance-associated mutations in RT only. Conf Retroviruses Opportun Infect 1999; Jan 31–Feb 4;6:160 (abstr 492).
29. DM Burger, RMW Hoetelmans, PWH Hugen, et al. Low plasma concentrations of indinavir are related to virological treatment failure in HIV-1-infected patients on indinavir containing triple therapy. Antiviral Ther 1998; 3:215–220.
30. GL Drusano, F Aweeka, J Gambertoglio, M Jacobson, M Polis, HC Lane, C Eaton, S Martin-Munley. Relationship between foscarnet exposure, baseline cytomegalovirus blood culture and the time to progression of cytomegalovirus retinitis in HIV-positive patients. AIDS 1996; 10:1113–1119.

13

Antifungal Pharmacodynamics

Michael E. Klepser
University of Iowa, Iowa City, Iowa

Russell E. Lewis
University of Houston College of Pharmacy, Houston, Texas

1 INTRODUCTION

Over the last two decades, advances in the characterization of antibacterial pharmacodynamics have greatly improved therapeutic strategies in the use of antimicrobial therapy. Progress in our understanding of antifungal pharmacodynamics, however, remains severely limited. Prospective clinical trials for serious fungal infections are difficult to complete and rarely evaluate multiple treatment strategies [1]. Moreover, the high mortality associated with systemic fungal disease lessens the likelihood that dose-ranging studies for antifungal agents will be pursued. Perhaps more surprising, however, is the profound lack of in vitro and animal data describing concentration–effect relationships for antifungals. This lack of even fundamental knowledge regarding the pharmacodynamics of antifungals can even be appreciated in the clinical literature, where optimal dosing strategies for amphotericin B remain largely undefined despite over 40 years of clinical use [2,3].

With the emergence of the AIDS epidemic, widespread use of broad-spectrum antibacterial therapy, and a growing population of immunocompromised patients, the spectrum of nosocomial pathogens has changed dramatically [4]. Fungi are now the fourth most commonly isolated nosocomial bloodstream pathogens in U.S. hospitals and have been identified as an independent risk factor for in-hospital death [5,6]. This staggering increase in the frequency of fungal infections coupled with the introduction of new antifungal agents has made the identification of optimal antifungal treatment strategies even more critical. Although still in its infancy, the study of antifungal pharmacodynamics is already providing important new information of the activity, dosing, and use of antifungals for treatment of candidiasis and cryptococcosis.

2 PROBLEMS WITH DESCRIBING ANTIFUNGAL PHARMACODYNAMICS

2.1 In Vitro Data

One of the primary factors that has hindered the study of antifungal pharmacodynamics over the last two decades was the lack of standardized methods for performing in vitro susceptibility testing of fungi. Prior to the 1980s, fungi were relatively infrequent pathogens and amphotericin B was the sole systemic antifungal therapy available; thus susceptibility testing of fungi was impractical and remained largely undeveloped. With the frequency of fungal infections increasing and the number of new antifungal agents growing, the development of standardized antifungal susceptibility testing methods has become a priority. Problems with inter- and intralaboratory reproducibility, however, hindered early efforts to develop antifungal susceptibility testing into a clinically useful tool. One study evaluating the interlaboratory reproducibility of antifungal susceptibility testing noted a 512-fold variation in MIC values among collaborating laboratories that used the same published but unstandardized methodology [7].

In the late 1990s, the National Committee for Clinical Laboratory Standards (NCCLS) approved standardized methods for in vitro antifungal susceptibility testing and susceptibility breakpoints for *Candida* species [8,9]. This step not only enabled the quantitative description of antifungal resistance but also provided the groundwork for performing in vitro pharmacodynamic work with antifungals.

2.2 Animal Models

Historically, animal (mostly rodent) models have been the preferred method of testing antifungal efficacy. Much of this deference to the use of animal models was a result of not having standardized in vitro susceptibility testing methods for fungi. Moreover, many fungal pathogens exhibit different morphology and growth characteristics in vivo from those of growth in culture media. *Candida albicans*, for example, generally does not form the hyphal structures in culture media that are seen with in vivo tissue invasion [10–12]. Published data from animal models, however, also suffer the limitation of unstandardized methodology and poor reproducibility [13]. Selection of the endpoint for evaluation of study results in vivo, i.e., survival versus mycology, can profoundly influence interpretation of data. Although survival is often the desired endpoint in vivo, animal studies are generally not conducted over a sufficient length of time to provide an adequate opportunity for relapse of infection once therapy is discontinued. Additionally, it is reasonable to theorize that if fungi are detectable in body tissues or fluids at the end of a treatment cycle these viable organisms may proliferate and cause relapse after antifungal therapy is withdrawn. Therefore, counts of viable fungi often provide the best information regarding in vivo antifungal efficacy. This can be problematic, however, for extrapolating pharmacodynamic parameters predictive of in vivo antifungal efficacy. Many antifungals possess fungistatic activity; thus the actual differences in counts of viable fungi in vivo may be too small to delineate pharmacodynamic relationships [13,14].

2.3 Clinical Data

Using clinical data to determine dose–response relationships for antifungals can be especially difficult. The multiplicity of non-drug factors that play a part in the development of severe fungal infections (i.e., previous chemotherapy, intravascular catheters, etc.) profoundly influence the overall effectiveness of antifungal therapy in the individual patient. Fungal infections are also a diagnostic challenge, and serial blood cultures are generally insensitive markers for diagnosis and response to antifungal therapy [15]. Moreover, monitoring of serum drug concentration for antifungals is rarely performed; thus comparison of different clinical studies is unfeasible.

Distinct diagnostic criteria compared to other systemic fungal infections generally make cryptococcal meningitis and/or oropharyngeal candidiasis best suited to the extrapolation of outcome data with respect to antifungal therapy. Cryptococcal meningitis, however, may be preferred for outcome measurement, because the mortality associated with oropharyngeal candidiasis is comparatively lower than that of other systemic infections.

3 PHARMACODYNAMICS

3.1 Amphotericin B

Despite the availability of better-tolerated agents, the broad spectrum of activity and potency of amphotericin B have maintained its role as the drug of choice for deep-seated mycoses. Amphotericin B is thought to act primarily by binding to ergosterol in the fungal cell membrane resulting in intercalation of the membrane and leakage of intracellular contents [3]. Amphotericin B has also been shown to induce oxidative damage to the cell membrane and to stimulate host immune responses [16], which may contribute to the overall elimination of fungal pathogens from the infected host.

Even with nearly 40 years of clinical use, relatively few pharmacodynamic data exist for this agent. This lack of data is surprising considering the numerous toxicities associated with amphotericin B therapy. The recent introduction of lipid formulations of amphotericin B, which have considerably different pharmacokinetic characteristics than those of the standard formulations, have further complicated issues regarding the optimal dosing of this agent.

3.1.1 In Vitro Data

In vitro data describing the pharmacodynamics of amphotericin B are relatively scarce. Although the NCCLS has proposed standardized methods for microbroth susceptibility testing of amphotericin B, these methods are still not well suited for detecting amphotericin B resistance and are still under active investigation [8,9,17,18].

Standardized methods for performing time-kill studies with amphotericin B against *Candida* and *Cryptococcus* spp., however, have been published [19]. These methods have been used to evaluate concentration–effect relationships of amphotericin B against *Candida albicans* [20] and *Cryptococcus neoformans* [21]. A representative graph from these studies is presented in Fig. 1. Against

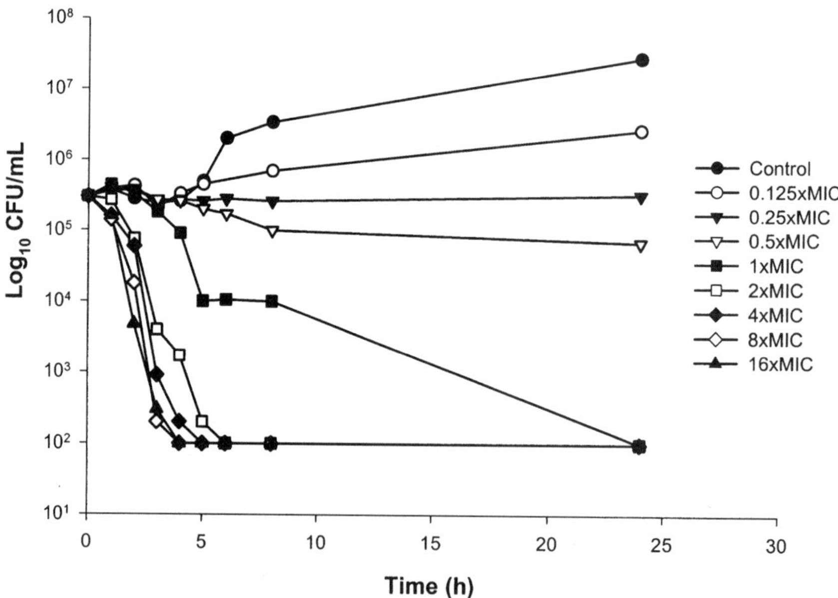

Figure 1 Representative graph of amphotericin B time-kill activity against *Candida* and *Cryptococcus* species. (From Refs. 20 and 21.)

both fungal species, amphotericin B at concentrations above the MIC produced rapid fungicidal activity. As concentrations of amphotericin B in the growth media increased, both the rate and extent of antifungal activity improved. This improvement in activity continued up to the maximal concentrations tested, 16–32 times the MIC of the test isolates. This concentration-dependent relationship of killing has also been reported by other investigators [22].

The postantifungal effect (PAE) of amphotericin B has also been evaluated for both *Candida* and *Cryptococcus* species [23]. Amphotericin B produces a prolonged PAE ranging from 0.5 to 10.6 h against *Candida* species and from 2.8 to 10.4 h against *C. neoformans*. Additionally, the authors noted that the PAE exerted by amphotericin B was dependent on the duration of exposure and the concentrations of drug tested.

According to these data, it appears that amphotericin B exhibits concentration-dependent antifungal activity in vitro. However, it is important to gauge in vitro results against clinically achievable drug concentrations. Examining the sigmoidal dose–response curves constructed from the time-kill data representative of fully susceptible *Candida* and *Cryptococcus* spp. (Fig. 2), one notes that the transitional portion of the dose response curve for amphotericin B against these isolates (in vitro) occurred over a concentration range of 0.25–2 times the

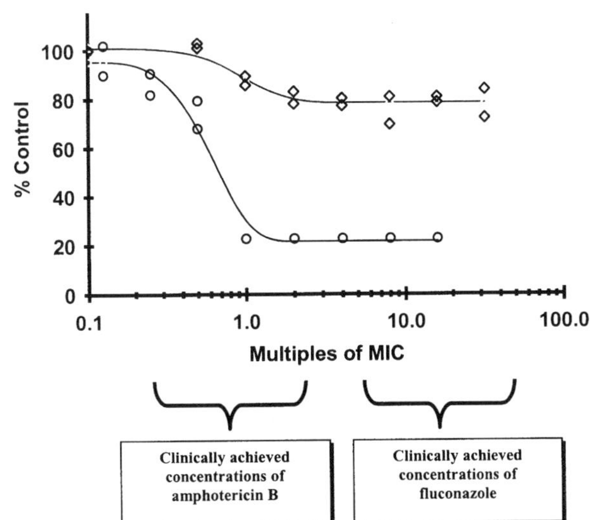

FIGURE 2 Representative sigmoidal dose–response curves of amphotericin B, ○, and fluconazole, ◇, against *Candida* and *Cryptococcus* spp. (From Refs. 20 and 21.)

MIC (0.2–2.0 μg/mL). This transitional portion represents a relatively broad range of serum concentrations that can be achieved with clinically used dosages of amphotericin B of 0.25–1.5 mg/kg q24h [3]. Therefore, these data predict over a range of clinically achieved concentrations that amphotericin B would be expected to exhibit concentration-dependent pharmacodynamics.

3.1.2 In Vivo Data

Currently, no studies, animal or human, specifically designed to evaluate the pharmacodynamic characteristics of amphotericin B have been published. However, some animal and clinical studies do exist that have evaluated multiple doses of amphotericin B under identical or similar testing conditions and can therefore be carefully evaluated for dose–response relationships. George et al. [24] used a rabbit model of aspergillosis to evaluate the efficacy of amphotericin B administered at 0.5 and 1.5 mg/(kg · day). These investigators employed both clinical (survival) and mycological (tissue burden) endpoints to evaluate the efficacy of the two dosing regimens. They reported that although there was no difference between the two amphotericin B regimens with respect to survival (both regimens yielded 100% survival), amphotericin B at 1.5 mg/(kg · day) resulted in fewer positive cultures and reduced fungal tissue burdens compared with the lower dose regimen.

Pharmacodynamic data from controlled human studies are lacking. Therefore, we are left to evaluate data from multiple studies in order to construct a picture of pharmacodynamic relationships. As mentioned, one of the best patient populations available for comparison among studies are patients with cryptococcal meningitis. Some of the primary reasons that this patient population lends itself to interstudy comparisons are the defined criteria used to diagnose and define disease, the ability to detect the pathogen relatively reliably, and the relatively standard endpoints used for clinical and microbiological outcomes. The major problem with extrapolating pharmacodynamic relationships from studies of cryptococcal meningitis, however, is the lack of data describing amphotericin B concentrations at the site of infection (cerebrospinal fluid). This could somewhat skew the dose–response relationships observed because distribution of amphotericin B into the CSF is generally poor (<10%) [3]. Several studies evaluating amphotericin B for the treatment of cryptococcal meningitis are presented in Table 1. Examination of these studies reveals a trend of improved outcomes with increasing doses of amphotericin B. It is interesting to note that mortality associated with cryptococcal meningitis decreased from 14% at a dose of 0.3 mg/kg per day to 2.9% at a dose of 1.0 mg/kg per day [25–27].

3.1.3 Summary

In vitro and in vivo data both reveal improved fungicidal activity with amphotericin B as concentrations or doses of the drug are increased. Therefore, in light of

TABLE 1 Use of Amphotericin B for the Treatment of Cryptococcal Meningitis

Investigators	Amphotericin B dose	Patient no.	Concurrent flucytosine use	Outcome: Negative CSF culture at 14 days (%)	Outcome: Clinical (mortality)	Comments
Saag, et al. (From Ref. 53)	0.3 mg/(kg · day)	63	Discretion of clinician	20%	9/63 (14%)	Mean amphotericin B dose used was 0.4–0.5 mg/(kg · day).
van der Horst et al. (From Ref. 26)	0.7 mg/(kg · day)	381	Yes (n = 202) No (n = 179)	60% 51%	11/202 (5.4%) 10/179 (5.6%)	Conducted by same investigators as Saag study. Attribute improved CSF sterilization to higher dose of amphotericin B.
de Lalla et al. (From Ref. 25)	1.0 mg/(kg · day)	35	Yes	Not reported	1/35 (2.9%)	—

the long half-life and PAE associated with the drug, it appears that the optimal dosing strategy for this agent would be to administer amphotericin B at relatively high doses (i.e., ≥0.8 mg/kg per day) at intervals of no less than every 24 h.

3.2 Azole Pharmacodynamics

Fluconazole has been the most widely studied of the azole antifungals. A synthetic triazole antifungal, fluconazole exhibits fungistatic activity against a variety of *Candida* species and *C. neoformans.*

3.2.1 In Vitro Data

Similar to amphotericin B, limited data are available regarding the pharmacodynamic characteristics of fluconazole. Klepser et al. [20,21] examined the fungistatic activity produced by fluconazole against *C. albicans* and *C. neoformans* using time-kill methods. According to their data, the fungistatic activity produced by fluconazole was maximized at concentrations of 2–4 times the MIC of the test isolates (Figs. 2 and 3). Similar findings have been reported by other investigators [22]. Additionally, using an in vitro dynamic model of infection, these

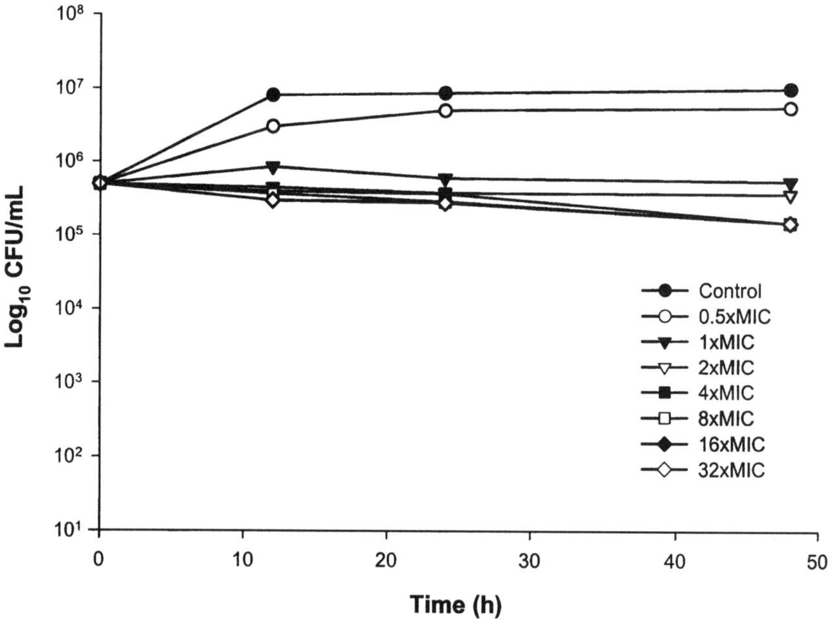

FIGURE 3 Representative graph of fluconazole time-kill activity against *Candida* and *Cryptococcus* spp. (From Refs. 20 and 21.)

investigators compared the activity of two fluconazole dosing regimens, 200 mg and 400 mg administered every 24 h, against *C. albicans* [28]. No differences with respect to the rate or extent of activity produced by the two fluconazole regimens were noted. It is important to note that the fluconazole MICs for the test isolates were 0.25 and 0.5 μg/mL. Given the long half-life of fluconazole, approximately 20–50 h, drug concentrations in the model for both regimens would be expected to remain above 10 times the MIC for each regimen and isolate tested.

Voriconazole is an investigational triazole antifungal with an enhanced spectrum of activity against *Candida*, *Cryptococcus*, and *Aspergillus* species. Using time-kill methods, Klepser et al. [29] examined the in vitro activity of voriconazole against *C. albicans*, *C. glabrata*, *C. tropicalis*, and *C. neoformans* over concentrations ranging from 0.125 to 16 times the MIC of test isolates. Against *C. albicans* and *C. neoformans*, voriconazole produced fungistatic activity that was maximized at concentrations between 1 and 4 times the MIC.

In vitro, fluconazole produces a short PAE against *Candida* species [30–33]. Against *C. albicans*, fluconazole produces a PAE of <0.5 h. The duration of the PAE is not increased with higher concentrations or by increasing the duration of exposure. Some investigators have noted that the PAE induced by fluconazole may increase if human serum is added to the in vitro system [30]. This observation led the investigators to suggest that the PAE induced by fluconazole may be significantly longer in vivo than in vitro.

3.2.2 In Vivo Data

Using a murine model of deep-seated *C. albicans* infection, Louie et al. [34] evaluated the pharmacodynamic characteristics of fluconazole. In this study, the investigators determined the range of concentrations over which response in the model was noted to change from minimal to maximal (transition portion of the dose–response curve). Then dose-fractionation studies were performed to evaluate the relationship between pharmacodynamic parameters such as peak/MIC and AUC/MIC ratios, and time above the MIC and outcome at concentrations near the transition portion of the dose–response curve. Upon analysis, the authors determined that a concentration-associated parameter, the AUC/MIC ratio, was best correlated with positive results. Although these in vivo data may appear to contradict previous in vitro findings, some limitations of this study warrant cautious interpretation of this study. First, the doses of fluconazole used in the study produced serum concentrations in the model that ranged from approximately 4 to 8 μg/mL, well below clinically observed concentrations even with low-dose, 200 mg daily, fluconazole. Second, viable colony counts of fungi in kidney homogenate served as the endpoint for the study, and the authors state that fungal densities were similar for groups that received the same daily dose of fluconazole. However, according to their data, there does not appear to be a difference among fungal densities in any of the dosing groups, suggesting poor sensitivity in the model. Finally, the authors specifically studied the transition portion of the dose–response curve. By definition, the measured response should increase as exposure to increased amounts of drug increase. This portion of the curve was noted to occur over a narrow range of concentrations. If one were to examine these data in the context of clinically achievable concentrations (Fig. 2), it would be apparent that this transition portion of the dose–response curve would be easily surpassed. Therefore, one might conclude that even though the activity noted in the transition portion of the curve may correlate with the AUC/MIC ratio, under clinical conditions activity would be dictated according to the concentration relationships of the flat portion or non-concentration-dependent portion of the curve against fully susceptible fungi (Fig. 2).

3.2.3 Clinical Studies

Clinical trials designed specifically to study the pharmacodynamic properties of fluconazole have not been completed. However, Witt et al. [35] examined the activity of fluconazole at doses ranging from 400 to 2000 mg in patients with cryptococcal meningitis. A total of 12, 15, 20, and 10 patients received intravenous fluconazole at doses of 400, 1200, 1600, and 2000 mg, respectively. The authors reported that no association was observed between the dose of fluconazole administered and outcome.

3.2.4 Summary

Although the fungistatic activity of fluconazole may improve as drug concentrations increase to 2–4 times the MIC of a given fungus, fluconazole appears to exhibit non-concentration-dependent characteristics over the range of concentrations yielded by clinically used doses. Therefore, it is not likely that the activity produced by fluconazole will be improved via the administration of larger than normal doses, i.e., 400 mg daily, unless the fungal pathogens exhibit relatively high MICs (>32–64 μg/mL) to fluconazole.

3.3 Flucytosine Pharmacodynamics

3.3.1 In Vitro Data

Flucytosine is a fluorinated pyrimidine that possesses antifungal activity against a variety of fungal species including *Candida* and *Cryptococcus*. In order to exert its antifungal activity, flucytosine must be converted to fluorouracil by cytosine deaminase located inside the fungal cell. The use of flucytosine is frequently limited secondary to its narrow therapeutic index, four times daily dosing interval, and rapid emergence of resistance if single-drug therapy is attempted.

As with the other antifungal agents discussed, few data currently exist regarding the pharmacodynamic characteristics of flucytosine. Lewis et al. [36] examined the influence of drug concentrations on the antifungal activity expressed by flucytosine using time-kill methods. Several *Candida* species and *C. neoformans* were tested at multiples of their flucytosine MICs ranging from 0.25 to 64 times the MIC. Against isolates of *C. albicans*, *C. glabrata*, *C. krusei*, and *C. tropicalis*, flucytosine exhibited fungistatic activity that improved as the concentration of flucytosine increased up to 16 times the MIC. In contrast, against *C. neoformans* there did not appear to be an identifiable relationship between concentration and increased antifungal activity once flucytosine concentrations exceeded the MIC of the isolate. It should be noted that even at 16 times the MIC of the test isolates, these concentrations are well within the range of clinically observed concentrations. In fact, steady-state serum and cerebrospinal fluid concentrations in humans average 50–100 μg/mL [26,37–39]. The MICs of the isolates used by Lewis et al. ranged from 0.06 to 4 μg/mL; therefore, clinically achievable concentrations would represent levels approximately 50–1600 times the MICs of these isolates. As a result, even though flucytosine does exhibit concentration-dependent activity in vitro, it is likely that concentration-independent activity would be observed clinically.

A measurable PAE has been reported for flucytosine [23,36]. In general, flucytosine produces an in vitro PAE ranging from 0.5 to approximately 4 h. The duration of the PAE is prolonged as the concentration of drug tested increases [36].

3.3.2 In Vivo Data

Using a murine model of disseminated candidiasis, Andes and colleagues examined the pharmacodynamic characteristics of flucytosine [40]. In their model the investigators determined that minimal concentration-dependent activity was noted. They determined that the time that concentrations remained above the MIC of the pathogen and the AUC/MIC ratio held the best correlation with observed effect. It is important to note, however, that the half-life of flucytosine in their model was approximately 0.35–0.45 h, significantly less than the 6 h half-life reported for humans.

3.3.3 Summary

Flucytosine exhibits non-concentration-dependent fungistatic activity over a range of clinically achievable concentrations. Therefore, given the relatively long half-life of this agent, its narrow therapeutic window, and correlation between time above the MIC and activity, it appears reasonable to advocate the use of low dose, 100 mg/(kg · day), regimens administered at extended intervals every 8–12 h. This strategy would appear to provide optimal activity while minimizing patient exposure to the drug.

3.4 Antifungal Combinations

With increasing reports of antifungal resistance and a limited number of therapeutic agents, the use of combination antifungal regimens to offset toxicity and improve efficacy has become common clinical strategy. Amphotericin B–flucytosine combination therapy has been proven to be an efficacious combination in the treatment of cryptococcal meningitis [26,38]. Some clinical data are available to suggest that azole-flucytosine combinations may be useful in the treatment of fungal peritonitis [41].

One of the most controversial topics in antifungal therapeutics, however, concerns azole-amphotericin B combinations. Considering the pharmacology of these two antifungals, this combination should result in antagonism. Theoretically, the inhibition of ergosterol synthesis by fluconazole should result in decreased binding and antagonism of amphotericin B activity. Results from many in vitro studies have supported this theory of azole-amphotericin B antagonism, yet the results of in vivo rodent and rabbit studies have been unequivocal [42]. Unlike many of the other azole antifungals, fluconazole exhibits reversible binding to the target enzyme, 14α-demethylase, and is relatively hydrophilic [43]. Based of these differences and data from in vivo models, several investigators have predicted that antagonism between amphotericin B and fluconazole would not occur in vivo [42,44–48].

If fluconazole does antagonize the activity of amphotericin B against yeast, two important pharmacodynamic questions need to be answered: (1) What is the time course (rate) for the development of antagonism—is pre-exposure to fluconazole necessary? (2) If antagonism does develop, to what extent will overall antifungal activity be lost? This second question is critical, because it may explain why many in vivo models have failed to show increased mortality with an amphotericin B-fluconazole combination.

Recently studies have been published examining these questions [28,49]. De novo ergosterol biosynthesis and incorporation into the fungal membrane in *Candida* species have been reported to occur over a period of approximately 6 h [50]. Considering the pharmacodynamics of each antifungal (Figs. 1–3), it appears that some amount of pre-exposure to fluconazole would be necessary to antagonize the activity of amphotericin B. Ernst and coworkers noted that the fungicidal activity of amphotericin B is dramatically decreased when isolates are pre-exposed to fluconazole for more than 8 h. The activity of amphotericin B against yeast exposed to fluconazole for at least 8 h was indistinguishable from that of fluconazole alone and was fungistatic ($\leq 2 \log_{10}$ decrease from starting inoculum). A limitation of these studies, however, was the static nature of drugs in the test conditions.

To test the likelihood of fluconazole antagonizing the fungicidal activity of amphotericin B over a range of dynamic concentrations, Lewis et al. [28]

developed an in vitro pharmacodynamic infection model of candidemia. In this model, the investigators simulated the human pharmacokinetic profile of five antifungal regimens plus control: (1) fluconazole 200 mg q24h, (2) fluconazole 400 mg q24h, (3) amphotericin B 1 mg/kg per day, (4) amphotericin B plus fluconazole (400 mg) simultaneously, and (5) amphotericin B administered 8 h after the fluconazole bolus. Similar to previous time-kill studies, amphotericin B administered 8 h after a fluconazole bolus drastically reduced amphotericin B fungicidal activity (Fig. 4).

Data from these pharmacodynamic studies have several implications. First, the time course and order of administration for amphotericin B and fluconazole are important for the development of antagonism. Therefore, traditional methods for screening antifungal antagonism that rely on static concentration of antifungals administered simultaneously (i.e., checkerboard testing) may not necessarily detect antagonism. Especially notable, the fungistatic activity of fluconazole seems to persist despite the loss of amphotericin B fungicidal activity (Fig. 4). If this antifungal activity persists in vivo, it is unlikely that studies using mortality as the principal endpoint would be able to detect antagonism of amphotericin B. This is also true clinically, as fluconazole has been shown to be as efficacious as moderate doses of amphotericin B for the treatment of systemic candidiasis in neutropenic and non-neutropenic patients [51,52].

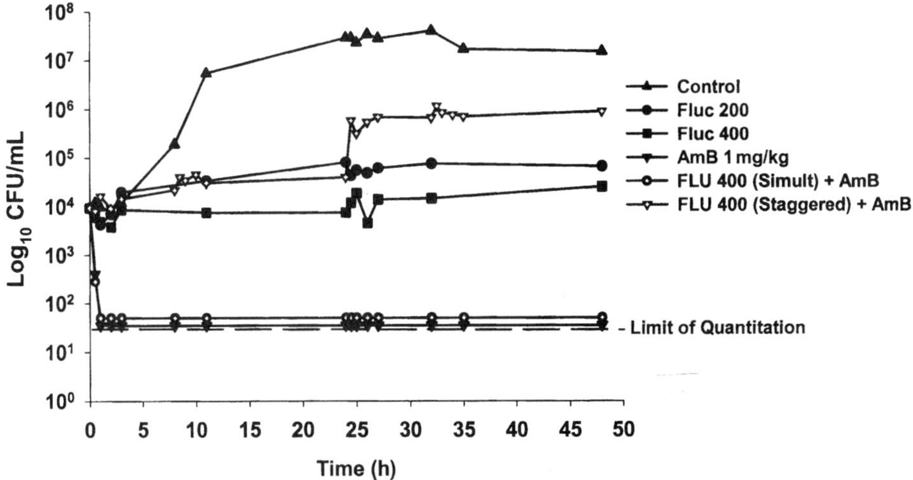

FIGURE 4 Representative graph of amphotericin B-fluconazole antifungal combination activity tested in an in vitro pharmacodynamic infection model against *Candida albicans*. (From Ref. 28.)

4 CONCLUSIONS

Clearly, the study of antifungal pharmacodynamics is still in its infancy. Nevertheless, early in vitro and in vivo work has provided some important new information on the activity, dosing, and use of antifungals for the treatment of candidiasis and cryptococcosis. The next challenge will be to bring pharmacodynamic data from benchtop and animal studies to the bedside. Other systemic mycoses critically need pharmacodynamic study. Aspergillosis, for example, has become a major cause of mortality among oncology patients, yet no clinical trials exist describing the optimal therapy for these fungal infections. Future progress in the field of antifungal pharmacodynamics will hopefully optimize our ability to treat mycoses despite a limited armamentarium.

REFERENCES

1. JE Edwards Jr, GP Bodey, RA Bowden, T Buchner, BE de Pauw, SG Filler, MA Ghannoum, M Glauser, R Herbrecht, CA Kauffman, S Kohno, P Martino, F Meunier, T Mori, MA Pfaller, JH Rex, TR Rogers, RH Rubin, J Solomkin, C Viscoli, TJ Walsh, M White. International Conference for the Development of a Consensus on the Management and Prevention of Severe Candidal Infections. Clin Infect Dis 1997;25:43–59.
2. MP Nagata, CA Gentry, EM Hampton. Is there a therapeutic or pharmacokinetic rationale for amphotericin B dosing in systemic Candida infections? Ann Pharmacother 1996;30:811–818.
3. HA Gallis, RH Drew,WW Pickard. Amphotericin B: 30 years of clinical experience. Rev Infect Dis 1990;12:308–329.
4. SN Banerjee, TG Emori, DH Culver, RP Gaynes, WR Jarvis, T Horan, JR Edwards, J Tolson, T Henderson, WJ Martone. Secular trends in nosocomial primary bloodstream infections in the United States, 1980–1989. National Nosocomial Infections Surveillance System. Am J Med 1991;91:86S–89S.
5. D Pittet, N Li, RF Woolson, RP Wenzel. Microbiological factors influencing the outcome of nosocomial bloodstream infections: A 6-year validated, population-based model. Clin Infect Dis 1997;24:1068–1078.
6. MA Pfaller, RN Jones, GV Doern, HS Sader, RJ Hollis, SA Messer. International surveillance of bloodstream infections due to Candida species: Frequency of occurrence and antifungal susceptibilities of isolates collected in 1997 in the United States, Canada, and South America for the SENTRY Program. The SENTRY Participant Group. J Clin Microbiol 1998;36:1886–1889.
7. DL Calhoun, GD Roberts, JN Galgiani, JE Bennett, DS Feingold, J Jorgensen, GS Kobayashi, S Shadomy. Results of a survey of antifungal susceptibility tests in the United States and interlaboratory comparison of broth dilution testing of flucytosine and amphotericin B. J Clin Microbiol 1986;23:298–301.
8. JH Rex, MA Pfaller, JN Galgiani, MS Bartlett, A Espinel-Ingroff, MA Ghannoum, M Lancaster, FC Odds, MG Rinaldi, TJ Walsh, AL Barry. Development of interpretive breakpoints for antifungal susceptibility testing: Conceptual framework and

analysis of in vitro–in vivo correlation data for fluconazole, itraconazole, and Candida infections. Subcommittee on Antifungal Susceptibility Testing of the National Committee for Clinical Laboratory Standards. Clin Infect Dis 1997;24:235–247.
9. National Committee for Clinical Laboratory Standards 1997. Reference method for broth dilution antifungal susceptibility testing of yeasts; approved standard. Villanova, PA: NCCLS.
10. RB Ashman, A Fulurija, TA Robertson, JM Papadimitriou. Rapid destruction of skeletal muscle fibers by mycelial growth forms of Candida albicans. Exp Mol Pathol 1995;62:109–117.
11. JC Parker Jr, JJ McCloskey, KA Knauer. Pathobiologic features of human candidiasis. A common deep mycosis of the brain, heart and kidney in the altered host. Am J Clin Pathol 1976;65:991–1000.
12. TJ Walsh,WG Merz. Pathologic features in the human alimentary tract associated with invasiveness of Candida tropicalis. Am J Clin Pathol 1986;85:498–502.
13. DM Dixon. In vivo models: evaluating antifungal agents. Methods Find Exp Clin Pharmacol 1987;9:729–738.
14. ME Klepser, RE Lewis, MA Pfaller. Therapy of Candida infections: Susceptibility testing, resistance, and therapeutic options. Ann Pharmacother 1998;32:1353–1361.
15. LA Mermel, DG Maki. Detection of bacteremia in adults: Consequences of culturing an inadequate volume of blood. Ann Intern Med 1993;119:270–272.
16. G Medoff. Controversial areas in antifungal chemotherapy: Short-course and combination therapy with amphotericin B. Rev Infect Dis 1987;9:403–407.
17. JH Rex, MA Pfaller, M Lancaster, FC Odds, A Bolmstrom, MG Rinaldi. Quality control guidelines for National Committee for Clinical Laboratory Standards—Recommended broth macrodilution testing of ketoconazole and itraconazole. J Clin Microbiol 1996;34:816–817.
18. JH Rex, MA Pfaller, MG Rinaldi, A Polak, JN Galgiani. Antifungal susceptibility testing. Clin Microbiol Rev 1993;6:367–381.
19. ME Klepser, EJ Ernst, RE Lewis, ME Ernst, MA Pfaller. Influence of test conditions on antifungal time-kill curve results: Proposal for standardized methods. Antimicrob Agents Chemother 1998;42:1207–1212.
20. ME Klepser, EJ Wolfe, RN Jones, CH Nightingale, MA Pfaller. Antifungal pharmacodynamic characteristics of fluconazole and amphotericin B tested against Candida albicans. Antimicrob Agents Chemother 1997;41:1392–1395.
21. ME Klepser, EJ Wolfe, MA Pfaller. Antifungal pharmacodynamic characteristics of fluconazole and amphotericin B against Cryptococcus neoformans. J Antimicrob Chemother 1998;41:397–401.
22. F Meunier, C Lambert, P Van der Auwera. In-vitro activity of SCH39304 in comparison with amphotericin B and fluconazole. J Antimicrob Chemother 1990;25:227–236.
23. JD Turnidge, S Gudmundsson, B Vogelman, WA Craig. The postantibiotic effect of antifungal agents against common pathogenic yeasts. J Antimicrob Chemother 1994;34:83–92.
24. D George, D Kordick, P Miniter, TF Patterson, VT Andriole. Combination therapy in experimental invasive aspergillosis. J Infect Dis 1993;168:692–698.
25. F de Lalla, G Pellizzer, A Vaglia, V Manfrin, M Franzetti, P Fabris, C Stecca. Amphotericin B as primary therapy for cryptococcosis in patients with AIDS: Reliability

of relatively high doses administered over a relatively short period. Clin Infect Dis 1995;20:263–266.
26. CM van der Horst, MS Saag, GA Cloud, RJ Hamill, JR Graybill, JD Sobel, PC Johnson, CU Tuazon, T Kerkering, BL Moskovitz, WG Powderly, WE Dismukes. Treatment of cryptococcal meningitis associated with the acquired immunodeficiency syndrome. N Engl J Med 1997;337:15–21.
27. MS Saag, GA Cloud, JR Graybill, JD Sobel, CU Tuazon, PC Johnson, WJ Fessel, BL Moskovitz, B Wiesinger, D Cosmatos, L Riser, C Thomas, R Hafner, WE Dismukes. A comparison of itraconazole versus fluconazole as maintenance therapy for AIDS-associated cryptococcal meningitis. National Institute of Allergy and Infectious Diseases Mycoses Study Group. Clin Infect Dis 1999;28:291–296.
28. RE Lewis, BC Lund, ME Klepser, EJ Ernst, MA Pfaller. Assessment of antifungal activities of fluconazole and amphotericin B administered alone and in combination against Candida albicans by using a dynamic in vitro mycotic infection model. Antimicrob Agents Chemother 1998;42:1382–1386.
29. ME Klepser, D Malone, RE Lewis, EJ Ernst, MA Pfaller. Evaluation of voriconazole pharmacodynamic characteristics using time-kill methodology. Antimicrob Agents Chemother 2000;44:1917–1920.
30. F Minguez, JE Lima, MT Garcia, J Prieto. Influence of human serum on the postantifungal effect of four antifungal agents on Candida albicans. Chemotherapy 1996; 42:273–279.
31. F Minguez, MT Garcia, JE Lima, MT Llorente, J Prieto. Postantifungal effect and effects of low concentrations of amphotericin B and fluconazole on previously treated Candida albicans. Scand J Infect Dis 1996;28:503–506.
32. F Minguez, ML Chiu, JE Lima, R Nique, J Prieto. Activity of fluconazole: Postantifungal effect, effects of low concentrations and of pretreatment on the susceptibility of Candida albicans to leucocytes. J Antimicrob Chemother 1994;34:93–100.
33. EJ Ernst, ME Klepser, MA Pfaller. Postantifungal effect of echinocaudin, azole, and polyene agents against Candida albicans and Cryptococcus neoformans. Antimicrob Agents Chemother 2000;44:1108–1111.
34. A Louie, GL Drusano, P Banerjee, QF Liu, W Liu, P Kaw, M Shayegani, H Taber, MH Miller. Pharmacodynamics of fluconazole in a murine model of systemic candidiasis. Antimicrob Agents Chemother 1998;42:1105–1109.
35. MD Witt, RJ Lewis, RA Larsen, EN Milefchik, MA Leal, RH Haubrich, JA Richie, JE Edwards Jr, MA Ghannoum. Identification of patients with acute AIDS-associated cryptococcal meningitis who can be effectively treated with fluconazole: The role of antifungal susceptibility testing. Clin Infect Dis 1996;22:322–328.
36. RE Lewis, ME Klepser, MA Pfaller. In vitro pharmacodynamic characteristics of flucytosine determined by time kill methods. Dicy Microbiol Infect Dis 2000;36: 101–105.
37. JE Bennett. Flucytosine. Ann Intern Med 1977;86:319–321.
38. JE Bennett, WE Dismukes, RJ Duma, G Medoff, MA Sande, H Gallis, J Leonard, BT Fields, M Bradshaw, H Haywood, ZA McGee, TR Cate, CG Cobbs, JF Warner, DW Alling. A comparison of amphotericin B alone and combined with flucytosine in the treatment of cryptoccal meningitis. N Engl J Med 1979;301:126–131.
39. P Francis, TJ Walsh. Evolving role of flucytosine in immunocompromised patients:

New insights into safety, pharmacokinetics, and antifungal therapy. Clin Infect Dis 1992;15:1003–1018.

40. DA Andes, M van Ogtrop. In vivo characterization of the pharmacodynamics of flucytosine in a neutropenic murine disseminated candidiasis model. Antimicrob Agents Chemother 2000;44:938–942.
41. G Barbaro, G Barbarini, G Di Lorenzo. Fluconazole vs itraconazole-flucytosine association in the treatment of esophageal candidiasis in AIDS patients. A double-blind, multicenter placebo-controlled study. The Candida Esophagitis Multicenter Italian Study (CEMIS) Group. Chest 1996;110:1507–1514.
42. AM Sugar. Use of amphotericin B with azole antifungal drugs: What are we doing? Antimicrob Agents Chemother 1995;39:1907–1912.
43. SM Grant, SP Clissold. Fluconazole. A review of its pharmacodynamic and pharmacokinetic properties, and therapeutic potential in superficial and systemic mycoses. Drugs 1990;39:877–916.
44. M Scheven, F Schwegler. Antagonistic interactions between azoles and amphotericin B with yeasts depend on azole lipophilia for special test conditions in vitro. Antimicrob Agents Chemother 1995;39:1779–1783.
45. M Scheven, C Scheven. Quantitative screening for fluconazole-amphotericin B antagonism in several Candida albicans strains by a comparative agar diffusion assay. Mycoses 1996;39:111–114.
46. M Scheven, L Senf. Quantitative determination of fluconazole-amphotericin B antagonism to Candida albicans by agar diffusion. Mycoses 1994;37:205–207.
47. AM Sugar. Interactions of amphotericin B and SCH 39304 in the treatment of experimental murine candidiasis: Lack of antagonism of a polyene-azole combination. Antimicrob Agents Chemother 1991;35:1669–1671.
48. AM Sugar, CA Hitchcock, PF Troke, M Picard. Combination therapy of murine invasive candidiasis with fluconazole and amphotericin B. Antimicrob Agents Chemother 1995;39:598–601.
49. EJ Ernst, ME Klepser, MA Pfuller. In vitro interaction of fluconazole and amphotericin B administered sequentially against candida albicans: effect of concentration and exposure time. Diag Microbiol Infect Dis 1998;32:205–210.
50. SL Kelly, J Rowe, PF Watson. Molecular genetic studies on the mode of action of azole antifungal agents. Biochem Soc Trans 1991;19:796–798.
51. EJ Anaissie, RO Darouiche, D Abi-Said, O Uzun, J Mera, LO Gentry, T Williams, DP Kontoyiannis, CL Karl, GP Bodey. Management of invasive candidal infections: Results of a prospective, randomized, multicenter study of fluconazole versus amphotericin B and review of the literature. Clin Infect Dis 1996;23:964–972.
52. JH Rex, JE Bennett, AM Sugar, PG Pappas, CM van der Horst, JE Edwards, RG Washburn, WM Scheld, AW Karchmer, AP Dine. A randomized trial comparing fluconazole with amphotericin B for the treatment of candidemia in patients without neutropenia. Candidemia Study Group and the National Institute. N Engl J Med 1994;331:1325–1330.
53. MS Saag, WG Powderly, GA Cloud, P Robinson, MH Grieco, PK Sharkey, SE Thompson, AM Sugar, CU Tuazon, JF Fisher, N Hyslop, JM Jacobson, R Hafner, WE Dismukes. Comparison of amphotericin B with fluconazole in the treatment of acute AIDS associated cryptococcal meningitis. N Engl J Med 1992;326:83–89.

14

Human Pharmacodynamics of Anti-Infectives: Determination from Clinical Trial Data

George L. Drusano
Albany Medical College, Albany, New York

1 INTRODUCTION

Determination of the relationship between drug exposure and response or between drug exposure and toxicity is key to achieving the ultimate aim of chemotherapy: obtaining the maximal probability of a good therapeutic response while engendering the smallest possible probability of toxicity.

In the area of anti-infective chemotherapy, there is a single difference from other areas of clinical pharmacological investigation. In other areas, we deal with receptors for the drug that are human in origin. There are true between-patient differences in receptor affinity for the drug that are, currently, not measurable. This unmeasured variance leads to difficulty in generating pharmacodynamic relationships.

In anti-infectives, however, we are dealing with an external invader. Whether we are dealing with bacteria, viruses, or fungi, we can, with few exceptions (e.g., hepatitis C virus), grow the offending pathogen and obtain a measure of the drug's potency for that particular pathogen. These measures have different names, depending on the pathogen [e.g., minimal inhibitory concentration (MIC), effective concentration that reduces growth by half (EC_{50}), minimal fungicidal (static) concentration (MFC)]. These measures of pathogen sensitivity to the drug can then be used to normalize the drug exposure in the patient relative to the invading pathogen. This markedly reduces the observed variability and improves the ability to define a relationship between exposure and response.

2 DETERMINANTS OF A PHARMACODYNAMIC RELATIONSHIP FOR ANTI-INFECTIVES

2.1 Endpoints

In order to determine a relationship between exposure and response or between exposure and toxicity, the first step is to identify an endpoint. Such endpoints differ according to what is being studied. Endpoints may be continuous in nature [e.g., change in glomerular filtration rate (GFR) after drug exposure], dichotomous or polytomous (e.g., success vs. failure; survival vs. death, a four-point pain scale), or time to an event (time to death, time to relapse, time to viral clearance). As will be discussed later, the endpoint chosen will in many ways determine a good deal of the rest of the analysis.

The first and most important step in defining a pharmacodynamic relationship is to obtain solid response endpoint data. If all other steps are performed well but the endpoint data are poorly defined, then the relationship will be poor at best and possibly misleading.

2.2 Pathogen Identification and Susceptibility Determination

If one is attempting to construct an effect relationship (i.e., between drug exposure and response), it is imperative that the offending pathogen be isolated and identified and that the susceptibility of that specific pathogen to the drug being used for therapy be measured. This is straightforwardly performed in many clinical antibacterial trials, because pathogen identification and MIC determination are integral parts of making a clinical study case both clinically and microbiologically evaluable for the Food and Drug Administration.

Amazingly little has been done regarding the EC_{50} of viruses and their influence on outcome in clinical trials of antiviral chemotherapy. It has only been recently, with the availability of commercial homologous recombination assays or rapid sequencing assays for HIV, that determination of drug susceptibility has become a part of the clinical trial arena. Nonetheless, EC_{50} has an important role to play, as demonstrated by the data in Figs. 1a–1f. In this evaluation the HIV protease inhibitor indinavir was administered as a single agent. Plasma concentrations were measured by HPLC, and EC_{50} values were determined for indinavir by the ACTG/DOD consensus assay. A sigmoidal E_{max} effect model was fit to

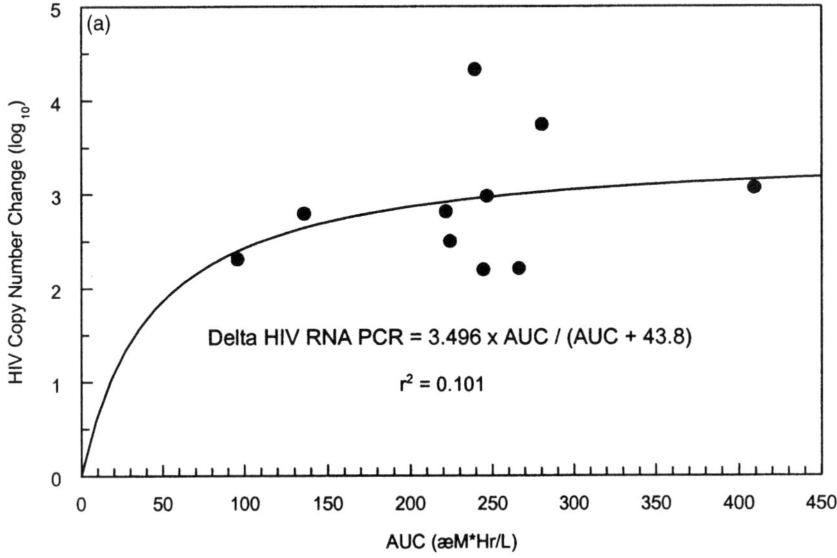

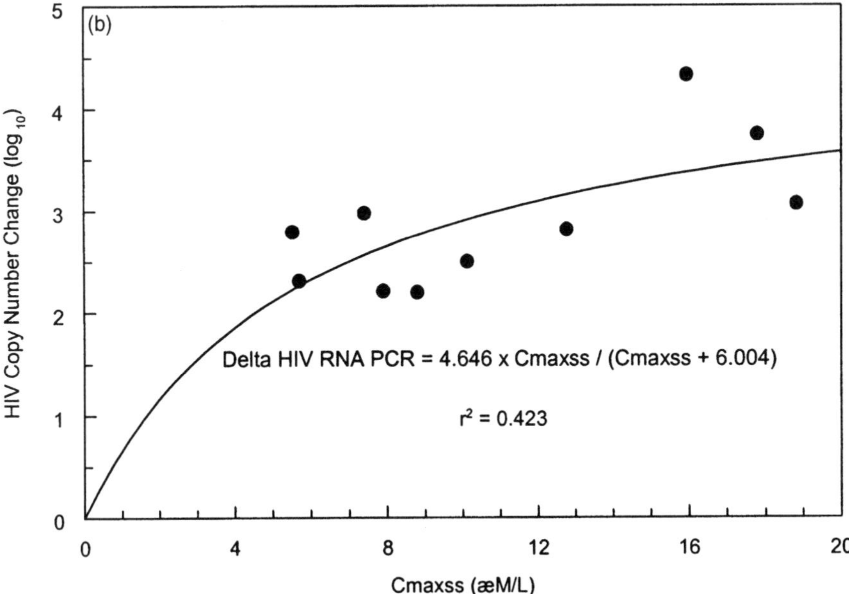

Figure 1 Pharmacodynamics of indinavir. E_{max} model of plasma copy number change. For part explanations, see text.

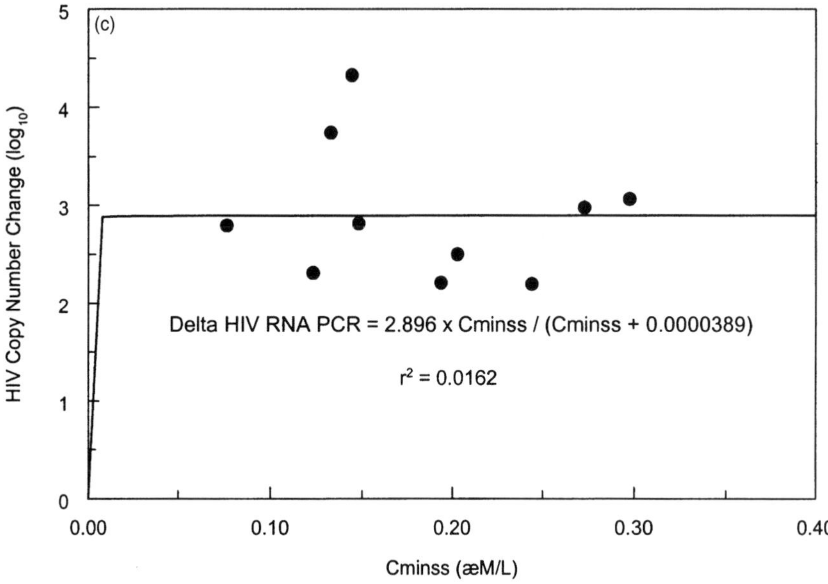

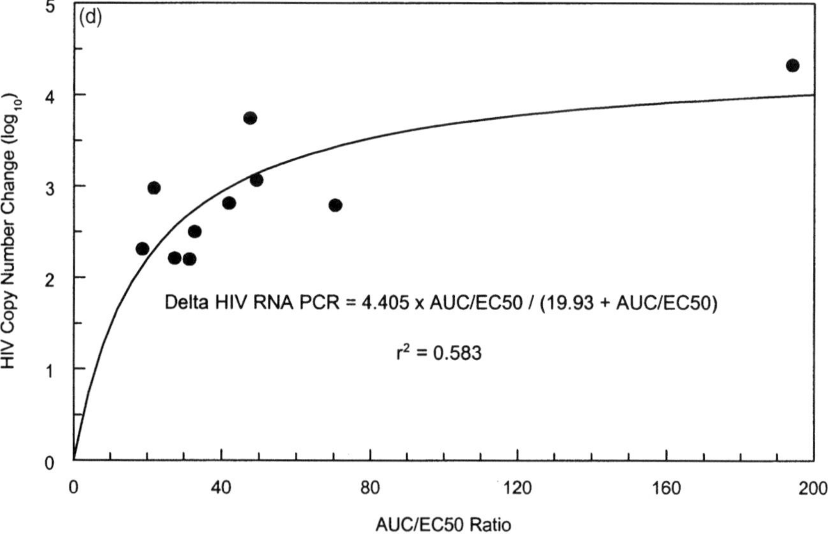

FIGURE 1 Continued

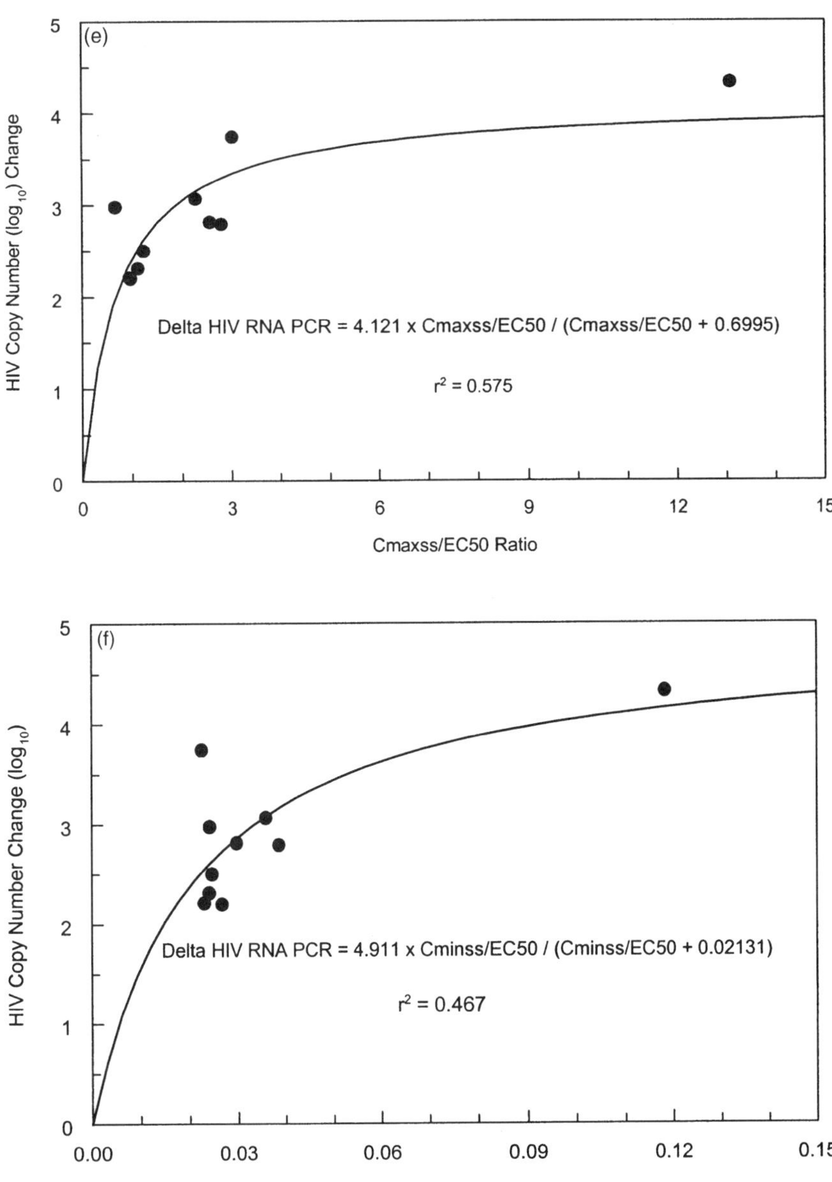

Figure 1 Continued

the data with area under the plasma concentration–time curve (AUC), peak concentration, and trough concentration each as the independent variable (Figs. 1a–1c). In Figs. 1d–1f, the drug exposures were normalized to the EC_{50} of that patient's virus [1]. It can be seen that the normalization improves the fit of the model to the data. It should be noted that the normalization transforms several points from well off the best-fit curve to an area where the fit improves. This is because of the added information gained from treating a very susceptible viral strain.

It should also be noted that because the drug was administered at essentially the same dose and schedule in all the patients there is significant co-linearity. That is, one cannot make the peak rise without also raising the trough and without increasing the AUC. Therefore one should not draw the inference from these data that the AUC/EC_{50} ratio is the pharmacodynamically linked variable for indinavir. Indeed, from other sources of data, the trough/EC_{50} ratio or (perhaps preferably) the time $> EC_{95}$ is the linked variable for protease inhibitors [2]. Clearly, normalization to a measure of potency for the viral isolate to indinavir improves the relationship between exposure and response.

Much the same is true for any type of pathogen. Our ability to grow the organism and identify its sensitivity to the therapeutic agent is key to our ability to formulate an exposure–response relationship.

However, the measure of sensitivity of the pathogen to the drug, although important, is not a sufficient condition for the development of a dynamics relationship. In order to have the highest probability of attaining a robust dynamics relationship, obtaining a good estimate of drug exposure for the individual patient is also critical. This was seen in a neutropenic rat model of fluoroquinolone pharmacodynamics [3]. Two stable mutants of a parental strain of *Pseudomonas aeruginosa* (MICs to the test fluoroquinolone of 1, 4, and 8 mg/L) were derived. Therapy with the same dose of drug produced a clear difference in response by MIC (80 mg/kg once daily as therapy with survivorships of 70%, 15%, and 0% for the groups challenged with MICs of 1, 4, and 8 mg/L, respectively). However, when the dose was altered (20 mg/kg once daily for the MIC of 1.0 mg/L challenge strain) so that the peak/MIC ratio and AUC/MIC ratio were the same as those seen for the challenge group with an MIC of 4.0 treated with 80 mg/kg once daily, the survivorship curves were identical. Because isogenic mutants were employed, this demonstrates that both pieces of information (drug exposure plus a measure of drug susceptibility) are necessary for the best pharmacodynamic relationships to be developed.

2.3 Drug Exposure in Clinical Trial Patients

Amazingly few pharmacodynamic relationships have been derived in the anti-infective arena. Part of the reason for this is that patients being treated for infections are often quite ill and unwilling or unable to undergo the rigors of a traditional pharmacokinetic evaluation. Often, dose has been employed as a surrogate for actual exposure estimates. This has proven to be a failed strategy. Dose is a poor measure of exposure. There are true between-patient differences in the pharmacokinetic parameter values such as clearance and volume of distribution. Such true differences (but unmeasured, when dose is used as a measure of exposure) translate into large differences in peak concentration, trough concentration, and AUC in a population of patients receiving the same dose. It should not be surprising that dose is a particularly poor measure of drug exposure and a poor exposure variable to employ in developing pharmacodynamic relationships.

Figure 2 demonstrates the inadequacy of examining just dose as a measure of drug exposure. This is the marginal density plot for clearance for levofloxacin. This drug was studied in 272 patients enrolled in the first study to prospectively develop a relationship between exposure and response [4]. This was done in a multicenter study that included 22 centers in the United States. In the study protocol, patients with serum creatinine values in excess of 2.0 mg/dL were excluded. Nonetheless, by inspection, the range of clearance exceeded tenfold. This also indicates that the range of AUC for a fixed dose would exceed tenfold. Obviously, any attempt to link exposure to outcome employing dose as the measure of exposure would be doomed to failure.

Over the past decade, a number of mathematical techniques have found their way into the toolbox of the kineticist or clinician wishing to construct such relationships. The first is optimal sampling theory. This technique allows identi-

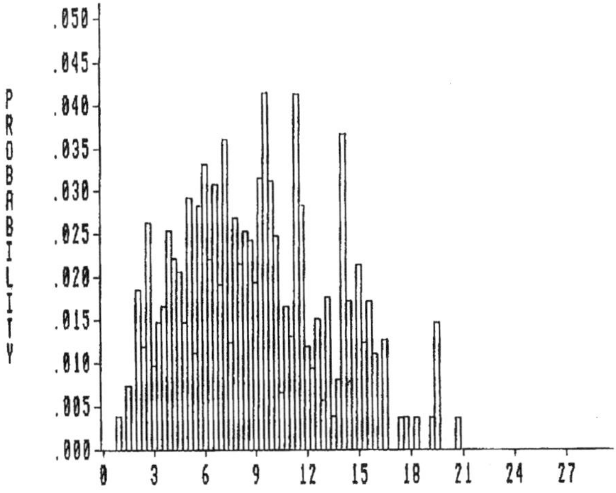

FIGURE 2 Approximate marginal density for clearance of levofloxacin.

fication of sample times that are laden with ''information.'' The definition of ''information'' is dependent upon the measure that is defined by the user. For instance, the most commonly employed measure is the determinant of the inverse Fisher information matrix. This is referred to as *D*-optimality. It has several properties that are desirable. The answers obtained are independent of how the system is parameterized and are also independent of units. This measure also has the remarkable property of replicativeness. That is, if one defines a four-parameter system, there will be exactly four optimal sampling times. If the investigator wishes to make the sampling scheme more robust to errors, *D*-optimality will tell the investigator to repeat one of the optimal sampling times. This is because *D*-optimality is deterministic and is based upon the (incorrect) assumption that there is only one true parameter vector, without true between-patient variability. Most other measures of information content (e.g., *C*-optimality, *A*-optimality) also suffer from being deterministic. Publications by D'Argenio [5] and Tod and Rocchisani [6] extended optimal sampling into the stochastic framework and allowed true between-subject variability in the parameter values. This allows the investigator to increase the number of samples and to have increasing amounts of information in the sampling scheme for patients whose values are more removed from the mean values.

Traditional (deterministic) optimal sampling has been well validated. Further, it is possible to employ traditional optimal sampling and still obtain sampling schedule designs robust for a large portion of the population.

One problem with optimal sampling strategy is that it assumes that the answer is already known, that is, that one knows the true mean parameter vector for the model system. This obviously places limitations on the use of optimal sampling strategy in the early phases of drug development when little is known regarding the ''true'' model to be employed for a specific drug and less is known regarding the true mean parameter vector. Nonetheless, with only a little information regarding these issues, optimal sampling has been employed successfully.

There was no validation of this technique in patients until a series of studies were published by Drusano and coworkers [7–10]. In what was, to our knowledge, the first clinical validation of optimal sampling theory, the drug ceftazidime was examined in young patients with cystic fibrosis receiving a single dose [7]. With the use of a Bayesian estimator, the optimal sampling subset of the full sampling set produced precise and unbiased estimates of the important pharmacokinetic parameter values.

This group then examined the drug piperacillin in a population of septic, neutropenic cancer patients [8]. Whereas the study with ceftazidime was performed with a single dose of drug, the study with piperacillin examined two issues: (1) whether optimal sampling would provide precise and unbiased estimates of parameter values in the steady-state situation and (2) whether obtaining duplicate samples obtained at the specified sample times would improve the precision of parameter estimation.

The results demonstrated that optimal sampling would, as expected, provide reasonably precise and unbiased parameter estimates. Further, this study also showed that resampling at the designated optimal times did *not* improve the precision of parameter estimation. The latter result was a bit of a surprise and flew in the face of the then-accepted theory regarding optimal sampling. Optimal sampling theory assumes that the mean parameter vector is known without error. Further, true between-patient variance is not incorporated into the optimal sampling time calculation. Given these limitations, it is not surprising that when queried regarding the next most optimal time to obtain a sample after the original optimal times have all been obtained, the theory forces one of the optimal times to be repeated (property of replication). This strategy may improve the precision for the mean patient, but in the clinical situation, where one is trying to construct a population model (part of the creation of a pharmacodynamic model), it is important to recognize that true between-patient variance exists for the parameter values.

If an investigator is to limit the number of plasma samples obtained to an optimal sampling set, it is important to know how robust optimal sampling is with regard to errors in nominal parameter values. This group also addressed this issue [10]. Theophylline has been demonstrated to have its clearance altered by smoking cigarettes. The degree of this alteration has been on the order of a 50% increase in the mean clearance of the population. It was felt that by studying a population of smokers as well as a population of nonsmokers and employing optimal sampling strategies for both smokers and nonsmokers they could examine how badly optimal sampling sets performed when systematic errors on the order of 50% (either high or low) were introduced into the nominal value for clearance. This study demonstrated that errors of this magnitude did not introduce significant bias or imprecision into the overall estimation of theophylline clearance. Further, because this study was performed in two stages, after the first stage they embedded a sampling set that was calculated by employing the patient's initial parameter values estimated from the full sample set obtained during the first stage. They demonstrated that the patient's own optimal samples provide excellent precision and minimal bias for the second stage of the study (patient by patient). Such a finding is important in that it means that toxic drugs can be adequately controlled with minimal sample acquisition if patients are to be dosed over a relatively long period of time (as is the case in antiretroviral chemotherapy). Likewise, obtaining information about the patient's parameter values for effect control with limited sample acquisition also becomes possible in the routine clinical situation.

Others have recognized the importance of optimal sampling theory in guiding the acquisition of plasma samples in the clinical trial setting for the develop-

Table 1 Precision (%) of Kinetic Parameters of Theophylline as Determined from Different Optimal Sampling Strategies Relative to Those Determined from the Full Sampling Strategy[a]

	V_c	V_{ss}	V_{area}	S_{Cl}	$T_{1/2\beta}$
Correct7	2.20	1.26	1.30	2.97	2.99
Wrong7	1.66	1.01	1.04	3.56	3.98
Patient's7	2.28	1.34	1.30	2.98	3.66
Patient's4	2.60	2.20	2.28	2.99	3.77

[a] Correct7 represents the 7 sample times derived from the "correct" prior population. Wrong7 represents the seven sample times derived from the "wrong" prior population. Patient's7 and Patient's4 represent the seven and four sample times derived from the patient's own prior parameter values.

ment of exposure–response relationships. Forrest's group [11] developed an optimal sampling strategy for ciprofloxacin that is useful in the environment of seriously ill hospitalized patients with lower respiratory tract infections. Fletcher and colleagues [12] adapted optimal sampling strategy to the AIDS arena for the development of concentration-controlled trials.

The second technique is population pharmacokinetic modeling. Credit for the initial development of this technique reflects to Sheiner, Beal, and colleagues [13–15]. After the initial development of the NONMEM system, other groups developed population modeling programs—Mallet (NPML) [16], Schumitzky et al. (NPEM) [17], the PPHARM system [18], Davidian and Gallant [19], Lindstrom and Bates [20], and Forrest et al. [21], among others. Population modeling allows the development of a mean parameter vector for the model without requiring that every patient have a robust sampling set. It also provides an estimate of the covariance matrix, allowing construction of parameter distributions and also allowing Monte Carlo simulation, which has recently been shown to be useful in evaluation of doses and schedules. Of course, the important issue with population modeling is that the data must be well timed. The looseness of execution often associated with performing population PK modeling is not an excuse for poor timing of sample collection. Such poor attention to detail can severely impact upon the estimates, rendering them either biased or imprecise. Nonetheless, it should be recognized that the ability to perform population modeling has resulted in nothing short of a revolution in our ability to obtain information about drug disposition in ill target patients. The data presented in Fig. 2 are from an analysis employing NPEM [4]. Ill patients with community-acquired infections were studied, with each patient having an optimal sampling set of seven plasma determinations, each guided by stochastic design theory.

Once population modeling has been performed, it is then useful to perform maximal *a posteriori* probability (MAP) Bayesian estimation. This allows point estimates of the model parameters to be obtained for all the patients in the population. Measures of drug exposure [peak concentration, trough concentration, area under the plasma concentration–time curve (AUC)] can be calculated and then normalized to the potency parameter (e.g., peak/MIC ratio, AUC/MIC ratio, time > MIC). It is now possible to examine the relationship between exposure and response and/or toxicity.

In the study cited above, a parameter vector was calculated for each patient by Bayesian estimation. The plasma drug concentrations were then simulated for the specific times they were obtained, and a predicted versus observed plot was produced. Figure 3 displays this analysis. The best-fit line was

$$\text{Observed} = 1.001 \times \text{predicted} + 0.0054, \qquad r^2 = 0.966;\ p \ll 0.001$$

Once robust estimates of parameter values are obtained for each patient, it is straightforward to attempt to link measures of exposure (peak concentration/MIC or AUC/MIC ratio, time > MIC, etc.) to outcomes. For continuous outcome variables (e.g., viral copy number, CD_4 counts), continuous functions, such as a traditional sigmoidal E_{max} effect function would be a natural choice (see Figs. 1a–1f).

However, clinical trials frequently have either dichotomous outcome variables (e.g., success/failure, eradication/persistence) or have time-to-event end-

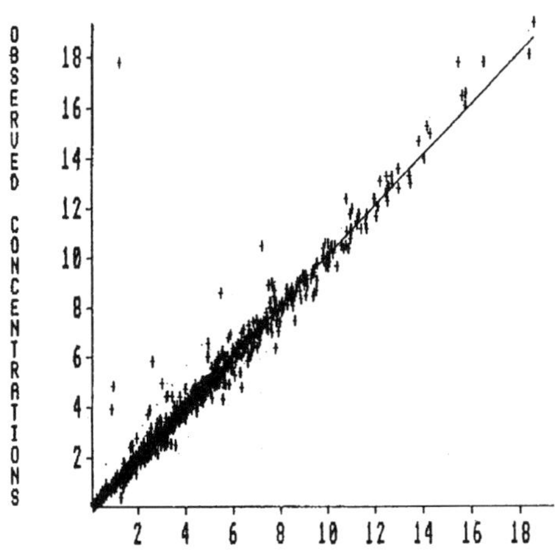

Figure 3 Scatterplot and least squares line for the entire population.

points (e.g., time to death, time to opportunistic infection, time to lesion change in CMV retinitis). For dichotomous outcome variables, logistic regression analysis is a natural choice. For the prospective study examining levofloxacin cited above, we had an analysis plan that tested 13 covariates univariately [4,22]. Model building then ensued from the covariates that significantly altered the probability of a good clinical or microbiological outcome (separate sets of analyses). The final models for clinical and microbiological outcomes are displayed graphically in Figs. 4 and 5, respectively.

It should also be noted that small boxes on the probability curve denote independent variable "breakpoints." These are arrived at through classification and regression tree (CART) analysis. These merely indicate that patients whose independent variable (here, peak concentration/MIC ratio) has a value equal to or greater than the breakpoint value have a significantly higher probability of obtaining a good outcome. CART is a useful adjunctive technique in pharmacodynamic analyses but should probably be seen as an exploratory tool and one for rational setting of breakpoints. Logistic regression should be seen as the primary tool for analysis with dichotomous endpoints.

In addition to modeling success/failure, logistic regression can also be employed to model the probability of occurrence of toxicity. An example can be seen in the analysis of aminoglycoside-related nephrotoxicity published by Rybak et al. [23]. These authors performed a prospective, randomized, double-blind trial in which patients received their aminoglycoside either once daily or twice daily.

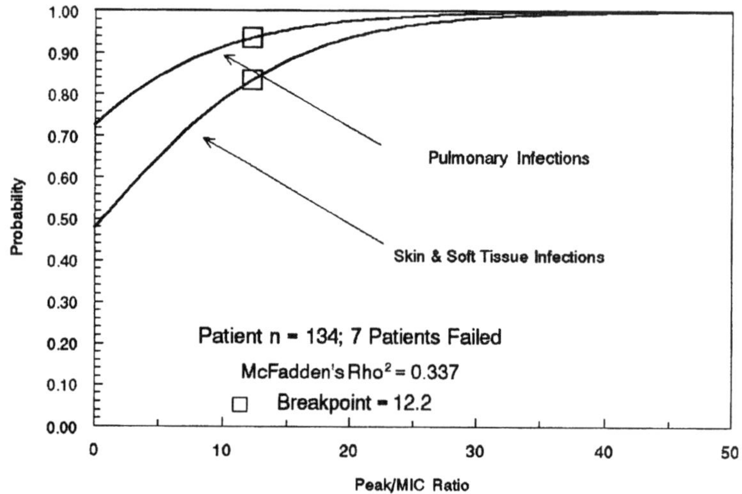

FIGURE 4 Logistic regression relationship between levofloxacin peak/MIC ratio and the probability of a good clinical outcome.

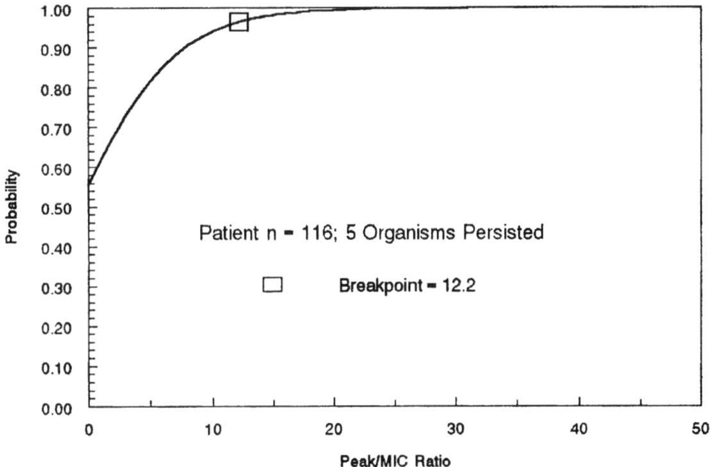

FIGURE 5 Logistic regression relationship between levofloxacin peak/MIC ratio and the probability of organism eradication.

In the final model, the schedule of administration, the daily AUC of aminoglycoside, and the concurrent use of vancomycin all independently influenced the probability of occurrence of aminoglycoside-related nephrotoxicity.

Sometimes, as with the therapy of cytomegalovirus retinitis, the endpoint examined is the time to an event, here the time to CMV lesion progression. In this circumstance, after having performed the Bayesian estimation, the measures of exposure may be employed as covariates in a Cox proportional hazards model analysis. This semiparametric approach is a useful way to approach such analyses. For those instances where fuller knowledge of the shape of the hazard function is available, fully parametric analyses (e.g., Weibull analysis) can be performed.

In an analysis of the use of foscarnet for the therapy of cytomegalovirus retinitis, Drusano et al. [24] performed a population pharmacokinetic analysis followed by Bayesian estimation. The exposures then became part of the pharmacodynamic analysis. Five covariates were examined: (1) baseline CD_4 count, (2) peak CD_4 count during therapy, (3) whether or not the patient had a baseline blood culture positive for CMV, (4) the peak concentration achieved, and (5) the AUC achieved. Trough concentrations were not considered, because they would generally be below the level of assay detection. In fact, all five covariates significantly shifted the hazard function. With model building, only AUC and the baseline CMV blood culture status remained in the final model. Figure 7 demonstrates the exposure response from the final Cox model.

Monte Carlo simulation has recently been demonstrated to be useful for the evaluation of doses and schedules for anti-infective agents. This technique

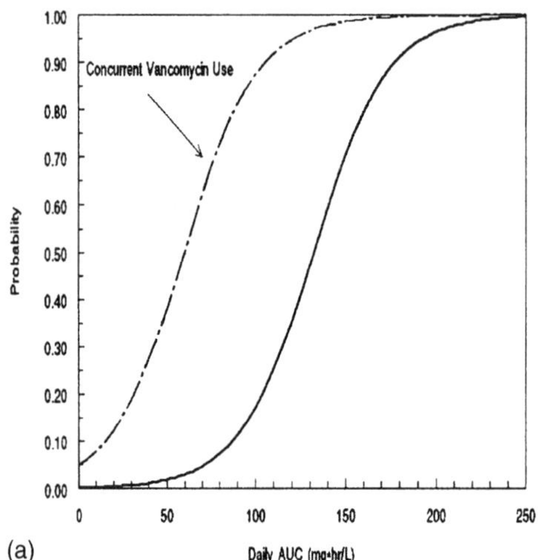

(a)

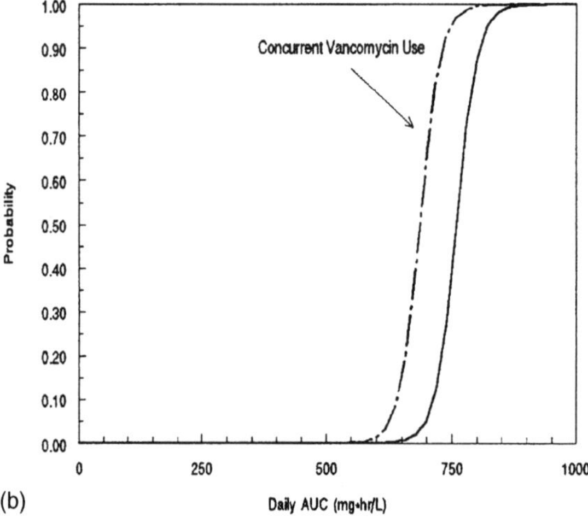

(b)

FIGURE 6 Probability of aminoglycoside toxicity. (a) Twice daily dosing—vancomycin use, and daily AUC. (b) Once daily dosing—vancomycin use and daily AUC.

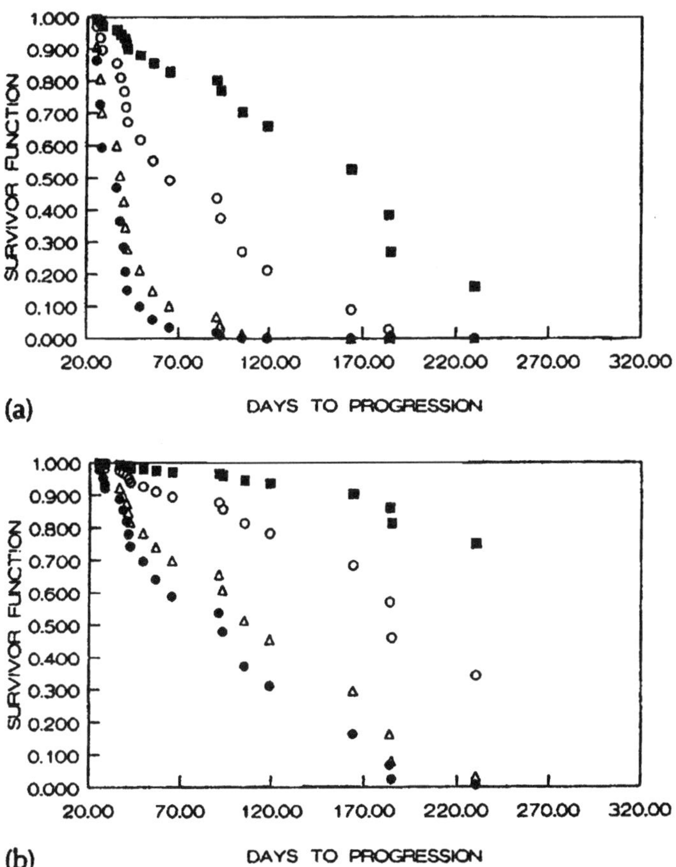

FIGURE 7 Exposure response of final Cox model. (a) Baseline cytomegalovirus blood culture negative; (b) baseline cytomegalovirus blood culture positive. (●) Lowest AUC observed in the population; (△, □, ■) 20th, 50th, and 80th percentiles, respectively, of AUC in the population.

was first applied for this purpose by Drusano at a meeting of the FDA Anti-Infective Drug Products Advisory Committee [25]. Two applications are demonstrated here. The first is for dose adequacy and for preclinical MIC breakpoint determination. The second is for the evaluation of the dosing schedule.

To evaluate the adequacy of a 500 mg dose of the fluoroquinolone levofloxacin, Drusano and Craig collaborated for the following analysis. The mean parameter vector and covariance matrix from the levofloxacin study cited earlier were employed to create a 10,000 subject Monte Carlo simulation. The AUC distribution for a 500 mg IV dose for these subjects was generated. The data

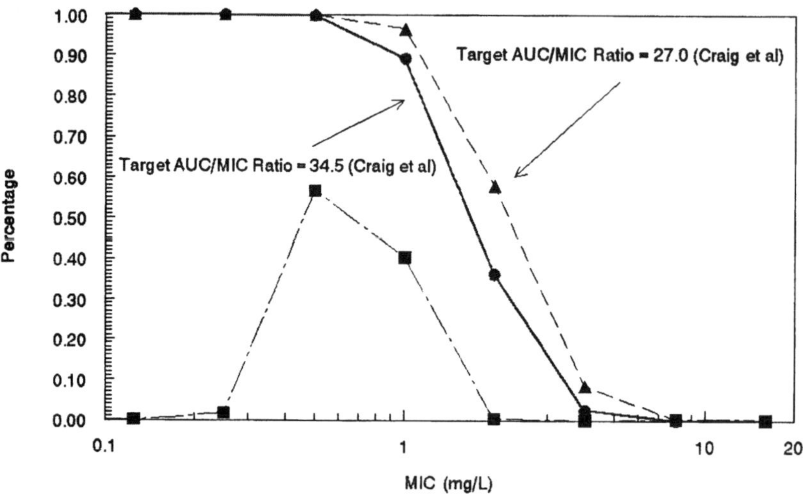

Figure 8 Levofloxacin 10,000-subject Monte Carlo simulation. Pneumococcal target attainment with a 500 mg qid dose. (●) 1 Log drop target; (▲) stasis target; (■) MIC distribution.

from the levofloxacin TRUST (Tracking Resistance in the United States Today) study was employed for the MIC distribution for *Streptococcus pneumoniae*. The key for this analysis was to set a ''target goal.'' Craig's mouse thigh model allowed setting the AUC/MIC target goal of 27.0 (total drug) associated with stasis and 34.5 (total drug) for a drop in the CFU of one $\log_{10}$ unit (associated with the shutoff of bacteremia) for levofloxacin [26]. Each of the 10,000 AUCs in the distribution were divided by the MIC range from 0.125 to 4.0 (in a twofold dilution series). The resultant values were compared to the target goals, and the frequency with which the target was achieved was ascertained. The outcome of this analysis is displayed in Fig. 8.

It is obvious that the goal attainment rate is 100% for both targets until an MIC of 0.5 mg/L is reached. At 1.0 mg/L, both target attainments decline, but

Table 2 Levofloxacin 10,000-Subject Monte Carlo Simulation: Target Attainment Over a 4296 Isolate Database of *Streptococcus pneumoniae*

Target	1 Log drop (34.5 AUC/MIC ratio)	Stasis (27 AUC/MIC ratio)
Attainment	94.7 ± 0.2%	97.8 ± 0.1%

Source: PK parameters, from Ref. 33; isolate MICs from the 1998–1999 TRUST study; target attainment data from Ref. 26.

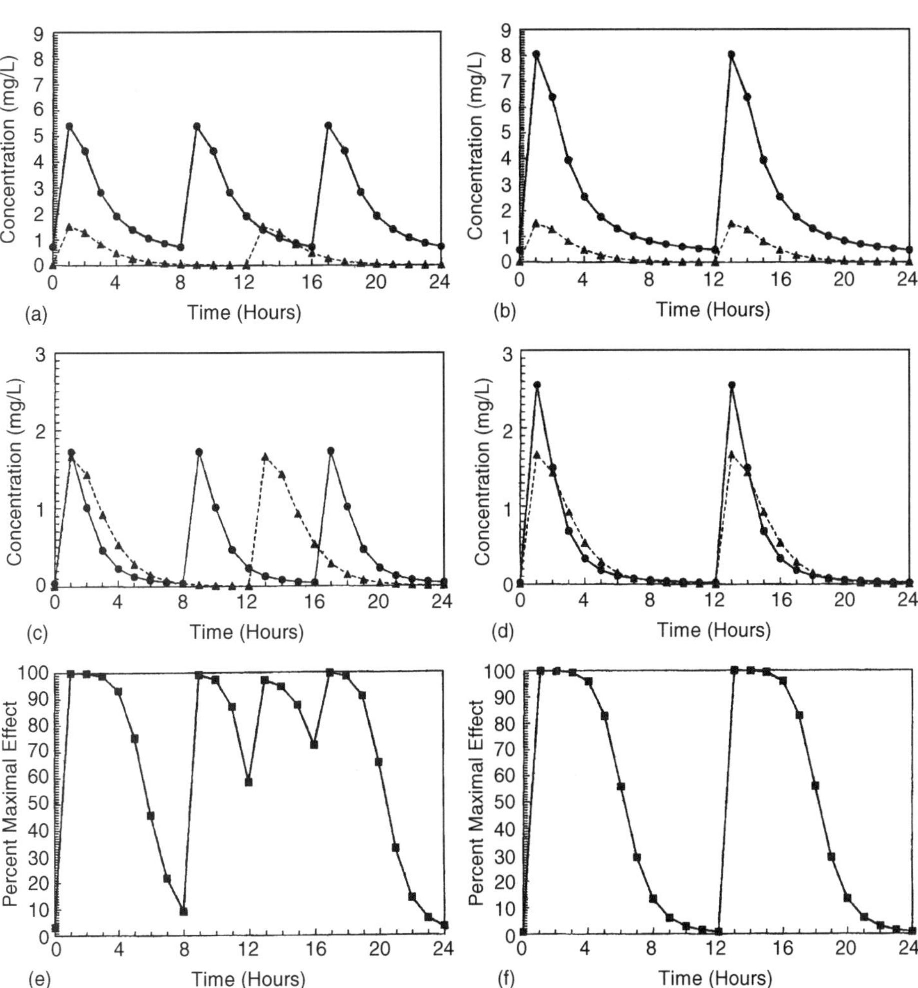

FIGURE 9 One randomly chosen concentration time profile resulting from Monte Carlo simulations of different dosage schedules for abacavir and amprenavir with 500 subjects. (a–d) Concentration–time profiles. (a, c) (●) Amprenavir 800 mg g8h; (▲) abacavir 300 mg q12h. (b, d) (●) Amprenavir 1200 mg q12h; (▲) abacavir 300 mg q12h. (e, f) Effect–time profiles for a specific patient.

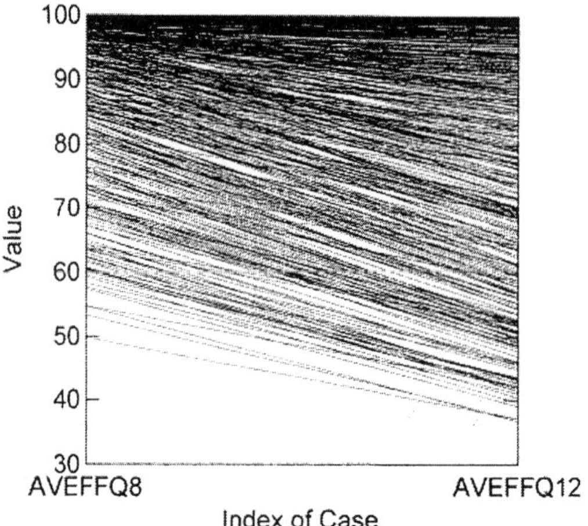

Figure 10 Average percent of maximal antiretroviral effect for combination therapy with abacavir plus amprenavir. Amprenavir schedule of administration was 800 mg (q8h) or 1200 mg (q12h). Abacavir schedule was 300 mg (q12h) in both groups. Results weere calculated from a Greco interaction model. Drug concentrations were from Monte Carlo simulation.

both are in excess of 90%. Only after this do we see a large decline in target attainment.

It is possible to remove the variability in the MIC by performing an expectation over the MIC distribution. In essence, we can multiply the target attainment rate by the fraction of the strains of pneumococcus represented at each levofloxacin MIC value. This gives us an estimate of the target attainment rate in a clinical trial, subject to the assumptions that the MIC distribution is representative of that seen in clinical trials and that the AUC distribution is likewise representative of a clinical trial. The target attainment rates are shown in Table 2.

This example demonstrates that a 500 mg dose of levofloxacin would likely be adequate for pneumococcal infections, given the distribution of the AUCs for the drug and the distribution of the MICs. This has been demonstrated in clinical trials of levofloxacin in community-acquired pneumonia [22,27].

It is also possible to examine schedule with this technique. Drusano et al. [28] examined the combination of abcavir plus amprenavir for HIV. The interaction of the two agents was quantitated in the presence of human binding proteins in vitro using the Greco interaction equation [29]. Population pharmacokinetic models were then derived from clinical trial data for both drugs. Monte Carlo simulations were derived of the effect–time curves for 500 subjects. In the simulations, doses of 300 mg of abacavir every 12 h (q12h) plus 800 mg of amprenavir every 8 h (q8h) were simulated, as well as doses of abacavir 300 mg every 12 h plus 1200 mg of amprenavir every 12 h. In Figs. 9a and 9b the mean concentration–time profiles are shown for the various simulations for 500 subjects. Figures 9c and 9d show one subject selected from the population. Figures 9e and 9f show the effect vs. time curves derived from that specific patient at steady state for the different schedules of administration.

The effect–time curves can be integrated over a 24 h steady-state interval

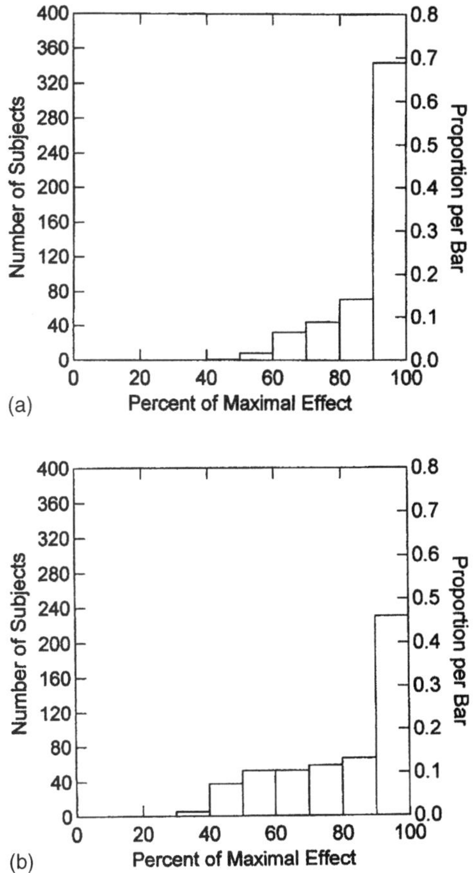

FIGURE 11 Frequency histograms for average percent of maximal effect for abacavir/amprenavir combination therapy. In (a), abacavir was 300 mg (q12h) and amprenavir dose was 800 mg (q8h). In (b), abacavir was 300 mg (q12h) and amprenavir was 1200 mg (q12h). Values were determined as in Figure 10.

and divided by the interval length (24 h). An average percent of maximal effect results from the calculation. These are plotted in Fig. 10 for the two schedules of administration for all 500 simulated subjects.

It is obvious from inspection that the schedule of administration that is more fractionated for the protease inhibitor (amprenavir q8h) is providing greater effects. This can clearly be seen in the frequency histograms presented in Fig. 11. Irrespective of how one tests the differences between regimens (frequency >90% maximal effect, frequency >70% maximal effect, difference between mean percent maximal effects), the more fractionated regimen is always statistically significantly superior.

Consequently, Monte Carlo simulation can be used for both dose and regimen evaluations and can also set preclinical and, after the human pharmacodynamic trials have been performed, clinical MIC breakpoints. It is obvious that there are other uses for this flexible and powerful technique for the clinical arena (e.g., drug penetration to the site of infection [30]).

Each of the foregoing examples leads to a simple paradigm. It is straightforward to attempt to define pharmacodynamic relationships in the clinical trial setting. The approach is set forth in Table 3. Once such relationships are defined, particularly when relationships are available for both efficacy and toxicity, as is the case for aminoglycoside antibiotics [23,31], the true goal of anti-infective chemotherapy (maximal effect with minimal toxicity) can be sought by using stochastic control techniques [32]. As part of the approach, it is clear that plasma concentration determination is a requirement. It should be brought home force-

TABLE 3 Paradigm for the Development of Exposure–Response Relationships for Anti-Infective Agents

1. Decide on an endpoint.
2. Make potency measurements on pathogens from trials (MIC, EC_{50}, etc).
3. Obtain exposure estimates for patients from those trials.
   a. Stochastic design for sampling scheme.
   b. Population pharmacokinetic modeling.
   c. MAP-Bayesian estimation for individual-patient exposure estimates.
4. Decide on an endpoint analysis (the following are examples only).
   a. Sigmoidal E_{max} analysis for a continuous variable.
   b. Logistic regression for dichotomous/polytomous outcomes.
   c. Cox proportional hazards modeling (or a variant) for time-to-event data.
   d. Classification and regression tree analysis for breakpoint determination.
5. Stochastic control when effect–toxicity relationships are available.

fully to pharmaceutical sponsors that the paradigm has shifted. We can successfully seek and generate such relationships. In the ''old days,'' the necessity for concentration determination was the death knell for the development of a compound. Now it is clear that for the patient's sake we can achieve maximal probability of a good clinical and microbiological outcome coupled with the minimal probability of toxicity and (perhaps) emergence of resistance by measuring drug concentrations in plasma. This should be the new (and positive) way of differentiating drugs. We should prefer those that provide us the possibility of having a rational basis for producing the best patient outcomes. Again, third party payors also need to understand that drugs with such relationships developed should have priority on clinical pathways, because they provide maximal probability of response with minimal probability of toxicity.

REFERENCES

1. GL Drusano. Antiviral therapy of HIV and cytomegalovirus. In: Symposium 130-A, S-121. 37th Interscience Conference on Antimicrobial Agents and Chemotherapy, Toronto, Canada, Sept 28–Oct 1, 1997. Am Soc Microbiol, Washington, DC.
2. GL Drusano, JA Bilello, SL Preston, E O'Mara, S Kaul, S Schittman, R Echols. Hollow fiber unit evaluation of BMS232632, a new HIV-1 protease inhibitor, for the linked pharmacodynamic variable. In: Session 171, Presentation 1662. 40th Interscience Conference on Antimicrobial Agents and Chemotherapy, Toronto, Canada, Sept 17–20, 2000. Am Soc Microbiol, Washington, DC.
3. GL Drusano, DE Johnson, M Rosen, HC Standiford. Pharmacodynamics of a fluoroquinolone antimicrobial in a neutropenic rat model of Pseudomonas sepsis. Antimicrob Agents Chemother 1993;37:483–490.
4. SL Preston, GL Drusano, AL Berman, CL Fowler, AT Chow, B Dornseif, V Reichl, J Natarajan, FA Wong, M Corrado. Levofloxacin population pharmacokinetics in hospitalized patients with serious community-acquired infection and creation of a demographics model for prediction of individual drug clearance. Antimicrob Agents Chemother 1998;42:631–639.
5. DZ D'Argenio. Incorporating prior parameter uncertainty in the design of sampling schedules for pharmacokinetic parameter estimation experiments. Math Biosci 1990; 99:105–118.
6. M Tod, J-M Rocchisani. Implementation of OSPOP, an algorithm for the estimation of optimal sampling times in pharmacokinetics by the ED, EID and API criteria. Comput Methods Programs Biomed 1996;50:13–22.
7. GL Drusano, A Forrest, MJ Snyder, MD Reed, JL Blumer. An evaluation of optimal sampling strategy and adaptive study design. Clin Pharmacol Ther 1988;44:232–238.
8. GL Drusano, A Forrest, KI Plaisance, JC Wade. A prospective evaluation of optimal sampling theory in the determination of the steady state pharmacokinetics of piperacillin in febrile neutropenic cancer patients. Clin Pharmacol Ther 1989;45:635–641.
9. GJ Yuen, GL Drusano, A Forrest, KI Plaisance, ES Caplan. Prospective use of opti-

mal sampling theory: Steady-state ciprofloxacin pharmacokinetics in critically ill trauma patients. Clin Pharmacol Ther 1989;46(4):451–457.
10. GL Drusano, A Forrest, JG Yuen, KI Plaisance. Optimal sampling theory: Effect of error in a nominal parameter value on bias and precision of parameter estimation. J Clin Pharmacol 1994;34:967–974.
11. AD Kashuba, CH Ballow, A Forrest. Development and evaluation of a Bayesian pharmacokinetic estimator and optimal, sparse sampling strategies for ceftazidime. Antimicrob Agents Chemother 1996;40:1860–1865.
12. SE Noormohamed, WK Henry, FS Rhames, HH Balfour Jr, CV Fletcher. Strategies for control of zidovudine concentrations in serum. Antimicrob Agents Chemother 1995;39:2792–2797.
13. TH Grasela, LB Sheiner. Population pharmacokinetics of procainamide from routine clinical data. Clin Pharmacokinet 1984;9:545–554.
14. SL Beal, LB Sheiner. Estimating population kinetics. CRC Crit Rev, Bioeng 1982; 8:195–222.
15. LB Sheiner, B Rosenberg, VV Marathe. Estimation of population characteristics of pharmacokinetic parameters from routine clinical data. J Pharmacokinet Biopharm 1977;5:445–479.
16. A Mallet. A maximum likelihood estimation method for random coefficient regression models. Biometrika 1986;73:645–656.
17. A Schumitzky, R Jelliffe, M Van Guilder. NPEM2: A program for pharmacokinetic population analysis. Clin Pharmacol Ther 1994;55:163.
18. F Mentre, R Gomeni. A two step iterative algorithm for estimation in non-linear mixed effects models with an evaluation in population pharmacokinetics. J Biopharm Stat 1995;5:141–158.
19. M Davidian, AR Gallant. Smooth nonparametric maximum likelihood estimation for population pharmacokinetics, with application to quinidine. J Pharmacokinet Biopharm 1992;20:529–556.
20. M Lindstrom, D Bates. Nonlinear mixed effects models for repeated measures data. Biometrics 1990;46:673–687.
21. A Forrest, CH Ballow, DE Nix, MC Birmingham, JJ Schentag. Development of a population pharmacokinetic model and optimal sampling strategies for intravenous ciprofloxacin. Antimicrob Agents Chemother 1993;37:1065–1072.
22. SL Preston, GL Drusano, AL Berman, CL Fowler, AT Chow, B Dornseif, V Reichl, J Natarajan, M Corrado. Prospective development of pharmacodynamic relationships between measures of levofloxacin exposure and measures of patient outcome: A new paradigm for early clinical trials. J Am Med Assoc 1998;279:125–129.
23. MJ Rybak, BJ Abate, SL Kang, MJ Ruffing, SA Lerner, GL Drusano. Prospective evaluation of the effect of an aminoglycoside dosing regimen on rates of observed nephrotoxicity and ototoxicity. Antimicrob Agents Chemother 1999;43:1549–1555.
24. GL Drusano, F Aweeka, J Gambertoglio, M Jacobson, M Polis, HC Lane, C Eaton, S Martin-Munley. Relationship between foscarnet exposure, baseline cytomegalovirus blood culture and the time to progression of cytomegalovirus retinitis in HIV-positive patients. AIDS 1996;10:1113–1119.
25. GL Drusano, SL Preston, C Hardalo, R Hare, C Banfield, D Andes, WA Craig. Use of pre-clinical data for the choice of a phase II/III dose for SCH27899 with applica-

tion to identification of a pre-clinical MIC breakpoint. Antimicrob Agents Chemother. 2001;45:13–22.

26. Craig WA. Personal communication.
27. TM File Jr, J Segreti, L Dunbar, R Player, R Kohler, RR Williams, C Kojak, A Rubin. A multicenter, randomized study comparing the efficacy and safety of intravenous and/or oral levofloxacin versus ceftriaxone and/or cefuroxim axetil in treatment of adults with community-acquired pneumonia. Antimicrob Agents Chemother 1997;41:1965–1972.
28. GL Drusano, DZ D'Argenio, SL Preston, C Barone, W Symonds, S LaFon, M Rogers, W Prince, A Bye, JA Bilello. Use of drug effect interaction modeling with Monte Carlo simulation to examine the impact of dosing interval on the projected antiviral activity of the combination of abacavir and amprenavir. Antimicrob Agents Chemother 2000;44:1655–1659.
29. GL Drusano, DZ D'Argenio, W Symonds, PA Bilello, J McDowell, B Sadler, A Bye, JA Bilello. Nucleoside analog 1592U89 and human immunodeficiency virus protease inhibitor 141W94 are synergistic in vitro. Antimicrob Agents Chemother 1998;42:2153–2159.
30. GL Drusano, SL Preston, M Van Guilder, D North, M Gombert, M Oefelein, L Boccumini, B Weisinger, M Corrado, J Kahn. A population pharmacokinetic analysis of the prostate penetration of levofloxacin. Antimicrob Agents Chemother 2000; 44:2046–2051.
31. AD Kashuba, AN Nafziger, GL Drusano, JS Bertino Jr. Optimizing aminoglycoside therapy for nosocomial pneumonia caused by gram-negative bacteria. Antimicrob Agents Chemother 1999;43:623–629.
32. A Schumitzky. Applications of stochastic control theory to optimal design of dosage regimens. In: DZ D'Argenio, ed. Advanced Methods of Pharmacokinetic and Pharmacodynamic Systems Analysis. Plenum, New York, 1991:137–152.
33. SL Preston, GL Drusano, AL Berman, CL Fowler, AT Chow, B Dornseif, V Reichl, J Natarajan, FA Wong, M Corrado. Levofloxacin population pharmacokinetics and creation of a demographic model for prediction of individual drug clearance in patients with serious community-acquired infection. Antimicrob Agents Chemother 1998;42:1098–1104.

15

Antibacterial Resistance

Philip D. Lister
Creighton University School of Medicine, Omaha, Nebraska

1 INTRODUCTION

Bacterial resistance to antibiotics is an inescapable response to the overuse of antimicrobial agents in the environment. It can arise from the selection of resistant subpopulations among susceptible strains or from the increased prevalence of strains expressing intrinsic or acquired resistance. The impact of antibiotic resistance on patients and society is overwhelming, as infections caused by resistant pathogens are associated with higher rates of morbidity and mortality than infections caused by pathogens [1,2]. Furthermore, microbial drug resistance has been projected to add between $100 million and $30 billion annually to health care costs [3]. Recognition of the factors associated with increasing resistance is essential for the development of new strategies to slow the evolution and progression of antimicrobial resistance among bacteria.

The heavy use and abuse of some antimicrobial agents have been directly linked to some of the more serious resistance problems challenging clinicians today [4,5]. Perhaps the best example is the association between excessive ceftazidime use and the development and spread of multidrug resistance among gram-negative bacteria [6,7]. With a diminishment in the number of novel agents entering the clinical arena, the judicious use of currently available antibiotics becomes essential if we are to preserve their clinical efficacy. Drug control strategies must not only involve tighter regulation on the use of antibiotics but also must involve a more scientific approach to dosing strategies. The field of antimicrobial pharmacodynamics strives to establish relationships between the pharmacokinetics of a drug and the effective treatment of infections. However, just as important are the relationships between pharmacokinetics and selection of resistance during therapy. This chapter will review some of the most critical resistance problems facing clinicians today, the problems encountered with accurate detection of resistance in the clinical laboratory, and the role of pharmacodynamic strategies in slowing the emergence of resistance among bacteria.

2 EMERGING RESISTANCE PROBLEMS IN INFECTIOUS DISEASES

2.1 Gram-Positive Bacteria

2.1.1 *Enterococcus* Species

Among the numerous species of enterococci, *E. faecalis* and *E. faecium* are the two most important clinically. In addition to causing serious hospital-acquired infections such as bacteremia and endocarditis [8], *E. faecalis* and *E. faecium* are two of the most intrinsically resistant bacteria challenging clinicians today [9]. These two pathogens naturally exhibit low-level resistance to the β-lactams, aminoglycosides, clindamycin, trimethoprim-sulfamethoxazole, and other classes of antimicrobial agents. When bacterial killing is required for clinical cure, the combination of a cell-wall-active agent (penicillin or vancomycin) with an aminoglycoside provides one of the true examples of antimicrobial synergy.

Unfortunately, *E. faecalis* and *E. faecium* have not been satisfied with their intrinsic resistance and have been acquiring high-level resistance to these antibiotics as well [9]. Once high-level resistance to either the β-lactams or aminoglycosides is acquired, synergistic killing is lost, therapy of serious infections is compromised, and the search for more effective antimicrobial agents or alternative combinations becomes essential.

2.1.2 *Staphylococcus aureus*

In contrast to the impressive intrinsic resistance displayed by the enterococci, *S. aureus* represents a prototype bacterium for rapid acquisition and development of resistance in response to antibiotics in the environment. Soon after penicillin became available for clinical use, Spink and Ferris [10] reported their isolation of a penicillin-resistant *S. aureus* that produced a penicillin-inactivating enzyme. Penicillinases in *S. aureus* are usually encoded on a plasmid and can spread easily among the genus. Currently, 70–90% of staphylococci are resistant to penicillin and the aminopenicillins [11]. To circumvent this problem, penicillinase-resistant penicillins such as methicillin and oxacillin were synthesized and introduced in the early 1960s. However, the first methicillin-resistant *S. aureus* (MRSA) was discovered as early as 1961 [12]. Resistance to this class of penicillins is not mediated through enzymatic inactivation but rather is mediated through the expression of a low-affinity penicillin binding protein, PBP2′ [13]. By the late 1980s, 25% of all staphylococcal isolates in the United States were resistant to methicillin [14], with prevalence rates varying markedly between geographical areas and between individual institutions.

Strains of MRSAs are frequently resistant to multiple antibiotics, including the penicillins, cephalosporins, cephamycins, carbapenems, β-lactamase–inhibitor combinations, aminoglycosides, macrolides, tetracyclines, and sulfonamides [11]. The glycopeptides vancomycin and teicoplanin remain the preferred therapy for MRSA infections. However, strains of *S. aureus* exhibiting intermediate resistance to both vancomycin and teicoplanin have been reported [15,16].

2.1.3 *Streptococcus pneumoniae*

Like *S. aureus*, *S. pneumoniae* has shown a remarkable ability to evolve and develop resistance to antibiotics in the environment. In contrast to *S. aureus*, however, the rate of resistance development is much slower among pneumococci. Clinical isolates of *S. pneumoniae* remained susceptible to penicillin until the 1960s, when the first intermediate-resistant isolates were reported in Boston in 1965 [17]. Thereafter, pneumococcal susceptibility to penicillin gradually decreased, with reports of intermediate resistance increasing globally and the first reports of high-level resistance and clinical failures with penicillin appearing in the literature [18–20]. In the United States, the prevalence of penicillin-nonsusceptible pneumococci steadily increased through the 1980s and 1990s, with 40% of pneumococci across the country having now lost their susceptibility to penicillin [21].

The mechanism of penicillin resistance among *S. pneumoniae* involves the acquisition of "resistant" PBP gene segments from other streptococci in the environment [22,23]. As susceptibility to penicillin decreases, a concurrent decrease in susceptibility to other penicillins, cephalosporins, cephamycins, and carbapenems is also observed [24]. In addition, penicillin-resistant pneumococci are increasing their resistance to other classes of antimicrobial agents, including the macrolides, tetracyclines, chloramphenicol, and trimethoprim-sulfamethoxazole [24]. The increased prevalence of multidrug-resistant pneumococci presents a therapeutic dilemma for the treatment to serious pneumococcal infections.

A summary of emerging resistance problems among gram-positive bacteria is provided in Table 1.

2.2 Gram-Negative Bacteria

2.2.1 *Haemophilus influenzae*

It is now well established that ampicillin resistance among *H. influenzae* strains can result from mutations affecting the PBP targets, decreased permeability

TABLE 1 Emerging Resistance Problems Among Gram-Positive Pathogens

Bacterial species	Class of antibiotics	Molecular mechanisms
Enterococcus faecium, Enterococcus faecalis	High-level β-lactam	Low-affinity PBPs β-lactamase inactivation
	Vancomycin	Production of altered cell-wall precursors that vancomycin binds with lower affinity
	Aminoglycosides	Inactivating enzymes
Staphylococcus aureus	Penicillin and aminopenicillins	Penicillinase
	All β-lactams	Acquired low-affinity PBP2′
	Vancomycin	Increased targets in outer cell wall
Streptococcus pneumoniae	β-Lactams	Acquired "resistant" PBP gene segments

through the outer membrane, and/or acquisition of plasmid-mediated β-lactamases [25]. Of these three resistance mechanisms, production of β-lactamase accounts for >90% of ampicillin resistance among *H. influenzae* globally, with TEM-1 being the most common enzyme produced [25]. On average, 30–37% of *H. influenzae* strains from every region of the United States produce β-lactamase [21]. Although β-lactamase-producing strains remain susceptible to the β-lactamase–inhibitor combinations and extended-spectrum cephalosporins, permeability and/or PBP changes can provide resistance to these agents as well [21,26]. In addition to β-lactam resistance, *H. influenzae* are developing impressive resistance to the macrolide antibiotics, with 54% of over 3000 isolates exhibiting resistance in a 1998 national survey [21].

2.2.2 *Escherichia coli* and *Klebsiella pneumoniae*

Strains of *E. coli* and *K. pneumoniae* have shown a remarkable ability to evolve and adapt to the threat of antibiotics in the environment, especially to the β-lactam class. Resistance to β-lactams among these two species is mediated primarily through the production of β-lactamases. Whereas both species encode for β-lactamase on their chromosome, plasmid-encoded β-lactamases are the predominant mechanism of resistance, with TEM-1 and SHV-1 being the most common enzymes produced [6]. TEM-1 and SHV-1 are considered broad-spectrum β-lactamases and account for the majority of *E. coli* and *K. pneumoniae* resistance to the penicillins and early narrow-spectrum cephalosporins. Two approaches used to circumvent β-lactamase-mediated resistance have been to develop ''enzyme-resistant'' cephalosporins and to combine an inhibitor of β-lactamases with enzyme-labile penicillins. *E. coli* and *K. pneumoniae* have evolved impressively in response to these two approaches and have rapidly developed resistance to the extended-spectrum ''third generation'' cephalosporins and the β-lactamase–inhibitor combinations.

In response to the β-lactamase–inhibitor combinations, *E. coli* and *K. pneumoniae* have mutated to either increase production of their plasmid-encoded β-lactamases [27,28] or decrease the sensitivity of their β-lactamases to inhibition by clavulanate, tazobactam, and sulbactam [29,30]. In response to the extended-spectrum cephalosporins (ceftazidime, cefotaxime, ceftriaxone) *E. coli* and *K. pneumoniae* have evolved through two distinct pathways. They have either mutated the active sites of their TEM-1 or SHV-1 enzymes to increase the hydrolysis of these drugs, or they have acquired plasmid-encoded AmpC cephalosporinases that originated from the chromosomal AmpCs of other species (see Sections 2.2.3 and 2.2.4) and are inherently capable of providing resistance to the extended-spectrum cephalosporins. The mutated variants of TEM-1 and SHV-1 have been termed extended-spectrum β-lactamases (ESBLs) because they have extended the resistance potential of *E. coli* and *K. pneumoniae* to include the extended-spectrum cephalosporins and aztreonam. Unfortunately, many strains producing these enzymes appear falsely susceptible to the newer cephalosporins and aztreonam in routine susceptibility tests [31,32], and the scope of this resistance problem remains largely unknown. Although most ESBL-producing bacteria are also resistant to ampicillin-sulbactam, amoxicillin-clavulanate, and ticarcillin-clavulanate, many remain susceptible to piperacillin-tazobactam. Similarly, many ESBL-producing *E. coli* and *K. pneumoniae* remain susceptible to the ''fourth generation'' cephalosporin cefepime. However, the clinical relevance of piperacillin-tazobactam and cefepime susceptibility has not been established, and there are concerns of false susceptibility similar to that observed with the extended-spectrum cephalosporins and aztreonam. Further complicating therapy of ESBL-producing bacteria is that these enzymes are encoded on plasmids that also carry genes encoding resistance to other classes of antimicrobial agents [33,34], Therefore, it is not uncommon to find ESBL-producing bacteria that are also resistant to the aminoglycosides, trimethoprim-sulfamethoxazole, chloramphenicol, and the tetracyclines. The most reliably active agents for treatment of ESBL-producing *E. coli* and *K. pneumoniae* are the carbapenems, cephamycins, and fluoroquinolones. However, strains of *K. pneumoniae* resistant to all available antimicrobial agents have been isolated [35] and may signal the beginning of the prophesied ''post-antibiotic era.''

2.2.3 Other Enterobacteriaceae

Although the predominant ESBL-producing bacteria are *E. coli* and *K. pneumoniae*, ESBLs have also been observed in species of *Enterobacter*, *Citrobacter*,

Proteus, *Salmonella*, *Serratia*, and other species of *Klebsiella* [6,36,37]. However, it is an inducible chromosomal AmpC cephalosporinase that is most commonly involved in the development of β-lactam resistance among some of these species [38]. Since the 1980s, Enterobacteriaceae possessing inducible AmpC cephalosporinases have played an important role in the emergence of resistance

TABLE 2 Emerging Resistance Problems Among Gram-Negative Pathogens

Bacterial species	Antibiotic class	Molecular mechanisms
H. influenzae	Penicillins	TEM-1 β-lactamase PBP affinity decrease Outer membrane permeability
K. pneumoniae, E. coli	Penicillins and narrow-spectrum cephalosporins	TEM-1 and SHV-1 β-lactamases
	β-Lactamase–inhibitor combinations	Inhibitor-resistant β-lactamases or hyperproduction of TEM-1/SHV-1
	Penicillins, cephalosporins, inhibitor–penicillin combinations, and monobactams	Extended-spectrum β-lactamases
	Cephamycins	Plasmid-encoded AmpC β-lactamase
E. cloacae, E. aerogenese, S. marcescens, C. freundii	Penicillins, cephalosporins, inhibitor–penicillin combinations, cephamycins and monobactams	Chromosomal AmpC β-lactamase
	Carbapenems	Carbapenemases AmpC + outer membrane porins
P. aeruginosa	Antipseudomonal penicillins	Plasmid-encoded β-lactamases
	Penicillins, cephalosporins, inhibitor–penicillin combinations, and monobactams	Chromosomal AmpC β-lactamase
	Multiple drug classes	Outer membrane porins Antibiotic efflux pumps

to the antipseudomonal penicillins, extended-spectrum cephalosporins, and aztreonam. Studies have shown that the rapid development of resistance to virtually all β-lactams is associated with mutant subpopulations that constitutively produce high levels of their AmpC cephalosporinase [39]. With one mutant cell being present among every 10^6–10^7 viable cells, high-level β-lactam resistance has been shown to emerge in anywhere from 19% to 80% of patients infected with isolates possessing an inducible AmpC cephalosporinase [6]. Although the emergence of AmpC-mediated resistance has been observed during therapy with many of the available β-lactam antibiotics, there appears to be a particular association with extended-spectrum cephalosporins, most particularly ceftazidime [2]. In contrast to the β-lactam class of drugs, carbapenem resistance is very rare among members of the Enterobacteriaceae. When resistance is observed, it is due to either the production of a β-lactamase capable of hydrolyzing carbapenem antibiotics (carbapenemase) or a reduction in the accumulation of drug in the periplasmic space [38,40,41].

2.2.4 *Pseudomonas aeruginosa*

Among the gram-negative bacterial species, *P. aeruginosa* is one of the most talented in terms of rapidly developing resistance to antibiotics. Similar to the Enterobacteriaceae, the mechanisms responsible for β-lactam resistance among *P. aeruginosa* often involve the production of β-lactamases, both plasmid- and chromosomally encoded, and the emergence of high-level β-lactam resistance during therapy is also primarily due to the selection of mutants that overproduce their chromosomal AmpC cephalosporinase [42]. In contrast to the Enterobacteriaceae, however, rates of imipenem resistance among *P. aeruginosa* can exceed 50% [43]. The β-lactams and carbapenem antibiotics are not the only classes that are impacted by *P. aeruginosa*'s ability to rapidly develop resistance. Due to its ability to rapidly alter outer membrane permeability, *P. aeruginosa* can develop resistance during the course of therapy with virtually any antibiotic.

A summary of emerging resistance problems among gram-negative bacteria is provided in Table 2.

3 DETECTION OF RESISTANCE IN THE CLINICAL LABORATORY

3.1 Clinical Relevance of Susceptibility Tests

The susceptibility of a bacterial pathogen to antibiotics is an important therapeutic guide for clinicians. However, antimicrobial susceptibility is just one piece of a complex puzzle determining clinical outcome. Just as important are the pharmacokinetics of the antibiotic at the site of infection, the physical and chemical environment at the site of infection, the pharmacodynamic interactions between the antibiotic and target bacterium, the immune status of the host, the need for surgical intervention, and the emergence of resistance during therapy. The interplay between some or all of these factors can lead to a clinical failure, even when the bacterium exhibits susceptibility to an antibiotic in vitro. Conversely, clinical success can sometimes be achieved in cases when the bacterial pathogen exhibits resistance in vitro. This is especially true when interpretive breakpoints for resistance are based upon serum pharmacokinetics yet the antimicrobial agents are known to concentrate to much higher levels at the site of infection.

There have been relatively few studies investigating the predictive value of susceptibility tests, and comparison of their data is difficult due to differences in susceptibility tests used, definitions of sensitivity or resistance, microorganisms studied, and criteria used for clinical success or failure [44]. Despite these problems, general conclusions can be reached. The correlation between in vitro susceptibility and favorable clinical outcome is moderately good at best, mostly due to the multitude of other factors that can significantly affect therapeutic success. Although the correlation between in vitro resistance and clinical failure is much stronger, the relationship is not 100% [44]. This is not surprising, however, considering that in vitro susceptibility assays are performed in the absence of host defense mechanisms and that interpretive breakpoints based on serum pharmacokinetics are inappropriate for drugs that concentrate to higher levels in tissues or urine. Despite these imperfections, there is a clinical relevance to the data obtained from in vitro susceptibility assays, especially when antimicrobial resistance is accurately detected. Unfortunately, most efforts directed toward improving susceptibility testing to date have focused on achieving a reproducible detection of *susceptibility*. As the threat of antimicrobial resistance continues to increase in our environment, it becomes essential that scientists shift the focus of susceptibility assays from the reproducible detection of susceptibility to the accurate detection of old and newly evolving resistance mechanisms. There are three general approaches that can be used to detect resistance in clinical isolates: (1) detection of resistance genes, (2) detection of gene products that mediate resistance, and (3) detection of phenotypic resistance through routine susceptibility assays. These three approaches will be reviewed in this chapter.

3.2 Methods for the Detection of Resistance Genes

One advantage of using genetic techniques to detect resistance is that they can give the clinician therapeutic guidance faster than routine culture and susceptibility methods. In addition, genetic techniques can sometimes be more accurate than susceptibility tests in defining the resistance mechanisms of a bacterium. For example, oxacillin resistance among strains of *S. aureus* can be mediated either through the production of PBP2′ or through the hyperproduction of a penicillinase [45]. It is not always possible to differentiate between these two resistance mechanisms based on routine susceptibility data, yet the therapeutic implications are important [46]. A genetically based assay that accurately detects *mecA* in staphylococci could provide important therapeutic information to the clinician and prevent the unnecessary use of vancomycin in some cases. It is important to note, however, that these genetically based assays are useful only when they detect a resistance gene in a bacterial isolate. A negative result is of little use to the clinician, because other unrelated resistance mechanisms may be operative in the bacterium. Therefore, a negative result should never be used as a confirmation of susceptibility.

Two approaches are currently used to detect resistance genes: (1) direct detection of genes with DNA probes and (2) amplification of genes using polymerase chain reaction (PCR) methodology. Variations of these methodologies are currently being developed to target resistance genes in numerous bacterial species. However, this section will only briefly review those genetic methods that target aminoglycoside and glycopeptide resistance in enterococci and β-lactam resistance mediated through *mecA* and β-lactamases (see Table 3).

3.2.1 Glycopeptide and Aminoglycoside Resistance

To date, there have been four different genotypes of vancomycin resistance, characterized *vanA*, *vanB*, *vanC*, and *vanD* [5]. Of these, *vanA* and *vanB* are the most important clinically, providing high-level vancomycin resistance among strains of *E. faecalis* and *E. faecium.* Gene probes and PCR assays have been designed to detect the *vanA*, *vanB*, *vanC* genotypes [47,48], and PCR assays are currently being evaluated for the identification of vancomycin-resistant enterococci in fecal samples [49].

Owing to the diversity of aminoglycoside-modifying enzymes among gram-negative bacteria, it is very difficult to find a consensus sequence that would allow for detection of multiple genes using one DNA probe or PCR primer set. In contrast, the genes encoding aminoglycoside-modifying enzymes in gram-positive bacteria are much more conserved. To date, most efforts have focused on detecting the genes encoding ANT(6) and AAC(6′)-APH(2″), which provide high-level aminoglycoside resistance to enterococci [50].

3.2.2 β-Lactam Resistance

Among gram-positive bacteria, most attention has focused on the genetic detection of *mecA*-mediated resistance in isolated colonies of staphylococci or blood culture [51,52]. These assays can require as few as 500 staphylococci to obtain a positive reaction using a PCR enzyme-linked colorimetric assay.

The enzymes that are responsible for β-lactam resistance among gram-negative bacteria are diverse not only in their function but also in their genetic code. DNA probes and PCR primer sets have already been prepared for several plasmid-encoded β-lactamases [53,54], and DNA probes have been used to detect

Table 3 Assays to Detect Antimicrobial Resistance Genes

Bacterial species	Resistance mechanism	Genes targeted
Enterococcus faecium, Enterococcus faecalis, Enterococcus spp.	Vancomycin resistance through VanA, VanB, or VanC	*vanA* *vanB* *vanC*
	High-level aminoglycoside through inactivating enzymes ANT(6) or AAC(6′)-APH(2″)	*ant*(6′) *aac*(6′)-*aph*(2″)
Staphylococcus aureus	β-Lactam resistance through production of low-affinity PBP2′	*mec*A
Escherichia coli *Klebsiella pneumoniae*	Resistance to penicillins and early cephalosporins through TEM-1 or SHV-1 β-lactamase	bla_{TEM} bla_{SHV}
Haemophilus influenzae	Resistance to penicillins through production of TEM-1 or ROB-1 β-lactamases	bla_{TEM} bla_{ROB}
Enterobacteriaceae	Resistance to penicillins, cephalosporins, inhibitor–penicillin combinations, and monobactams through production of ESBLs	Oligonucleotide typing to detect nucleotide changes at critical basepairs of bla_{TEM} and bla_{SHV}

the bla_{TEM} gene (TEM-1) in urethral exudates, urine, and spinal fluid [55–57]. However, because of the diversity of β-lactamase produced by gram-negative bacteria, samples may need to be tested with multiple probes or PCR primer sets. For example, to accurately detect β-lactamase-mediated resistance in *E. coli* and *K. pneumoniae*, probes or primer sets for TEM-1, SHV-1, and a multitude of other β-lactamases may need to be tested on a single isolate. Similarly, to accurately detect β-lactamase-mediated resistance among *H. influenzae*, probes or primer sets for TEM-1 or ROB-1 should be evaluated, even though TEM-1 is by far the most predominant enzyme. Even with the development of probes to every known β-lactamase gene, this genetically based approach would not detect resistance mediated by porin or PBP changes, and thus a negative result should be used as a confirmation of susceptibility.

The ever-evolving family of ESBLs presents an additional problem for genetically-based assays. Because these enzymes have evolved over time through point mutations within the active sites of TEM-1 and SHV-1 [33,37], probes and primer sets designed for bla_{TEM} and bla_{SHV} will detect an ESBL gene. However, these probes cannot differentiate an ESBL-encoding gene from a gene encoding TEM-1 or SHV-1. Considering the therapeutic implications associated with ESBLs, it is critical that any genetically-based assays demonstrate this differentiation capability. Mabilat and Courvalin [58] described an oligonucleotide-based hybridization method that can differentiate β-lactamase genes based on nucleotide changes at critical basepairs. However, because of the logistics and labor-intensive nature of this technology, oligonucleotide typing presents a greater benefit for epidemiological studies at this time. As technologies continue to evolve, the direct detection of ESBLs may become a reality in the clinical laboratory.

3.3 Methods For Detection of Gene Products That Mediate Resistance

Similar to the genetically-based methods discussed above, methods that directly detect the active products of resistance genes can provide valuable therapeutic information to the clinician faster than routine culture and susceptibility methods. A positive result from these tests can guide the clinician by inferring resistance to those drugs known to be affected by the expressed resistance mechanism. However, similar to genetically based methods, a negative result does not ensure the lack of resistance, as other mechanisms of resistance may be operative. A summary of the methods used for direct detection of β-lactamases and chloramphenicol acetyltransferase (CAT) is provided in Table 4.

3.3.1 Direct Detection of β-Lactamases

There are three direct β-lactamase detection assays used clinically: (1) iodometric assay, (2) acidometric assay, and (3) chromogenic assay. The iodometric and acidometric assays are based upon the colorimetric detection of penicillinoic acid produced from β-lactamase hydrolysis of penicillin [59,60]. In the acidometric assay, hydrolysis of citrate-buffered penicillin causes a decrease in pH and a color change of phenol red to yellow. In the iodometric assay, penicillinoic acid reduces iron and prevents the interaction of iron with starch. Without the hydrolysis of penicillin to penicillinoic acid, iron and starch interact and the medium turns bluish purple. In the chromogenic assay, the chromogenic cephalosporin nitrocefin can either be incorporated into liquid suspension or impregnated into sterile paper disks. Hydrolysis of nitrocefin results in an electron shift and a red product [61]. The disk chromogenic assay, commercially known as the cefinase disk, is the most common method used for β-lactamase detection in clinical laboratories.

Table 4 Assays to Detect Gene Products that Mediate Antimicrobial Resistance

Bacterial species	Resistance mechanism	Methodology
Haemophilus influenzae, Moraxella catarrhalis, Enterococcus spp., *Neisseria gonorrheae, Staphylococcus aureus*	Plasmid-encoded β-lactamase	*Acidometric* detection of penicillinoic acid from β-lactamase hydrolysis of penicillin. Decrease in pH changes phenol red to yellow. *Iodometric* detection of penicillinoic acid, which reduces iron and prevents interaction with starch. Lack of iron–starch interaction prevents color change. *Chromogenic* nitrocefin, in suspension or impregnated into paper disks, is hydrolyzed by β-lactamase, and electron shift results in red color product.
Haemophilus influenzae, Streptococcus pneumoniae, Salmonella spp.	Chloramphenicol acetyltransferase (CAT)	Acetyl coenzyme A is converted to hydrogen sulfide coenzyme A during the reaction of CAT with chloramphenicol. Free sulfhydryl of coenzyme A is detected by a color change in the reaction medium.

The direct detection of β-lactamase in species of staphylococci, enterococci, *H. influenzae*, *Neisseria gonorrhea*, and *Moraxella catarrhalis* indicates resistance to all penicillin antibiotics but does not indicate resistance to all the cephalosporins. Furthermore, a negative reaction does not rule out penicillin resistance, because some strains are resistant to penicillins through altered PBPs and/or decreased permeability [62]. Another consideration is the inducibility of penicillinase production in staphylococci. Unlike the constitutive production of β-lactamase by *H. influenzae*, most staphylococci produce detectable levels of their penicillinase only after induction with a β-lactam drug [63]. Therefore, any negative results from uninduced cultures of staphylococci must be repeated with cultures grown in the presence of subinhibitory concentrations of a β-lactam antibiotic.

3.3.2 Detection of CAT

The majority of chloramphenicol resistance is mediated through the enzyme chloramphenicol acetyltransferase (CAT) [64]. A rapid method for detecting CAT in cultures of *H. influenzae* has been described [65] and is available commercially as a kit. This assay has also been used to detect the production of CAT in *S. pneumoniae* [66] and *Salmonella* spp. [67]. In this assay, acetyl coenzyme A is converted to hydrogen sulfide coenzyme A during the reaction of CAT with chloramphenicol. The free sulfhydryl of coenzyme A then reacts with 5,5′-dithiobis(2-nitrobenzoic acid), and a resultant color change from pale yellow to deep yellow is observed. Similar to β-lactamase detection assays, a negative result does not ensure that the bacterium is susceptible to chloramphenicol.

3.4 Susceptibility Methods for Phenotypic Detection of Resistance

Assays that evaluate the growth of bacteria on or in antibiotic-containing media have been the standard approach to susceptibility testing for decades. These assays can be either qualitative, quantitative, or semiquantitative. Qualitative assays provide susceptible, intermediate, and resistance phenotypes but do not provide information on how susceptible or resistant a bacterium is to antibiotics. In contrast, quantitative assays provide a minimum inhibitory concentration (MIC) and thus provide information on the degree of susceptibility or resistance. Semiquantitative assays fall between the qualitative and quantitative methods—they evaluate susceptibility using a short range of antibiotic concentrations around an important ''breakpoint'' concentration or a single concentration that can differentiate between mechanisms of resistance.

3.4.1 In Vivo Correlation of Susceptibility Assays

The primary criticism of any in vitro susceptibility test is that the in vivo environment is not simulated and that the assays are artificially evaluating antimicrobial susceptibility. The four most important criticisms focus on the growth of bacteria in nutrient-rich media, the size of starting inocula, the absence of serum proteins that bind antibiotics, and the lack of pharmacodynamic correlations.

Growth In or On Artificial Media. When the interactions of an antibiotic with a bacterium are evaluated in vitro, the bacteria are usually growing logarithmically in or on nutrient-rich media. This is in contrast to the slow growth or stasis governed by the nutrient-deprived environment of most infections. Therefore, cells that are growing rapidly in vitro may appear more susceptible to growth-phase-dependent antibiotics, such as β-lactam antibiotics, than they would actually be in the infected patient. In addition, other factors such as pH, osmolarity, and levels of gas exchange, which can play an important role in the interactions of antibiotics with bacteria, may also be misrepresented in broth cultures and in the growing bacterial colony [68].

Inoculum Size. Because the load of bacteria can vary substantially from patient to patient and between different sites of infection, it is difficult to define a clinically relevant inoculum. Therefore, scientists have chosen to focus their attention on standardizing inocula so that the reproducibility of data is maximized [69,70]. Unfortunately, accurate reproducibility is best achieved through reducing the inoculum size to provide a more uniform bacterial population. By reducing the inoculum size, one also increases the apparent activity of some antibiotics [68,71] and limits the ability to detect resistant subpopulations that may cause therapeutic failure [72, 73].

Regardless of the inoculum size selected, however, the methods used to achieve the standard inoculum are also important. Standard inocula can be obtained either by growing the bacteria in broth to a desired turbidity or through the suspension of colonies from agar cultures to achieve a desired turbidity. It has been suggested that inocula be prepared from at least four or five colonies to ensure that all phenotypes are present [74]. However, others have suggested that five colonies is less than adequate to represent the clinical situation [75].

Protein Binding. The degree of protein binding can vary widely between and within the different classes of antibiotics. For example, just among the β-lactam antibiotics, percent protein binding can range from <5% to >90% [76]. Although the degree of protein binding has been shown to influence the movement of antibiotics from the bloodstream to extravascular spaces [77], the impact of protein binding on antibacterial activity remains unsettled. The interaction between antibiotics and serum proteins is a dynamic reversible process, with drug molecules constantly binding and unbinding at a rapid rate [78]. In studies with ciprofloxacin and ofloxacin, which exhibit 20–40% binding to serum proteins, the addition of 40–50% serum to MIC assays did not affect the potency of these fluoroquinolones [79–82]. In studies with trovafloxacin, which exhibits 70% protein binding, intra- and interspecies variations have been observed, ranging from no effect at all to significant reductions in potency in the presence of serum proteins [83]. Just as conflicting are data from studies with cefonicid, which is highly protein-bound and exhibits a significant decrease in in vitro potency in the presence of serum proteins [84]. Although protein binding has been used to explain clinical failures with cefonicid when the pathogens are susceptible in vitro [85], the efficacy of cefonicid against *K. pneumoniae* was actually enhanced by the administration of excess serum albumin to mice [86]. The best explanation for this observation is that the binding of cefonicid to the excess serum albumin extended its elimination half-life and increased the time for which concentrations remained above the MIC.

Pharmacodynamic Correlations. One of the major drawbacks of most susceptibility assays is that they evaluate only the inhibition of visible growth. With the exception of broth dilution methodologies, susceptibility assays cannot differentiate bacteriostasis from bactericidal killing, and this differentiation can be critical for successful treatment of some serious infections. Another drawback of in vitro susceptibility assays is that they evaluate antibiotic–bacterium interactions using static concentrations over limited periods of time. In contrast, during the treatment of an infection, bacteria are exposed to constantly changing concentrations of antibiotic over several days. Therefore, important pharmacodynamic interactions may be missed during routine susceptibility assays, especially the outgrowth of slow-growing mutant subpopulations that could result in therapeutic failure in the patient.

Whereas it is obvious that in vitro susceptibility assays are far from perfect and fall far short of mimicking the in vivo environment, the data obtained from them can be useful if their limitations are recognized and more attention is directed toward their accurate detection of antibacterial resistance. The salient aspects of currently used quantitative, semi quantitative, and qualitative assays will be reviewed.

3.4.2 Quantitative Assays

The four quantitative assays used in research and clinical laboratories are the macrobroth dilution assay, microbroth dilution assay, agar dilution assay, and E-test. These assays provide MIC data that can be directly compared to achievable drug concentrations in the patient, especially at the site of infection. Therefore, quantitative assays provide clinicians with the type of information that allows them to optimize therapeutic strategies to not only help the patient but also slow the emergence of resistance.

Macrobroth Dilution. The macrobroth dilution assay is the most conservative of the quantitative assays and is considered the gold standard against which all susceptibility tests are evaluated. One advantage of macrobroth dilution assays is that they allow evaluation of bacterial killing as well as evaluation of the MIC. However, because of the laboriousness of this method, its use in clinical laboratories is not practical. To perform a macrobroth dilution assay, twofold serial dilutions of antibiotic are prepared in 1–3 mL of broth media, and each tube is inoculated with 5×10^5 colony-forming units (CFU) per milliliter of the test bacterial culture [87]. Therefore, the total number of bacteria inoculated into each tube ranges from 5×10^5 to 1×10^6 CFU. Although the macrobroth dilution assay is the most reliable for detecting resistance among clinical isolates, the starting inoculum is often insufficient to evaluate the presence of mutant subpopulations that could cause therapeutic failures.

Microbroth Dilution. Because of the laboriousness of macrobroth dilution assays, a microbroth dilution version was developed. This assay is performed in small plastic trays with individual wells containing 50–100 μL of media and twofold serial dilutions of antibiotic. Although microdilution assays also use starting inocula of approximately 10^5 CFU/mL, the total number of bacteria inoculated into each well is only 10^4 CFU. Considering the established relationship between inoculum size and susceptibility, it is not surprising that bacteria appear to be more susceptible in microdilution assays than in macrodilution assays. Furthermore, with an even lower starting inoculum, microdilution assays are even less likely to detect resistant subpopulations that could cause therapeutic failure.

Agar Dilution. The basic principle of the agar dilution assay is similar to that of broth dilution methods, with the exception that drug is incorporated into an agar medium and bacteria are inoculated on top of the agar. One major limitation of agar dilution assays is that they can only evaluate the inhibition of visible growth and cannot distinguish bacteriostasis from bacterial killing. Like microbroth dilution assays, agar dilution assays are hindered by a starting inoculum of only 10^4 CFU, which make bacteria appear more susceptible than with macrobroth methods [88–90]. Furthermore, the detection of resistant subpopulations is even less likely with agar dilution assays than with either of the broth dilution methods. The reason for this is that one resistant cell will grow into only a single colony on an agar plate, and this single mutant colony would likely be ignored. In contrast, one mutant cell in a broth culture would eventually grow to turbidity and would not likely be ignored.

E-test. The E-test is a quantitative assay that represents a marriage between agar dilution and the disk diffusion assay discussed in Section 3.4.5. In this test, a standard inoculum of bacteria (0.5 McFarland turbidity) is used to create a confluent lawn of growth on an agar plate. Onto this lawn of bacteria are placed plastic-coated strips impregnated with a continuous and exponential gradient of antibiotic concentrations. As antibiotic diffuses from the E-test strip into the agar medium, it interacts with the lawn culture of bacteria. In either the absence of drug or presence of subinhibitory drug concentrations, confluent growth is observed. However, near the E-test strips an elliptical zone of inhibition is observed, reflecting the increasing concentrations of antibiotic along the strip. The MIC is obtained from the point of intersection between the ellipse of growth inhibition and the antibiotic gradient on the E-test strip. Unlike in the other dilution-based methods, the E-test inoculum is not measured by the number of viable bacteria per milliliter or spot. However, the density of the inoculum still plays a critical role in the data obtained. If the inoculum is too light, an unwanted advantage is provided to the drug diffusing from the E-test strip, thus resulting in larger zones of inhibition and lower MICs. Even with the strictest of standard procedures, bacteria appear more susceptible with E-test methodology than with broth dilution assays.

Problems Associated with Interpretive Breakpoints. Once an MIC is obtained from a quantitative assay, the next step is to determine the susceptible, intermediate, or resistant phenotype of the bacterium. These phenotypes are determined by comparing MICs to established interpretive breakpoints. When drug pharmacokinetics are considered during the establishment of interpretive criteria, breakpoints are based on the serum pharmacokinetics of the drug. There are two critical flaws with this approach. The first problem is that some are known to concentrate to much higher levels in tissues and urine than their peak concentrations in serum. Therefore, establishing susceptible breakpoints based on the serum pharmacokinetics of a drug that concentrates outside the bloodstream may incorrectly classify bacteria as nonsusceptible when in fact therapeutic levels would be achieved at the site of infection. The second problem is just the converse of the first, in that drug access to the central nervous system and other restricted areas is often limited and only a fraction of serum antibiotic is able to penetrate. Therefore, establishing breakpoints based on serum pharmacokinetics may actually overestimate the activity of some drugs for treatment of infections in inaccessible sites. This is best illustrated by the problems encountered with establishing interpretive breakpoints for cephalosporins in the treatment of pneumococcal meningitis. As susceptibility to cephalosporins began to decrease with increasing problems of penicillin resistance, clinical failures with cephalosporins in the treatment of meningitis were observed despite in vitro susceptibility based on the established interpretive breakpoints. Therefore, it was apparent that the original interpretive breakpoints for cephalosporins did not relate to pneumococcal infections within the central nervous system, and re-evaluation was necessary.

Even when interpretive breakpoints do correlate with the pharmacokinetics of a drug, problems with detection of resistance can occur. The best example to illustrate this problem is the dilemma of detecting ESBL-mediated resistance among *E. coli* and *K. pneumoniae*. As previously discussed, the MICs of ceftazidime and cefotaxime against ESBL-producing *E. coli* and *K. pneumoniae* are often in the susceptible or intermediate range [91]. Therefore, current interpretive criteria do not reliably identify ESBL-producing bacteria as resistant, and the results can be detrimental to the infected patient. To address this problem, new assays and screening criteria are being developed to increase the detection of ESBL-mediated resistance in the clinical laboratory. However, similar problems will likely occur with other antibiotics and bacterial species as mechanisms of antimicrobial resistance continue to evolve and spread in the environment.

3.4.3 Automated Susceptibility Systems

There are a number of semiautomated or fully automated systems available for susceptibility testing in clinical laboratories. Most of these involve the automated monitoring of bacterial growth in drug-free and drug-containing wells. Data are analyzed using algorithms that are then converted into quantitative results. To evaluate multiple drugs and drug classes on a single susceptibility card, these systems are limited in the number of drug concentrations that can be tested. Therefore, susceptibility is measured with just a narrow range of drug concentrations around a critical ''breakpoint'' concentration, and semiquantitative data are obtained. The major drawback of these systems is that they rely on the assumption that the breakpoint concentrations selected have clinical relevance. Therefore, any errors in selecting the appropriate ''breakpoint'' concentrations can provide potentially harmful susceptibility data for patients. Another disadvantage of breakpoint assays is they have no way of detecting declining susceptibility in the environment. Only when susceptibility crosses the critical breakpoint is resistance detected. This creates a problem for the detection of those resistance mechanisms that fail to increase MICs above the susceptible breakpoint, i.e., ESBLs. One final problem associated with automated susceptibility systems is that they are designed to provide rapid results within hours rather than the usual overnight incubations associated with routine dilution assays. This rapid approach has been shown to be unreliable in detecting resistance to some antibiotics, and research continues to solve these problems.

3.4.4 Resistance Screening Assays

Similar to the automated susceptibility systems, resistance screening assays are semiquantitative assays that evaluate growth or lack of growth at a single drug concentration. In contrast to automated systems, however, the concentrations chosen for these assays are not ''breakpoint'' concentrations, but rather concentrations that allow for differentiation between resistance mechanisms, intrinsic and high-level resistance, and truly susceptible and falsely susceptible populations. A summary of the screening assays for *mecA*-mediated methicillin resistance among staphylococci, vancomycin and high-level aminoglycoside resistance among enterococci, and ESBL-mediated resistance among *E. coli*, *K. pneumoniae*, and *K. oxytoca* is provided in Table 5.

TABLE 5 Screening Assays to Detect or Differentiate Mechanisms of Antimicrobial Resistance

Bacterial species	Resistance mechanism	Methodology
Staphylococcus spp.	β-Lactam resistance due to low affinity PBP2′ from *mec*A	Inoculate 10^4 CFU/spot onto surface of agar supplemented with 4% sodium chloride and 6 μg/mL of oxacillin. Any growth after 24 h of incubation at 37°C is indicative of *mecA-mediated resistance to all β-lactams.*
Enterococcus faecium, Enterococcus faecalis	Vancomycin resistance due to VanB or VanC	Inoculate 10^4 CFU/spot onto surface of agar supplemented with 6 μg/mL of vancomycin. Any growth after 24 h of incubation at 37°C is indicative of vancomycin resistance.
	High-level aminoglycoside resistance	*Agar screen*: Inoculate 10^6 CFU/spot onto surface of agar supplemented with 500 μg/mL of gentamicin or 2000 μg/mL of streptomycin. Any growth after 24–48 h of incubation at 37°C is indicative of high-level aminoglycoside resistance. *Microdilution broth screen*: Inoculate 5×10^5 CFU/mL into broth containing 500 μg/mL of gentamicin or 1000 μg/mL of streptomycin. Presence of visible growth after 24 h of incubation is indicative of high-level aminoglycoside resistance.
Escherichia coli, Klebsiella pneumoniae, Klebsiella oxytoca	Extended-spectrum β-lactamases	Inoculate 5×10^5 CFU/mL into broth containing 1 μg/mL of cefpodoxime, ceftazidime, cefotaxime, ceftriaxone, or aztreonam. Presence of visible growth after 24 h of incubation is suggestive of ESBL production. Confirmatory assay required.

MRSA Screen. The therapeutic importance of differentiating between different mechanisms of methicillin resistance in staphylococci has been discussed. Because hyperproduction of β-lactamase or alterations in PBPs unrelated to *mecA* result in borderline resistance, strains expressing these mechanisms of resistance are typically inhibited by concentrations of oxacillin that do not inhibit the growth of MRSA expressing PBP2′. An agar-based oxacillin screening assay has been described that differentiates *mecA*-mediated resistance from other mechanisms of oxacillin/methicillin resistance [87]. In this assay, agar supplemented with 4% sodium chloride and 6 μg/mL of oxacillin is inoculated with 10^4 CFU of bacteria, as in agar dilution methodology. Growth on this agar screen indicates that the isolate is expressing *mecA*. Although this screening assay is not 100% accurate, it does allow for the differentiation of the majority of MRSA and can be used to guide appropriate therapy.

High-Level Aminoglycoside Resistance Screen. Enterococci are intrinsically resistant to aminoglycosides with MICs in the range of 8–256 μg/mL [9]. Although intrinsic resistance prevents aminoglycosides from being used as single agents for serious enterococcal infections, it does not interfere with their synergistic interactions with cell-wall-active agents. In contrast, the acquisition of high-level resistance is characterized by much higher MICs and does interfere with synergistic killing. Broth- and agar-based screening assays have been developed to detect high-level aminoglycoside resistance among enterococcal isolates [87]. Due to cross-resistance, the only two aminoglycosides that need to be tested are gentamicin and streptomycin. In the agar screening methodology, 500 μg/mL of gentamicin or 2000 μg/mL of streptomycin is incorporated into agar medium, and 10^6 CFU/spot of enterococcal isolates is inoculated onto the agar surface, much as in agar dilution methodology. After 24–48 h of incubation, the presence of more than one colony or hazy growth indicates high-level resistance to aminoglycosides. For broth screening purposes, a microdilution theme is used, and high-level aminoglycoside resistance is detected by the visible growth of a 5×10^5 CFU/mL inoculum in the presence of 500 μg/mL of gentamicin or 1000 μg/mL of streptomycin.

Vancomycin Resistance Screen. Because vancomycin resistance can be low level with strains expressing the VanB and VanC phenotypes, routine susceptibility methods may fail to detect these resistance mechanisms [92,93]. Therefore, an agar screening method is used that evaluates the growth of enterococcal isolates on agar containing 6 μg/mL of vancomycin [87,93]. After 24 h of incubation, the presence of more than one colony indicates resistance to vancomycin.

ESBL Screen. Although MICs of extended-spectrum cephalosporins and aztreonam against ESBL-producing bacteria do not always exceed susceptible breakpoints, they are elevated compared to those of strains lacking ESBLs. The NCCLS recommends a broth-based screening assay for *E. coli*, *K. pneumoniae*, and *K. oxytoca* that evaluates the growth of these three species in the presence of 1 μg/mL of cefpodoxime, ceftazidime, cefotaxime, ceftriaxone, or aztreonam [94]. Visible growth after 16–20 h of incubation is suggestive of ESBL production, and this phenotype must then be confirmed. Confirmation of ESBL production involves the measurement ceftazidime-clavulanate and cefotaxime-clavulanate MICs and comparison with the MICs obtained with each cephalosporin alone. A threefold or greater difference confirms the production of an ESBL. Similar assays are being developed for some automated systems and the E-test assay.

3.4.5 Qualitative Assays

Qualitative assays provide simple "yes" or "no" susceptibility information through establishment of susceptible, intermediate, or resistant phenotypes. However, quantitative information on the level of susceptibility is not provided.

Disk Diffusion Assay. The disk diffusion assay is well standardized, reproducible, and inexpensive and is relatively easy to perform. Because of these qualities, the disk diffusion is the most common susceptibility assay used in clinical laboratories. Although similar in methodology to the E-test, disk diffusion assays use paper disks impregnated with a single drug concentration rather than the range of antibiotic concentrations associated with E-test strips. This difference results in circular zones of growth inhibition, the size of which ultimately determines the susceptibility phenotype of the bacterium. Although the susceptibility of a bacterium to an antibiotic influences the size of the inhibition zone, the inoculum, incubation temperature, incubation time, and media consistency and depth are all important factors that influence the size of growth inhibition zones.

The NCCLS establishes the interpretive breakpoint criteria from which the sizes of growth inhibition zones are translated into susceptible, intermediate, and resistant phenotypes. These breakpoints are established through error-rate-bounded analysis of disk diffusion and MIC data for hundreds of bacterial isolates. The ultimate goal of any disk diffusion assay is to achieve 100% correlation between the phenotypes determined by "gold standard" MIC assays and those obtained with the disk diffusion assay. Because 100% correlation is not often attainable, it becomes important to limit or prevent any false susceptibility errors with the disk diffusion assay. False susceptibility errors occur when a bacterium appears susceptible by disk diffusion assay but is found to be truly resistant by MIC methods. This type of error has also been referred to as a "fatal error" because of the life-threatening problems it can present to patients with serious infections. What level of false susceptibility error rates is acceptable with the disk diffusion assay has been a controversial subject for many years.

Special Disk Diffusion Assays for Detection of ESBLs. Similar to problems encountered with dilution-based quantitative assays, the disk diffusion assay

TABLE 6 Modified Disk Diffusion Assays for Confirmation of ESBL-Mediated Resistance

Detection assay	Methodology	Interpretation
Three-dimensional disk diffusion assay	The test bacterial isolate is inoculated on top of an agar plate similar to standard disk diffusion methodology. In addition, a concentrated suspension of the bacterial culture is inoculated into a slit prepared in the agar with a scalpel. Commercial disks of cefotaxime, ceftazidime, ceftriaxone, and aztreonam are placed proximate to the slit in the agar. Plates are incubated for 18–24 h.	If the bacterial isolate produces an ESBL, the enzyme will inactivate drug diffusing from the commercial disks through the "wall" of bacteria in the agar slit. This interaction will result in a truncated zone of growth inhibition.
Double-disk diffusion	The test bacterial isolate is inoculated on top of an agar plate similar to standard disk diffusion methodology. Commercial disks of cefotaxime, ceftazidime, ceftriaxone, and aztreonam are placed proximate to commercial disks of amoxicillin-clavulanate (source of clavulanate acid). Plates are incubated for 18–24 h.	If the bacterial isolate produces an ESBL, the enzyme will be inhibitied by the clavulanate diffusing from the amoxicillin-clavulanate. The inhibition of the ESBL by clavulanate will enhance the activity of the test drugs, resulting in an enhancement of the zone of growth inhibition between the amoxicillin-clavulanate disk and the disks containing the cephalosporins or aztreonam. Since the optimum distance between disks varies with each test strain and drug, multiple distances between disks should be evaluated to prevent false negative results.
NCCLS ESBL assay	The test bacterial isolate is inoculated on top of an agar plate similar to standard disk diffusion methodology, and commercial disks containing cefotaxime and ceftazidime are placed onto the lawn culture. In addition, commercial cefotaxime and ceftazidime disks are impregnated with 10 μg of clavulanate and placed onto the lawn culture. Plates are incubated for 18–24 h.	If the bacterial isolate produces an ESBL, the zone of growth inhibition around the cephalosporin-clavulanate disks will be increased 5 mm compared to the zones around the disks containing cephalosporins alone.

is unreliable in detecting ESBL-mediated resistance. Up to 75% of ESBL-producing strains appear susceptible to cefotaxime and 43% appear susceptible to ceftazidime according to disk diffusion methodology [31,95]. Three modifications of the disk diffusion assay have been shown to provide improved detection of ESBLs in clinical isolates (see Table 6).

The three-dimensional assay [32] is performed much like the standard disk diffusion assay. The one exception is that the bacterial inoculum is introduced into a slit in the agar as well as on top of the agar. Commercial disks containing extended-spectrum cephalosporins or aztreonam are placed in close proximity to the slit in the agar. If the inoculated organism produces an ESBL, drug is inactivated before it can diffuse through the concentrated culture in the agar slit, and truncated zones of inhibition are observed. The three-dimensional assay reliably detects >90% of ESBL-mediated resistance but is currently not suited for routine laboratory use.

The double-disk diffusion assay [31] is based upon the sensitivity of ESBLs to inhibition by clavulanic acid. In this assay, disks containing extended-spectrum cephalosporins or aztreonam are placed proximate to a disk containing clavulanic acid. The inhibition of ESBLs by clavulanic acid results in an enhancement of the inhibition zone around commercial ceftazidime, cefotaxime, ceftriaxone, or aztreonam disks. Although this assay substantially improves the detection of ESBLs, the optimum distance between disks required for detection varies substantially from strain to strain. Therefore, multiple assays must be run with varying distances between the clavulanate- and drug-containing disks. Of even more concern are the reports of ESBLs that also exhibit resistance to clavulanate inactivation. The increased prevalence of these enzymes threatens the future usefulness of the double-disk assay and any other ESBL detection assays that require clavulanate inhibition of the enzymes.

The NCCLS has approved a set of disk diffusion screening assays to detect ESBLs in *E. coli*, *K. pneumoniae*, and *K. oxytoca* [94]. For initial screening, zones of inhibition around cefpodoxime, ceftazidime, cefotaxime, ceftriaxone, or aztreonam disks are evaluated for diameters that fall below ESBL-indicative breakpoints. ESBL production is then confirmed by a special assay in which 10 μg of clavulanate is added to commercial disks of ceftazidime and cefotaxime, and a 5 mm increase in the zone of inhibition around the cephalosporin-clavulanate disks compared to the cephalosporins alone confirms ESBL production.

4 PHARMACODYNAMICS AND ANTIMICROBIAL RESISTANCE

The field of antimicrobial pharmacodynamics strives to establish relationships between the pharmacokinetics of a drug, its interaction with target bacteria, and the effective treatment of infections. As previously discussed, the emergence of resistance can result in therapeutic failure when the original isolate is susceptible by routine assays. Therefore, the relationship between antimicrobial pharmacodynamics and suppression of resistant subpopulations is also critical for optimizing therapy of many infections.

Resistance to antimicrobial agents can develop through two distinct pathways: (1) acquisition of new genes encoding resistance-mediating proteins and (2) evolutionary mutations in existing genes. The impact of optimizing antimicrobial pharmacodynamics on each of these pathways is very different. Although the optimization of antimicrobial pharmacodynamics can slow the evolution of most mutation-mediated resistance mechanisms, there are many acquired resistance mechanisms that cannot be treated with safe doses of antibiotic. Therefore, the goal of pharmacodynamics should be to optimize therapy such that mutational resistance is prevented. This section will differentiate acquired from mutational resistance and discuss the pharmacodynamic parameters that can impact the emergence of mutational resistance during therapy.

4.1 Acquired Versus Mutational Resistance

4.1.1 Acquired Resistance

Acquired resistance, as the name suggests, represents the development of resistance in a bacterium through the acquisition of a new gene or set of genes from other bacteria in the environment. Examples of acquired resistance mechanisms include plasmid-encoded β-lactamases, plasmid-encoded aminoglycoside-inactivating enzymes, acquired vancomycin resistance, and methicillin resistance mediated through *mecA*. The common theme with these resistance problems is that they are passed from bacterium to bacterium on transferable genetic elements, i.e., plasmids or transposons. Once a bacterium acquires one of these resistance mechanisms, the level of resistance that is expressed usually exceeds the levels of antibiotic that can be safely achieved in serum or other sites of infection. For example, acquisition of the TEM-1 β-lactamase by an *E. coli* can increase the MIC of ampicillin from 2 to 256 μg/mL [96]. Similarly, acquisition of the genes responsible for vancomycin resistance can increase the MIC of vancomycin against enterococci from 2 to 512 μg/mL [97]. Although acquisition of new genes usually results in an instantaneous conversion to high-level resistance, there are exceptions to this rule. It has been well established that penicillin resistance among pneumococci is mediated through the acquisition of PBP gene segments from other resistant streptococci in the environment. However, development of high-level penicillin resistance does not result from a single transfer event but rather requires multiple steps affecting multiple PBPs.

4.1.2 Mutational Resistance

In contrast to acquired resistance, mutational resistance is mediated through genetic changes (point mutations) within a bacterium's own chromosome. These evolutionary mutations can alter the binding of a drug to its target, decrease the accumulation of a drug at the site of action, or disrupt the regulatory genes controlling the production of resistance-mediating enzymes. Similar to acquired resistance mechanisms, mutational events can result in instantaneous high-level resistance or gradual decreases in susceptibility, requiring multiple steps to achieve clinically significant resistance. Whether high-level resistance is achieved with a single point mutation or requires multiple mutational events depends upon the specific drug and the specific target bacterium. In fact, differences between drugs within the same family can be observed. This point is best illustrated using the example of β-lactam resistance in gram-negative bacteria as mediated through derepression of the *ampC* operon.

As previously discussed, derepression of the *ampC* results from point mutations within a regulatory gene, *ampD*, resulting in a loss of the negative control of *ampC* transcription [38]. Once negative control is lost, AmpC production increases significantly, and the bacteria become resistant to virtually all β-lactam antibiotics. Such mutations occur in one out of every 10^6–10^7 viable bacteria. Therefore, one or more highly resistant mutants are likely to be present at the start of therapy of some infections. If these mutants are not eliminated by the host or killed by the antibiotic, they can eventually become the predominant population and lead to therapeutic failure. Clinical failure due to the emergence of this resistance problem has been observed in 19–80% of patients infected with bacteria possessing inducible AmpC cephalosporinases [6]. Although almost any β-lactam antibiotic can select for these mutants, there appears to be a particular association with the ''third generation'' cephalosporin ceftazidime [2].

In contrast, a single mutational event is not always sufficient to provide resistance to the ''fourth generation'' cephalosporin cefepime, especially among the Enterobacteriaceae. In a 1994 survey of five medical centers in the United States, cefepime was tested against 256 ceftazidime-resistant clinical isolates [98]. Among the *Enterobacter* in this study, almost all species were 100% susceptible to cefepime. The only exception was *E. cloacae,* of which 94% of the ceftazidime-resistant isolates remained susceptible to cefepime. In a separate study, 100% of *Enterobacter* strains with proven *ampC* derepression were susceptible to cefepime [99]. The activity of cefepime against ceftazidime-resistant *Enterobacter* spp. can be explained by the differing number of mutational steps required to achieve resistance with each of these drugs. In contrast to the single mutational event required for ceftazidime resistance, it takes two independent mutational events to achieve cefepime resistance among *Enterobacter* spp. [100]. First, the level of AmpC production must be increased through derepression of the *ampC* operon, and then the penetration of cefepime through the outer membrane must be slowed or prevented through a second mutational event. Since each of these mutational steps occurs in one out of every 10^6–10^7 viable bacteria, it is unlikely that resistance will develop in a ceftazidime-susceptible enterobacter during the course of therapy with cefepime. This hypothesis is supported by data from a murine infection model [101]. However, once an enterobacter mutates to a state of *ampC* derepression and bacterial numbers increase above 10^6, the chances of selecting the second permeability mutation increases and emergence of cefepime resistance becomes a real threat.

Differences between antibiotics in the number of mutational steps required to achieve clinically relevant resistance is not unique to the β-lactam class, as similar observations have been reported with other drug classes as well, particularly the fluoroquinolones [102]. Although appropriate dosing of antibiotics does not often impact problems associated with acquired resistance, pharmacodynamics can play an influential role in slowing the development of mutational resistance, especially when first step mutations do not result in high-level resistance. Therefore, the relationship between antimicrobial pharmacodynamics and the emergence of mutational resistance is essential for developing optimum therapeutic strategies.

4.2 Antimicrobial Pharmacodynamics and Emergence of Resistance

The three best characterized pharmacodynamic parameters influencing the clinical efficacy of antibiotics are the time antibiotic concentrations remain above the MIC ($T >$ MIC), the ratio of peak concentrations to the MIC (peak/MIC), and ratio of the area under the concentration curve to the MIC (AUC/MIC). Which pharmacodynamic parameter is most predictive of clinical efficacy depends upon the class of drugs being used. For example, with β-lactam antibiotics the $T >$ MIC is the pharmacodynamic parameter that most influences clinical outcome, whereas with fluoroquinolones the most important parameter can either be the peak/MIC ratio or the AUC/MIC ratio. Further complicating therapeutic strategies is the observation that the pharmacodynamic parameter that most influences overall efficacy may not be the most important parameter impacting the emergence of resistance during therapy. With the data accumulated to date, it appears that the peak/MIC ratio is the most critical pharmacodynamic parameter dictating whether resistance will emerge during therapy with virtually all drug classes.

4.2.1 Peak/MIC Ratio and Emergence of Resistance During Therapy

The likelihood of a bacterium undergoing two mutational events during the course of therapy is very small. Therefore, to prevent the emergence of resistance during therapy, the pharmacodynamic focus must be on effectively treating both the original isolate and any first-step mutants present within the initial bacterial population. This demands that the concentration of antibiotic at the site of infection exceed the MIC for the first-step mutant. Since neither $T >$ MIC nor AUC/MIC directly addresses this need, the peak/MIC ratio becomes the pharmacodynamic parameter that can most impact selection of resistance. Indirect evidence to support this hypothesis has come from studies in an animal model of infection [103]. Using a neutropenic rat model of *Pseudomonas* sepsis, Drusano and colleagues evaluated the effects of dose fractionation of lomefloxacin on survival. Although the emergence of resistance was not directly evaluated in this study, the peak/MIC ratio was most closely linked to survival when the ratios exceeded 10/1. Their hypothesis to explain these results was that sufficient peak/MIC ratios resulted in suppression of mutant subpopulations, thus preventing death due to the emergence of resistance. Similar conclusions were reached in a study of levofloxacin in the treatment of human infections [104].

The best evidence supporting the importance of peak/MIC ratios in preventing the emergence of resistance comes from studies with in vitro pharmacokinetic models. The flexibility provided by these models allows for the design of experiments to specifically address this issue. Using a two-compartment pharmacokinetic model, Blaser et al. [105] varied the pharmacokinetics of enoxacin and netilmicin such that bacteria were exposed to varying peak/MIC ratios while maintaining a constant total drug exposure over 24 h. These investigators observed the outgrowth of resistant subpopulations when simulated peak/MIC ratios failed to exceed 8/1. Similarly, Marchbanks et al. [106] used a two-compartment pharmacokinetic model to simulate ciprofloxacin doses of 400 mg TID (peak/MIC ratio = 4/1) and 600 mg BID (peak/MIC ratio = 6/1) and observed outgrowth of resistant subpopulations of *P. aeruginosa.* When the same daily dose of 1200 mg was simulated as a single injection, the 11/1 peak/MIC ratio prevented the outgrowth of resistant subpopulations. However, in the same study, peak/MIC ratios of only 6/1 were sufficient to prevent the emergence of resistant subpopulations of *S. aureus*. Similarly, Lacy et al. [107] observed differences between levofloxacin and ciprofloxacin and the emergence of resistance in experiments with *S. pneumoniae.* Although these investigators simulated peak/MIC ratios of ≤5/1 with both fluoroquinolones, they observed the emergence of resistance only in studies with ciprofloxacin. Resistance did not emerge in studies with levofloxacin despite peak/MIC ratios as low as 1/1. These data suggest that although the peak/MIC ratio exerts an important influence on the emergence of resistance during therapy, the minimum peak/MIC ratio needed to prevent this problem will likely vary depending upon the drug used and the bacterium targeted. This conclusion is supported with data from my own pharmacodynamic studies of *P. aeruginosa.*

4.2.2 Studies with Levofloxacin Against *P. aeruginosa*

A two-compartment pharmacokinetic model was used to simulate the serum pharmacokinetics of a once daily 500 mg dose of levofloxacin and evaluate pharmacodynamic interactions against a panel of six *P. aeruginosa* strains. Three of the strains evaluated were fully susceptible to levofloxacin (MIC = 0.5 μg/mL), and three strains were borderline susceptible (MIC = 2 μg/mL). The peak concentration simulated for the 500 mg dose was 6 μg/mL, which provided peak/MIC ratios of 13/1 for the fully susceptible strains and 3/1 for the borderline-susceptible strains. Levofloxacin was dosed into the model at 0 and 24 h. The pharmacodynamics of levofloxacin against representative susceptible and borderline-susceptible strains of *P. aeruginosa* are shown in Fig. 1. In studies with the fully susceptible strains, levofloxacin exhibited rapid and significant bactericidal activity, with viable counts falling to undetectable levels (<10 CFU/mL) within 4–12 h after the first dose. In studies with the borderline-susceptible strains, levofloxacin also exhibited significant bacterial killing. However, killing was observed only over the initial 6–8 h, with viable counts increasing rapidly thereafter due to the outgrowth of resistant subpopulations. By 24 h, viable counts in the levofloxacin-treated cultures were approaching those in the drug-free control cultures. The MICs of levofloxacin against the resistant subpopulations ranged from 8 to 16 μg/mL. Therefore, emergence of resistance could have been predicted because peak concentrations with each dose of levofloxacin never exceeded the MICs for these mutant subpopulations.

4.2.3 Studies with Ceftazidime and Ticarcillin Against *P. aeruginosa*

A two-compartment pharmacokinetic model was used to investigate the relationships between mutational frequencies, pharmacodynamics, and the emergence of resistance during the treatment of *P. aeruginosa* with ticarcillin and ceftazidime. Mutational frequency studies were performed in agar by exposing logarithmic phase cultures of *P. aeruginosa* 164 to ticarcillin and ceftazidime at concentrations two-, four-, and eightfold above their respective MICs. The initial MICs for ticarcillin and ceftazidime against *P. aeruginosa* 164 were 16 μg/mL and 2 μg/mL, respectively. Analysis of mutational frequencies showed there was one resistant mutant present among every 10^6–10^7 parent cells, with MICs of ticarcillin and ceftazidime against these mutants increasing to >512 μg/mL and 32 μg/mL, respectively. Using a two-compartment pharmacokinetic model, the kinetics of a 3.0 g QID dose of ticarcillin and 2.0 g TID dose of ceftazidime were simulated, and their pharmacodynamics against *P. aeruginosa* 164 were evaluated over 24 h. With peak concentrations of 260 μg/mL for ticarcillin and 140 μg/mL for ceftazidime, peak/MIC ratios were 16/1 for ticarcillin and 70/1 for ceftazidime. The observed pharmacodynamic interactions are shown in Fig. 2. In studies with ceftazidime, viable counts decreased over 3 logs throughout the 24 h experimental period and no resistant mutants were detected on drug selection plates. The lack of resistance emergence was not unexpected, because peak concentrations achieved with the 2.0 g dose of ceftazidime were fourfold above the 32 μg/mL MIC of first-step mutants. In contrast, outgrowth of a resistant mutant was observed in studies with ticarcillin, despite simulated peak/MIC ratios of

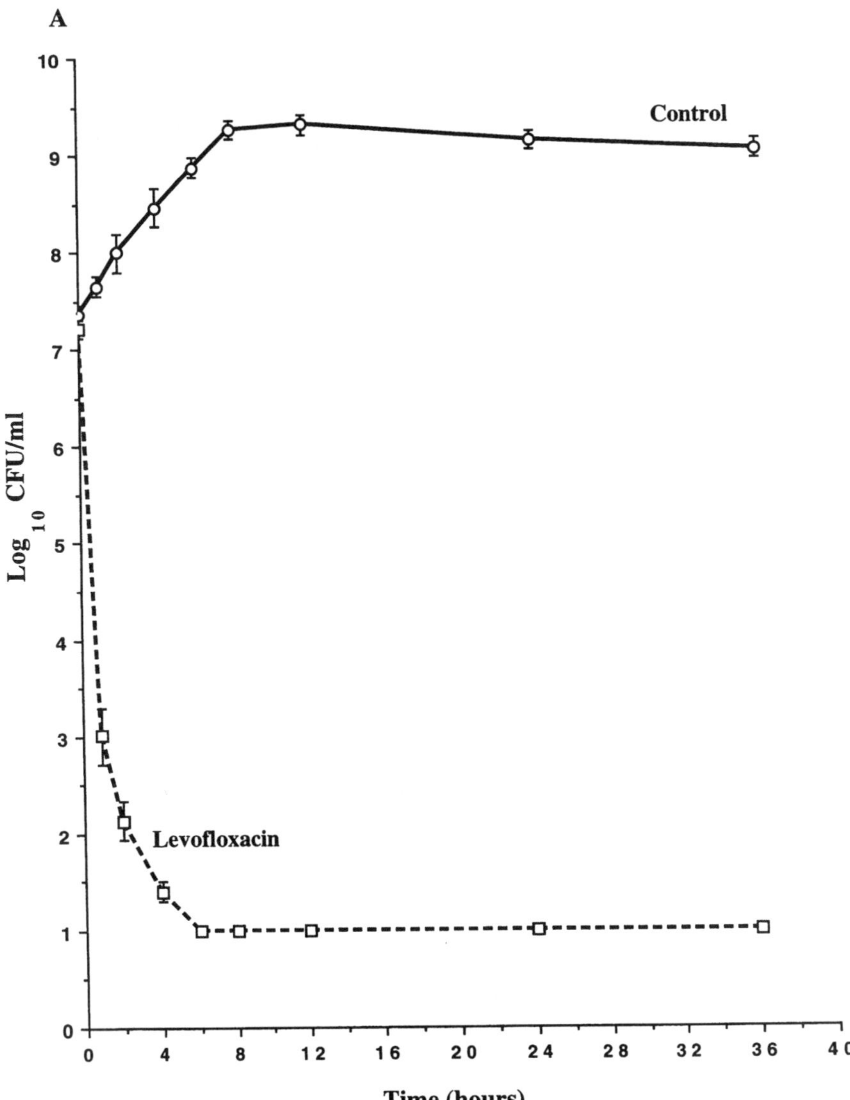

FIGURE 1 Pharmacodynamics of (A) levofloxacin against *P. aeruginosa* GB240 and (B) *P. aeruginosa* GB65 in an in vitro pharmacokinetic model. Levofloxacin MICs were 0.5 μg/mL for *P. aeruginosa* GB240 and 2.0 μg/mL for *P. aeruginosa* GB65. Levofloxacin was dosed at 0 and 24 h, and the pharmacokinetics of a 500 mg dose were simulated. Each datum point represents the mean number of viable bacteria per milliliter of culture for duplicate experiments. Error bars show standard deviations.

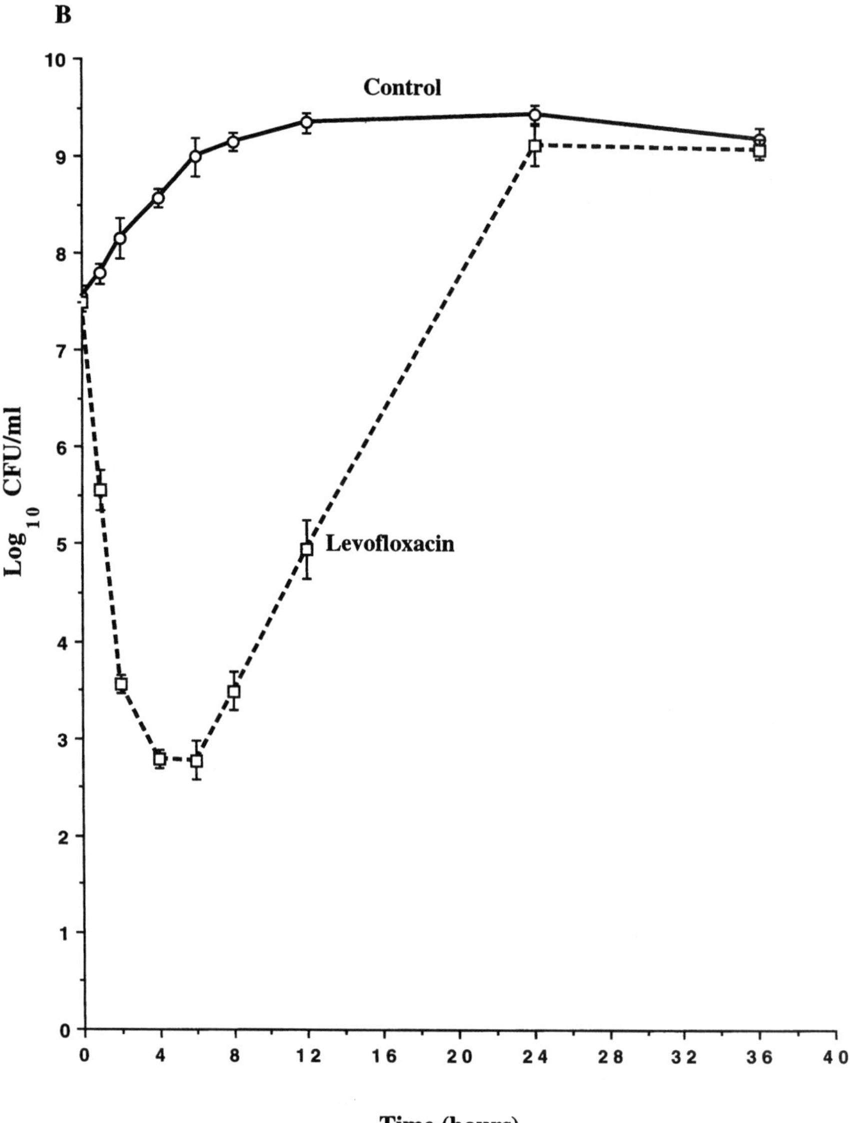

FIGURE 1 Continued

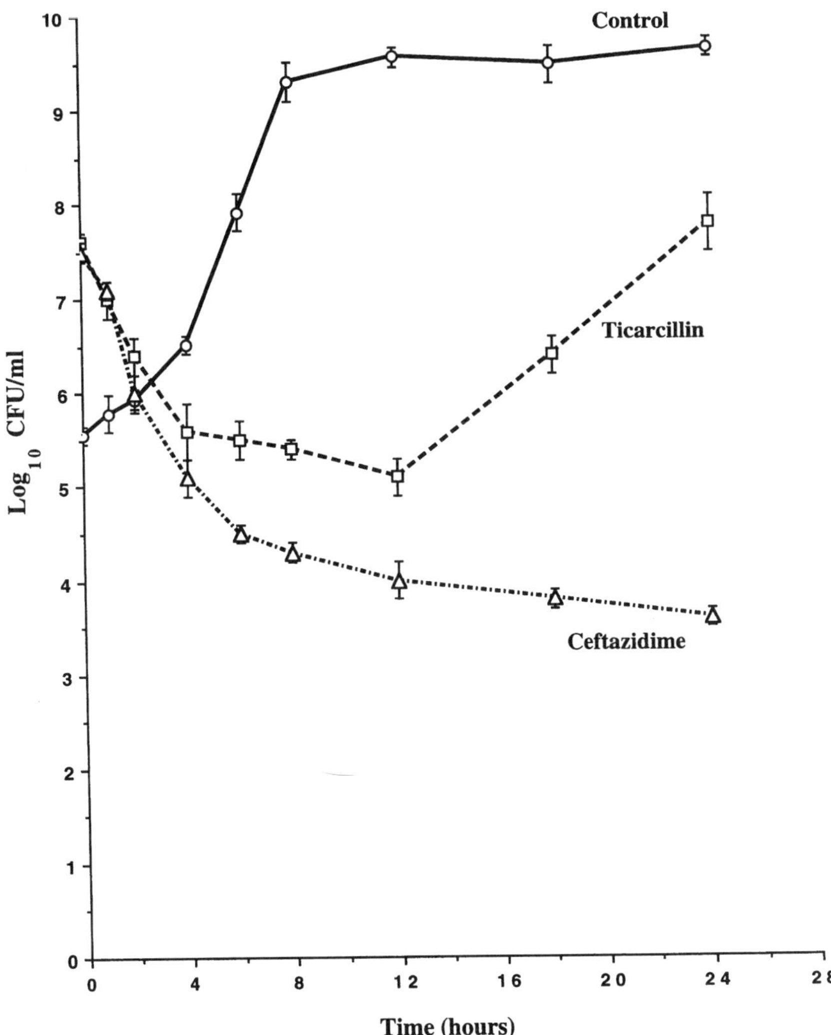

FIGURE 2 Pharmacodynamics of ticarcillin and ceftazidime against *P. aeruginosa* 164 in an in vitro pharmacokinetic model. Ticarcillin and ceftazidime MICs were 16 μg/mL and 2.0 μg/mL, respectively. Ticarcillin was dosed at 0, 6, 12, and 18 h, and the pharmacokinetics of a 3.0 g dose were simulated over each 6 h dose interval. Ceftazidime was dosed at 0, 8, and 16 h, and the pharmacokinetics of a 2.0 g dose were simulated over each 8 h dose interval. Each datum point represents the mean number of viable bacteria per milliliter of culture for duplicate experiments. Error bars show standard deviations.

16/1 against *P. aeruginosa* 164. The outgrowth of these mutant subpopulations could have been predicted, because peak concentrations of ticarcillin never exceeded the MIC against the resistant subpopulation.

These pharmacodynamic data and data from other investigators highlight the importance of the peak/MIC ratio in dictating whether emergence of resistance will complicate therapy. Unfortunately, these studies also demonstrate that the optimum peak/MIC ratio needed to prevent the emergence of resistance varies between different drug classes and with different bacteria–drug combinations. Furthermore, these studies suggest that optimization of therapy cannot just be directed toward the ''parent'' isolate. Rather, optimization of therapy to prevent emergence of resistance during therapy requires a greater understanding of the quantitative influence that different resistance mechanisms exert on susceptibility. In other words, the relationship between peak concentrations and the MIC against first-step mutants is more important in preventing the emergence of resistance than targeting peak/MIC ratios based on MICs against the original isolate.

5 CONCLUDING REMARKS

Antibacterial resistance is an inevitable consequence of the overuse of antibiotics in the environment. The emergence of multidrug resistance among prominent gram-positive and gram-negative pathogens presents serious therapeutic problems, not only for clinicians but also for the clinical microbiologists who have to reliably detect new resistance mechanisms in the laboratory. Where assays fail to detect resistance, new assays are being developed and provide some hope for the future. However, the reliable detection of resistance gains nothing for the clinician faced with dwindling therapeutic options. How, then, do we curve the evolution of antibiotic resistance among bacteria and once again take control of the ongoing resistance battle?

As the number of stronger or truly novel antimicrobial agents achieving FDA approval declines, scientists must continue to develop strategies to slow the emergence of resistance in the environment. One approach is to control the use of antibiotics and to rotate antibiotics before resistance becomes a problem. This theory is referred to as antibiotic cycling [108]. A further step that can be taken is to pharmacodynamically optimize antimicrobial therapy such that the evolution of mutational resistance is slowed. This requires dosing antibiotics such that peak concentrations at the site of infection exceed the MICs of the parent and any resistant subpopulations that might be present. Through the combination of judicious antimicrobial use and pharmacodynamically based optimization of dosing, the evolution of antibiotic resistance can be slowed and the ''postantibiotic era'' need not become a reality.

REFERENCES

1. SD Holmberg, SL Solomon, PA Blake. Health and economic impacts of antimicrobial resistance. Rev Infect Dis 1987;9:1065–1078.
2. JW Chow, MJ Fine, DM Shlaes, JP Quinn, DC Hooper, MP Johnson, R Ramphal, MM Wagener, DK Miyashiro, VL Yu. *Enterobacter* bacteremia: Clinical features and emergence of antibiotic resistance during therapy. Ann Int Med 1991;115:585–590.
3. CE Phelps. Bug/drug resistance: Sometimes less is more. Med Care 1989;27:194–203.
4. JE McGowan. Antimicrobial resistance in hospital organisms and its relations to antibiotic use. Rev Infect Dis 1983;5:1033–1048.
5. DCE Speller. The clinical impact of antibiotic resistance. J Antimicrob Chemother 1988;22:583–586.
6. CC Sanders, WE Sanders Jr. β-lactam resistance in gram-negative bacteria: Global trends and clinical impact. Clin Infect Dis 1992;15:824–839.
7. KS Thomson, AM Prevan, CC Sanders. Novel plasmid-mediated β-lactamases in Enterobacteriaceae: Emerging problems for new β-lactam antibiotics. In: JS Remington, MN Swartz, eds. Current Clinical Topics in Infectious Diseases. Cambridge, MA: Blackwell Science, 1996:151–163.
8. J Robert, C Moellering. *Enterococcus* species, *Streptococcus bovis*, and *Leuconostoc* species. In: GL Mandell, JE Bennett, R Dolin, eds. Principles and Practice of Infectious Diseases. 4th ed. New York: Churchill Livingstone, 1995:1826–1835.
9. GM Eliopoulos. Antibiotic resistance in *Enterococcus* species: An update. In: JS Remington, ed. Current Clinical Topics in Infectious Diseases. Cambridge, MA: Blackwell Science, 1996:21–51.
10. WW Spink, V Ferris. Quantitative action of penicillin inhibitor from penicillin-resistant strains of staphylococci. Science 1945;102:221.
11. RN Jones, EN Kehrberg, ME Erwin. Prevalence of important pathogens and antimicrobial activity of parenteral drugs at numerous medical centers in the United States. I. Study on the threat of emerging resistances: Real or perceived? Diagn Microbiol Infect Dis 1994;19:203–215.
12. M Barber. Methicillin-resistant staphylococci. J Clin Pathol 1961;14:385.
13. BM Hartman, A Tomasz. Low-affinity penicillin binding protein associated with beta-lactam resistance in *Staphylococcus aureus*. J Bacteriol 1984;158:513.
14. RN Jones, AL Barry, RV Gardiner. The prevalence of staphylococcal resistance to penicillinase-resistant penicillins. A retrospective and prospective trial of isolates from 40 medical centers. Diagn Microbiol Infect Dis 1989;12:383–394.
15. K Kiramatsu, H Hanaki, T Ino, K Yabuta, T Oguri, FC Tenover. Methicillin-resistant *Staphylococcus aureus* clinical strain with reduced vancomycin susceptibility. J Antimicrob Chemother 1997;40:135–136.
16. CDC. *Staphylococcus aureus* with reduced susceptibility to vancomycin–United States, 1997. MMWR 1997;46:765–766.
17. JW Kislak, LMB Razavi, AK Daly, M Finland. Susceptibility of pneumococci to nine antibiotics. Am J Med Sci 1965;250:262–268.

18. PC Applebaum, A Bhamjee, JN Scragg, AJ Hallett, AF Bowen, RC Cooper. *Streptococcus pneumoniae* resistant to penicillin and chloramphenicol. Lancet 1977;ii: 995–997.
19. S Naraqi, GP Kirkpatrick, S Kabins. Relapsing pneumococcal meningitis: Isolation of an organism with decreased susceptibility to penicillin G. J Pediatr 1974;85: 671–673.
20. VJ Howes, RG Mitchell. Meningitis due to relatively penicillin-resistant pneumococcus. Br Med J 1976;1:996.
21. JE Mortensen, MR Jacobs, LM Koeth. Susceptibility of *Streptococcus pneumoniae* and *Haemophilus influenzae* in 1997: Results of a hospital-based U.S. study. In: Abstracts of the 38th Interscience Conference on Antimicrobial Agents and Chemotherapy, Abstr C-19. Washington, DC: Am Soc Microbiol, 1998.
22. CG Dowson, A Hutchison, JA Brannigan, RC George, D Hansman, J Linares, A Tomasz, JM Smith, BG Spratt. Horizontal transfer of penicillin-binding protein genes in penicillin-resistant clinical isolates of *Streptococcus pneumoniae*. Proc Nat Acad Sci USA 1989;86:8842–8846.
23. CG Dowson, TJ Coffey, C Kell, RA Whiley. Evolution of penicillin resistance in *Streptococcus pneumoniae*: The role of *Streptococcus mitis* in the formation of a low affinity PBP2B in *Streptococcus pneumoniae*. Mol Microbiol 1993;9:635–643.
24. PD Lister. Multiply-resistant pneumococcus: Therapeutic problems in the management of serious infections. Eur J Clin Microbiol Infect Dis 1995;14(1):18–25.
25. AL Smith. Antibiotic resistance in *Haemophilus influenzae*. In: EM Ayoub, GH Cassell, WC Branche, TJ Henry, eds. Microbial Determinants of Virulence and Host Response. Washington, DC: Am Soc Microbiol, 1990:321–343.
26. JH Jorgensen, GV Doern, C Thornsberry. Susceptibility of multiply-resistant *Haemophilus influenzae* to newer antimicrobial agents. Diagn Microbiol Infect Dis 1988;9:27–32.
27. CC Sanders, JP Iaconis, GP Bodey, G Samonis. Resistance to ticarcillin-potassium clavulanate among clinical isolates of the family *Enterobacteriaceae*: Role of PSE-1 β-lactamase and high levels of TEM-1 and SHV-1 and problems with false susceptibility in disk diffusion tests. Antimicrob Agents Chemother 1988;32:1365–1369.
28. KS Thomson, DA Weber, CC Sanders, J Eugene, W Sanders. β-Lactamase production in members of the family Enterobacteriaceae and resistance of β-lactam–enzyme inhibitor combinations. Antimicrob Agents Chemother 1990;34:622–627.
29. CJ Thomson, SGB Amyes. TRC-1: Emergence of a clavulanic acid-resistant TEM β-lactamase in a clinical strain. FEMS Microbiol Lett 1992;91:113–118.
30. J Blazquez, M Baquero, R Canton. Characterization of a new TEM-type β-lactamase resistant to clavulanate, sulbactam, and tazobactam in a clinical isolate of *Escherichia coli*. Antimicrob Agents Chemother 1993;37:2059–2063.
31. V Jarlier, M-H Nicolas, G Fournier, A Philippon. Extended broad-spectrum β-lactamases conferring transferable resistance to newer β-lactam agents in Enterobacteriaceae: Hospital prevalence and susceptibility patterns. Rev Infect Dis 1988;10:867–878.

32. KS Thomson, CC Sanders. Detection of extended-spectrum β-lactamases in members of the family *Enterobacteriaceae*: Comparison of the double-disk and three-dimensional tests. Antimicrob Agents Chemother 1992;36:1877–1882.
33. A Philippon, R Labia, GA Jacoby. Extended-spectrum β-lactamases. Antimicrob Agents Chemother 1989;33:1131–1136.
34. GA Jacoby. Genetics of extended-spectrum β-lactamases. Eur J Clin Microbiol Infect Dis 1994;(suppl 1)13:2–11.
35. PA Bradford, C Urban, N Mariano, SJ Projan, JJ Rahal, K Bush. Imipenem resistance in *Klebsiella pneumoniae* is associated with the combination of ACT-1, a plasmid-mediated AmpC β-lactamase, and the loss of an outer membrane protein. Antimicrob Agents Chemother 1997;41:563–569.
36. GA Jacoby, AA Medeiros. More extended-spectrum β-lactamases. Antimicrob Agents Chemother 1991;35:1697–1704.
37. SK DuBois, MS Marriott, SGB Amyes. TEM- and SHV-derived extended-spectrum β-lactamases: Relationship between selection, structure and function. J Antimicrob Chemother 1995;35:7–22.
38. CC Sanders. β-Lactamases of gram-negative bacteria: New challenges for new drugs. Clin Infect Dis 1992;14:1089–1099.
39. CC Sanders. Chromosomal cephalosporinases reponsible for multiple resistance to newer β-lactam antibiotics. Ann Rev Microbiol 1987;41:573–593.
40. Y Yang, P Wu, DM Livermore. Biochemical characterization of a β-lactamase that hydrolyzes penems and carbapenems from two *Serratia marcescens* isolates. Antimicrob Agents Chemother 1990;34:755–758.
41. E-H Lee, MH Nicholas, MD Kitzkis, G Pialou, E Collatz, L Gutmann. Association of two resistance mechanisms in a clinical isolate of *Enterobacter cloacae* with high-level resistance to imipenem. Antimicrob Agents Chemother 1991;35:1093–1098.
42. WE Sanders, CC Sanders. Inducible β-lactamases: Clinical and epidemiological implications for use of newer cephalosporins. Rev Infect Dis 1988;10:830–838.
43. JP Quinn, AE Studemeister, CA DiVincenzo, SA Lerner. Resistance to imipenem in *Pseudomonas aeruginosa*: Clinical experience and biochemical mechanisms. Rev Infect Dis 1988;10:892–898.
44. WE Sanders, CC Sanders. Do in vitro antimicrobial susceptibility tests accurately predict therapeutic responsiveness in infected patients? In: V Lorian, ed. Significance of Medical Microbiology in the Care of Patients. 2nd ed. Baltimore, MD: Williams and Wilkins, 1982:325–340.
45. HF Chambers. Methicillin-resistant staphylococci. Clin Microbiol Rev 1988;1:173–186.
46. RM Massanari, MA Pfaller, DS Wakefield, GT Hammons, LA McNutt, RF Woolson, CH Helms. Implications of acquired oxacillin resistance in the management and control of *Staphylococcus aureus* infections. J Infect Dis 1988;158:702–709.
47. S Dutka-Malen, S Evers, P Courvalin. Detection of glycopeptide resistance genotypes and identification to the species level of clinically relevant enterococci by PCR. J Clin Microbiol 1995;33:24–27.

48. N Clark, RC Cooksey, BC Hill, JM Swenson, FC Tenover. Characterization of glycopeptide-resistant enterococci from U.S. hospitals. Antimicrob Agents Chemother 1993;37:2311–2317.
49. S Sachiko, N Clark, D Rimland, FS Nolte, FC Tenover. Detection of vancomycin-resistant enterococci in fecal samples by PCR. J Clin Microbiol 1997;35:2325–2330.
50. JAMvd Klundert, JS Vliegenthart. PCR detection of genes coding for aminoglycoside modifying enzymes. In: DH Persing, TF Smith, FC Tenover, TJ White, eds. Diagnostic Molecular Microbiology: Principles and Applications. Washington, DC: Am Soc Microbiol, 1993:547–552.
51. K Ubukata, S Nakagami, A Nitta, A Yamane, S Kawakami, M Sugiura, A Konno. Rapid detection of the *mec*A gene in methicillin-resistant staphylococci by enzymatic detection of polymerase chain reaction products. J Clin Microbiol 1992;30: 1728–1733.
52. K Murakami, W Minamide, K Wada, E Nakamura, H Teraoka, S Wantanabe. Identification of methicillin-resistant strains of staphylococci by polymerase chain reaction. J Clin Microbiol 1991;29:2240–2244.
53. G Arlet, A Philippon. Construction by polymerase chain reaction and use of intragenic DNA probes for three main types of transferable beta-lactamases (TEM, SHV, CARB). FEMS Microbiol Lett 1991;66:19–25.
54. RC Levesque, A Medeiros, GA Jacoby. Molecular cloning and DNA homology of plasmid-mediated β-lactamase genes. Mol Gen Genet 1987;206:252–258.
55. GI Carter, KJ Towner, NJ Pearson, RCB Slack. Use of a non-radioactive hybridization assay for direct detection of gram-negative bacteria carrying TEM beta-lactamase genes in infected urine. J Med Microbiol 1989;28:113–117.
56. PL Perine, PA Totten, KK Holmes, EH Sng, AV Ratman, R Widy-Wersky, H Nsanze, E Habte-Gabr, WG Westbrook. Evaluation of a DNA hybridization method for detection of African and Asian strains of *Neisseria gonorrhoeae* in men with urethritis. J Infect Dis 1985;152:59–63.
57. FC Tenover, MB Huang, JK Rasheed, DH Persing. Development of PCR assays to detect ampicillin resistance genes in cerebrospinal fluid samples containing *Haemophilus influenzae*. J Clin Microbiol 1994;32:2729–2737.
58. C Mabilat, P Courvalin. Development of ''oligotyping'' for characterization and molecular epidemiology of TEM β-lactamases in members of the family *Enterobacteriaceae*. Antimicrob Agents Chemother 1990;34:2210–2216.
59. BW Catlin. Iodometric detection of *Haemophilus influenzae* beta-lactamase: Rapid, presumptive test for ampicillin resistance. Antimicrob Agents Chemother 1975;7: 265–270.
60. J Escamilla. Susceptibility of *Haemophilus influenzae* to ampicillin as determined by use of a modified one-minute beta-lactamase test. Antimicrob Agents Chemother 1976;9:196–198.
61. CH O'Callaghan, A Morris, SM Kirby, AH Shingler. Novel method for detection of β-lactamase by using a chromogenic cephalosporin substrate. Antimicrob Agents Chemother 1972;1:283–288.
62. GV Doern, HH Jorgensen, C Thornsberry, DA Preston, T Tubert, JS Redding, LA Maher. National collaborative study of the prevalence of antimicrobial resistance

among clinical isolates of *Haemophilus influenzae*. Antimicrob Agents Chemother 1988;32:180–185.
63. KGH Dyke. Beta-lactamases of *Staphylococcus aureus*. In: JMT Hamilton-Miller, JT Smith, eds. Beta-Lactamases. London: Academic Press, 1979:291–310.
64. MC Roberts, CD Swenson, LM Owens, AL Smith. Characterization of chloramphenicol resistant *Haemophilus influenzae*. Antimicrob Agents Chemother 1980; 18:610–615.
65. P Azemun, T Stull, M Roberts, AL Smith. Rapid detection of chloramphenicol resistance in *H. influenzae*. Antimicrob Agents Chemother 1981;20:168–170.
66. HW Matthews, CN Baker, C Thornsberry. Relationship between in vitro susceptibility test results for chloramphenicol and production of chloramphenicol acetyltransferase by *Haemophilus influenzae*, *Streptococcus pneumoniae*, and *Aerococcus* species. J Clin Microbiol 1988;26:2387–2390.
67. L de la Maza, SIL Miller, MJ Ferraro. Use of commercially available rapid chloramphenicol acetyl-transferase test to detect resistance in *Salmonella* spp. J Clin Microbiol 1990;28:1867–1869.
68. D Amsterdam. Susceptibility testing of antimicrobials in liquid media. In: V Lorian, ed. Antibiotics in Laboratory Medicine. Baltimore: Williams and Wilkins, 1991: 53–105.
69. D Greenwood. *In vitro veritas*? Antimicrobial susceptibility tests and their clinical relevance. J Infect Dis 1981;144:380–385.
70. CC Sanders. ARTs versus ASTs: Where are we going? J Antimicrob Chemother 1991;28:621–622.
71. KS Thomson, JS Bakken, CC Sanders. Antimicrobial susceptibility testing within the clinic. In: MRW Brown, P Gilbert, eds. Microbiological Quality Assurance: A Guide Towards Relevance and Reproducibility of Inocula. New York: CRC Press, 1995.
72. JH Jorgensen. Antimicrobial susceptibility testing of bacteria that grow aerobically. In: JA Washington, ed. Infectious Disease Clinics of North America: Laboratory Diagnosis of Infectious Diseases. Philadephia: WB Saunders, 1993:393–409.
73. CC Sanders, KS Thomson, PA Bradford. Problems with detection of β-lactam resistance among nonfastidious gram-negative bacilli. Infect Dis Clin N Am 1993;7: 411–425.
74. C Thornsberry. Antimicrobial susceptibility testing: General considerations. In: A Balows, WJ Hausler, KL Herrmann, HD Isenberg, HJ Shadomy, eds. Manual of Clinical Microbiology. Washington, DC: Am Soc Microbiol, 1991:1059–1064.
75. RB Thomson, TM File, RA Burgoon. Repeat antimicrobial susceptibility testing of identical isolates. J Clin Microbiol 1989;27:1108–1111.
76. WA Craig, B Suh. Protein binding and the antimicrobial effects: Methods for determination of protein binding. In: V Lorian ed. Antibiotics in Laboratory Medicine. Baltimore: Williams and Wilkins, 1991:367–402.
77. R Wise, AP Gillet, B Cadge. Influence of protein binding on the tissue levels of 6 β-lactams. J Infect Dis 1980;142:77.
78. M Barza, H Vine, L Weinstein. Reversibility of protein binding of penicillins: An in vitro study employing a rapid diafiltration process. Antimicrob Agents Chemother 1972;1:427–432.

79. J Blaser, MN Dudley, D Gilbert, SH Zinner. Influence of medium and method on the in vitro susceptibility of *Pseudomonas aeruginosa* and other bacteria to ciprofloxacin and enoxacin. Antimicrob Agents Chemother 1986;29:927–929.
80. NX Chin, HC Neu. Ciprofloxacin, a quinolone caraboxylic acid compound active against aerobic and anaerobic bacteria. Antimicrob Agents Chemother 1984;25: 319–326.
81. JF Chantot, A Bryskier. Antibacterial activity of ofloxacin and other 4-quinolone derivatives: In vitro and in vivo comparison. J Antimicrob Chemother 1985;16: 475–484.
82. T Kumada, HC Neu. In vitro activity of ofloxacin, a quinolone carboxylic acid compared to other quinolones and other antimicrobial agents. J Antimicrob Chemother 1985;16:563–574.
83. J Child, J Andrews, F Boswell, N Brenwald, R Wise. The in-vitro activity of CP 99,219, a new naphthyridone antimicrobial agent: A comparison with other fluoroquinolone agents. J Antimicrob Chemother 1995;35:869–876.
84. MN Dudley, CH Nightingale, R Quintiliani, RC Tilton. In vitro activity of cefonicid, ceforanide, and cefazolin against *Staphylococcus aureus* and *Staphylococcus epidermidis* and the effect of human serum. J Infect Dis 1983;148:178.
85. HF Chambers, J Mills, TA Drake, MA Sande. Failure of a once-daily regimen of cefonicid for treatment of endocarditis due to *Staphylococcus aureus*. Rev Infect Dis 1984;6 (suppl 4):S870–S874.
86. D Andes, R Walker, S Ebert, WA Craig. Increasing protein binding of cefonicid enhances its in-vivo activity in an animal infection model. Abstr A81. Program and Abstracts of the 34th Interscience Conference on Antimicrobial Agents and Chemotherapy. Washington, DC. Am Soc Microbiol, 1994:146.
87. National Committee for Clinical Laboratory Standards. Methods for dilution antimicrobial susceptibility tests for bacteria that grow aerobically. Approved Standard M7-A4. Villanova, PA: National Committee for Clinical Laboratory Standards, 1997.
88. PA Bradford, CC Sanders. Use of a predictor panel for development of a new disk for diffusion tests with cefoperazone-sulbactam. Antimicrob Agents Chemother 1992;36:394–400.
89. FH Kayser, G Morenzoni, F Homberger. Activity of cefoperazone against ampicillin-resistant bacteria in agar and broth dilution tests. Antimicrob Agents Chemother 1982;22:15–22.
90. M Rylander, JE Brorson, J Johnsson, R Norrby. Comparison between agar and broth minimum inhibitory concentrations of cefamandole, cefoxitin, and cefuroxime. Antimicrob Agents Chemother 1979;15:572–579.
91. JM Casellas, M Goldberg. Incidence of strains producing extended spectrum β-lactamases in Argentina. Infection 1989;17:434–436.
92. DF Sahm, L Olsen. In vitro detection of enterococcal vancomycin resistance. Antimicrob Agents Chemother 1990;34:1846–1848.
93. BM Willey, BN Kreiswirth, AE Simior, G Williams, SR Scriver, A Phillips, DE Low. Detection of vancomycin resistance in *Enterococcus* species. J Clin Microbiol 1992;30:1621–1624.

94. National Committee for Clinical Laboratory Standards. Performance Standards for Antimicrobial Susceptibility Testing; Ninth Informational Supplement M100-S9. Wayne, PA: National Committee for Clinical Laboratory Standards, 1999.
95. A Philippon, SB Redjeb, G Fournier, AB Hassen. Epidemiology of extended spectrum β-lactamases. Infection 1995;17:347–354.
96. PA Bradford, CC Sanders. Development of test panel of β-lactamases expressed in a common *Escherichia coli* host background for evaluation of new β-lactam antibiotics. Antimicrob Agents Chemother 1995;39:308–313.
97. DM Schlaes, A Bouvet, C Devine, JH Schlaes, S Al-Obeid, R Williamson. Inducible, transferable resistance to vancomycin in *Enterococcus faecalis* A256. Antimicrob Agents Chemother 1989;33:198–203.
98. RN Jones, SA Marshall. Antimicrobial activity of cefepime tested against Bush group 1 β-lactamase-producing strains resistant to ceftazidime: A multi-laboratory national and international clinical isolate study. Diagn Microbiol Infect Dis 1994; 19:33–38.
99. AF Ehrhardt, CC Sanders. β-lactam resistance amongst *Enterobacter* species. J Antimicrob Chemother 1993;32(suppl B):1–11.
100. CC Sanders. Cefepime: The next generation? Clin Infect Dis 1993;17:369–379.
101. B Marchou, M Michea-Hamzehpour, C Lucain, J-C Pechere. Development of β-lactam-resistant *Enterobacter cloacae* in mice. J Infect Dis 1987;156:369–373.
102. KS Thomson, CC Sanders. Dissociated resistance among fluoroquinolones. Antimicrob Agents Chemother 1994;38:2095–2100.
103. GL Drusano, DE Johnson, M Rosen, HC Standiford. Pharmacodynamics of a fluoroquinolone antimicrobial agent in a neutropenic rat model of *Pseudomonas* sepsis. Antimicrob Agents Chemother 1993;37:483–490.
104. SL Preston, GL Drusano, AL Berman, CL Fowler, AT Chow, B Dornsief, V Reichl, J Natarajan, M Corrado. Pharmacodynamics of levofloxacin: A new paradigm for early clinical trials. JAMA 1998;279:125–129.
105. J Blaser, BB Stone, MC Groner, SH Zinner. Comparative study with enoxacin and netilmicin in a pharmacodynamic model to determine importance of ratio of antibiotic peak concentration to MIC for bactericidal activity and emergence of resistance. Antimicrob Agents Chemother 1987;31:1054–1060.
106. CR Marchibanks, JR McKiel, DH Gilbert, NJ Robillard, B Painter, SH Zinner, MN Dudley. Dose ranging and fractionation of intravenous ciprofloxacin against *Pseudomonas aeruginosa* and *Staphylococcus aureus* in an in vitro pharmacokinetic model. Antimicrob Agents Chemother 1993;37:1756–1763.
107. MK Lacy, W Lu, X Xu, PR Tessier, DP Nicolau, R Quintiliani, CH Nightingale. Pharmacodynamic comparisons of levofloxacin, ciprofloxacin, and ampicillin against *Streptococcus pneumoniae* in an in vitro pharmacokinetic model. Antimicrob Agents Chemother 1999;43:672–677.
108. CC Sanders, WE Sanders. Cycling of antibiotics: An approach to circumvent resistance in specialized units of the hospital. Clin Microbiol Infect 1998;1:223–225.

16

Basic Pharmacoeconomics*

Mark A. Richerson
Medical Service Corps, United States Navy, and Department of Defense Pharmacoeconomic Center, Fort Sam Houston, Texas

Eugene Moore
Department of Defense Pharmacoeconomic Center, Fort Sam Houston, Texas

1 INTRODUCTION

Changes in the economic structure of the U.S. health care delivery system have driven the need for pharmacists, physicians, and others in health care to develop expertise in evaluating the economic implications of selecting among competing health care programs and drug therapies. With the enactment of the Tax Equity and Fiscal Responsibility Act (TEFRA) of 1983, most hospital departments, including pharmacy, laboratory, and radiology, have transitioned from revenue-generating departments to cost centers within their institutions [1]. Finite economic resources for health care, combined with the increasing prevalence of managed care, rapidly emerging new medical technologies, and increasing demand on the part of health care consumers, has resulted in a need for decision makers to carefully allocate these limited resources to those programs and products that provide the most value in terms of health benefits.

* All views expressed are those of the authors and do not necessarily represent those of the Departments of the Army, Navy, Air Force, or those of the Department of Defense.

The medical community, the pharmaceutical industry, nursing, and other allied health fields have increasingly discovered the usefulness of various health economic methodologies as they relate to making informed health care allocation decisions. As a result, readers must understand how to interpret the ever-increasing amount of economic data appearing in the medical literature. In a briefing to the Office of Health Economics (OHE), Prichart [2] described the Health Economics Evaluations Database (HEED) and the growth of health economics evaluations appearing in the literature. In 1998, the HEED database contained over 14,000 references. Between 1992 and 1996, there was a near doubling of the references added each year to the database [2].

So, how is a chapter concerning itself with pharmacoeconomic analysis relevant to a book about the pharmacodynamic properties of antimicrobials? Interestingly, when the subject matter of published economic evaluations was examined, it was discovered that diseases of the circulatory system, neoplasm, and infectious/parasitic diseases were the top three disease states studied between 1992 and 1996. Furthermore, in examining drug expenditures by therapeutic category, it was found that annual total spending on antimicrobials rose 4% between 1999 and 2000 and was ranked fourth within the 16 therapeutic categories evaluated (exceeded only by spending on cardiovascular, alimentary, and central nervous system agents). Patients with complaints associated with respiratory tract infection constitute a large portion of those visiting primary care providers in the United States. The 1995 National Ambulatory Medical Care Survey (NAMCS) identified acute respiratory tract infection as the most frequent principal diagnosis (31,856,976 in 1995) provided by office-based physicians [3]. Taking into consideration the unique pharmacodynamic characteristics of various antimicrobials can lead to economic efficiencies in the treatment of a variety of infectious disease states.

The purpose of this chapter is to provide the reader with an understanding of the basic principles of pharmacoeconomic analysis. Specifically, we will describe the elements that define a pharmacoeconomic evaluation and the major types of analysis and attempt to demonstrate how these forms of analysis have been applied to the decision-making process.

2 CHARACTERISTICS OF A PHARMACOECONOMIC ANALYSIS

Pharmacoeconomics is a discipline concerned with comparing the *costs* and *consequences* of two or more competing alternatives. The four major types of analysis include the evaluation of cost minimization, cost effectiveness, cost vs. benefit, and cost vs. utility. Most often, pharmacoeconomic analysis is concerned with the selection of particular drugs, treatment protocols, or therapeutic options. In addition to the four basic types of analysis, other frequently encountered types of analysis include cost analysis and cost–consequence analysis. These types of evaluations are frequently referred to as partial evaluations. The basic difference between complete and partial evaluations is that partial analyses focus on either cost or consequence and may or may not describe a comparison between competing products or services. The focus of this chapter will be on the complete forms of pharmacoeconomic analysis. Although the major types of analysis differ in how the therapeutic outcomes are quantified, they all share one common element, the inclusion of a cost measure.

2.1 Cost and Perspective

Costs in health care economics studies are generally described as being direct, indirect, or intangible. Direct costs are further divided between direct medical costs and direct non-medical costs. Direct medical costs are the costs of those items that are used up in the course of providing medical services. In the case of pharmacoeconomic studies, direct medical costs are typically associated with the cost of drugs, medical supplies, laboratory tests, hospitalizations, and patient visits. Other direct medical costs that are particularly relevant when comparing competing antimicrobials include the additional costs associated with therapeutic drug concentration monitoring, treatment failure, and adverse drug events.

Direct non-medical costs include out-of-pocket expenses incurred by the patient, or by the patient's family, in the course of obtaining health care. For example, lost wages that a patient experiences while taking time away from work to attend a doctor's appointment is considered a direct non-medical cost. Indirect costs, from an economist's viewpoint, are those costs that result from lost productivity. The inclusion of indirect costs is controversial for a variety of reasons, particularly the difficulty in placing a precise dollar value on productivity. What is the dollar value of lost productivity associated with treatments directed toward children or stay-at-home spouses? Including indirect costs assumes that a patient's medical condition by itself would not have resulted in lost productivity. There are a number of methods, each associated with trade-offs, to address these issues. No single method is universally accepted, and a tremendous amount of controversy remains about when and how to include indirect cost in health care economic studies.

Intangible costs refer to those costs incurred outside the medical system. Drummond et al. [4] describe a scenario where an occupational health program changes the production cost of automobiles. The increased costs associated with the program are ultimately passed on to the purchasers of cars, far removed from the company's new health program. These costs are typically omitted from pharmacoeconomic evaluations, because it is generally understood that they are usually insignificant and that there is little to be gained by attempting to include them in an analysis.

The perspective of the ultimate user of the analysis should determine which types of costs are included in the study. From a managed care organization's perspective, direct medical costs (cost of providing medical personnel, equipment, and supplies) may be of primary importance. In addition to direct medical costs, an analysis completed from a governmental or societal perspective may need to include patients' out-of-pocket expenses and lost productivity. The major message for the reader is that the perspective of the analysis and the costs included in the study must be fully understood before generalizing the results to any one particular setting.

Evaluations of long-term drug therapies, such as those for hypertension and dyslipidemia, require that health care costs incurred over the multiple years of the study be discounted and reported in the current year's value. Discounting, in addition to accounting for inflation, considers the opportunity costs associated with investment in one option versus another. As a rule of thumb, discounting is required when completing an analysis that spans more than a one-year time frame. The evaluation of competing therapy options for acute infectious disease processes is somewhat straightforward in that the entire episode spans periods ranging from a few days to a few weeks, and discounting is generally not required. On the other hand, in an analysis of a more chronic infection, human immune deficiency infection, for example, the economic evaluation is likely to require discounting in order to express future expenditures in the most current year's dollar values [5].

2.2 Major Types of Pharmacoeconomic Evaluation

As stated previously, the four major types of pharmacoeconomic evaluation include cost-minimization, cost effectiveness, cost-benefit, and cost-utility analysis. Each type is unique in the way in which consequences, or outcomes, are measured and compared. A *cost-minimization* pharmacoeconomic evaluation refers to the comparison of two or more drug alternatives where the choice of any one agent will result in exactly the same outcome as selection of any of the others. Clearly, the focus in this type of analysis becomes cost, and the alternative associated with the lowest cost is generally the preferred agent. This does not mean that the analysis is concerned with drug acquisition cost only. Other costs to consider, depending on the perspective taken in the analysis, might include drug administration cost, cost associated with therapeutic drug monitoring, and the cost of treating an adverse drug event. Comparison of a brand name drug product and an FDA-approved AB rated generic product serves as a classic example of a cost-minimization study. The comparison of two or more antimicrobials for which randomized clinical trials have demonstrated equal efficacy serves as another example. It cannot be overemphasized, however, that sufficient information must be available to demonstrate equal treatment outcomes with all the agents being compared. Too often, equal efficacy is assumed without sufficient supportive evidence.

Cost-effectiveness studies employ an analytical technique that compares both costs and outcomes of competing agents or services. This form of analysis differs from the others in that outcomes are measured in some form of naturalistic unit. For example, when comparing two drugs used to treat hypertension, the outcome of interest may be reduction in systolic and diastolic pressure. In a cost-effectiveness analysis comparing two antimicrobials used to treat acute sinusitis, the outcome of interest is likely to be cure. Quenzer et al. [6] used complication-free cure as the outcome measure of interest when comparing the cost effectiveness of various antimicrobials used to treat lower respiratory tract infections. They contended that from the perspective of a managed care organization, patient satisfaction, indirectly measured by a complication-free episode of care, was an important outcome of interest. Life years saved is a frequently encountered outcome measure, particularly when comparing drugs used for the treatment of chronic diseases.

The term ''cost-effective'' has a very specific set of meanings. As Lee and Sanchez [7] point out, the term has frequently been misused in the literature. It is commonly misinterpreted to mean that the least costly product (frequently based on drug acquisition cost only) or decision is the product or decision of choice. From a pharmacoeconomic decision-making perspective, however, there are three different situations that arise in which one decision is more cost-effective than another. The most intuitive situation occurs when product A is preferred over product B because it results in lower costs while also being clinically more effective than product B. Product A would be the decision of choice and would be considered dominant to product B. Another fairly straightforward example is a situation where product B is discovered to be equally as effective as product A, yet product A results in lower costs. Again, product A would be preferred. The final description of cost effectiveness is frequently overlooked. In a situation where product A is both more costly and more effective than product B, product A may still be the most cost-effective choice because the extra clinical benefit associated with product A may be judged to be worth the additional incremental costs. This illustrates the point that although pharmacoeconomic analysis can contribute to more informed decisions, value judgments will continue to be necessary in many situations.

Cost-benefit analysis expresses the benefits (or consequences) of a decision choice in terms of dollar value. By measuring the cost and benefits in the same units (currency), it forces decision makers to make explicit decisions about whether the benefits of a drug or program choice are worth the investment (cost). This form of analysis possesses the advantage of allowing comparison of any combination of drugs and program options available in a particular institution. Cost-benefit analysis is particularly useful in situations where the health care system is funding multiple competing programs or where treatment options are competing for the same finite amount of money. As long as the benefits of each choice can be expressed in currency, any combination of programs, services, or therapies can be compared. One of the most difficult barriers to using this form of analysis is the need to place an acceptable dollar value on a particular level of health.

Cost-utility is a form of analysis where the outcome of interest is the patient's preference, or that of a population of patients, for a particular state of health status or improvement in health status. Utility scores are further multiplied by expected life years to yield quality-adjusted life years (QALY) gained. In terms of methodologies, a cost-utility analysis is conducted in much the same fashion as a cost-effectiveness analysis. Unlike cost-effectiveness analysis, where two or more alternatives are compared for the same condition, cost-utility analysis allows the comparison of different programs or treatment options directed toward different medical conditions, as long as those programs or treatment options result in changes in patient quality of life. The role of cost-utility analysis is controversial, and the measurement methods continue to evolve. Although there are a variety of methods and measure tools designed to collect utility scores, none have been universally accepted.

3 OUTCOMES IN PHARMACOECONOMIC ANALYSIS

Pharmacoeconomics is a discipline concerned with the *costs* and *consequences* of selections of particular drugs, treatment protocols, or therapeutic options [8]. Frequently the consequences of such selections in health care are termed *outcomes*. An outcome, in the strictest definition, is the final consequence of an action [9]. In health care economic research and decision making, there are usually different types of outcome measures, describing different markers of interest, that can be studied or analyzed for a given disease state [10,11]. Outcome measures can describe the efficacy of a drug or treatment option, the effectiveness, or the economic benefit. Outcome measures can be surrogate or intermediate (e.g., a laboratory value) or absolute (e.g., absence of disease). The best or most valid outcome to study varies with the disease state being analyzed and with the interests (perspective) of the persons conducting the study. Outcomes may be clinical, economic, or humanistic [1,3,4].

3.1 Outcome Measures in the Treatment of Infectious Disease

Outcome measures of drug therapy in any disease state are generally driven by pharmacodynamic considerations. In the case of infectious disease, pharmacodynamics refers to the relationship between the concentration of the drug at its target tissues and its microbiological effect [12]. The microbiological effect of interest is, of course, the eradication of the pathogenic invasion and "cure" of the infection. For any given antimicrobial drug, administration will result in its selective distribution to tissues in concentrations that vary according to pharmacokinetic properties of the drug and the drug–host–disease interaction [5]. There is also a specific minimum concentration at which the drug will produce its antimicrobial action with respect to a given pathogen. In vitro this is called the minimum inhibitory concentration (MIC) and is a measure of the drug's *efficacy* [5]. A drug's MIC is inversely related to its antimicrobial activity. The lower a drug's MIC, the greater the drug's activity against the given pathogen. An antimicrobial drug's *effectiveness* is determined by the interplay between its pharmacokinetics and its pharmacodynamics. The drug must distribute to the target tissues (site of infection) in concentrations that meet or exceed the MIC, be capable of killing the pathogen, and do so without causing serious adverse events in the patient. The result is a measurable outcome for the treatment of the infectious disease. Examples of outcome measures in infectious disease are provided in Table 1.

In general, outcomes measurement in pharmacoeconomic analysis of infectious disease therapy is fairly straightforward. The acute nature of most infectious diseases (HIV being the exception) makes it easy to define a desired outcome. An acute infection is a short-duration event, with obvious measurable signs of

TABLE 1 Types of Outcomes in Pharmacoeconomic Analysis

Type of outcome	Examples applicable to infectious disease
Clinical	Cure of infection (confirmed by culture)
	Absence of opportunistic infection (in immunocompromise)
	Resolution of febrile illness
	Resolution of pneumonia symptoms (decreased sputum production, "clearing" of sputum color)
Economic	Decreased length of stay (LOS)
	Decreased total health care cost
	Decreased drug acquisition cost
	Decreased intensity of care (nursing and ancillary services, supplies)
	Decreased resource utilization
Humanistic	Years of life added
	Quality-adjusted life years saved
	Decreased incidence of adverse drug reaction
	Decreased pain and suffering
	Quality of life

morbidity and in many cases the potential for death or serious complications if inadequately treated. The treatment goal is resolution of the infection and, in the case of hospitalized patients, discharge or stepdown to a less intensive therapy. The outcome measure that provides the most valuable information in a pharmacoeconomic analysis is cure of the infection. Indeed, most research studies in drug therapy of infectious diseases measure efficacy and/or effectiveness by the probability that the therapy will result in elimination of the infection. In a sense, cure of the infection can be seen as the effectiveness measure that is of greatest interest to the patient. It's frequently the reason for the encounter with the health care system in the first place!

The health care system or the payer, while concerned with clinical outcomes, may also be interested in economic outcomes [1]. An economic analysis done from the payer's perspective may focus on decreasing hospital lengths of stay or intensity of care. These variables are directly related to the drug's clinical outcomes (i.e., drugs with greater efficacy might produce more desirable economic outcomes), but the decision maker's focus might be on the economic outcome for obvious reasons. In general, payers look to increase economic efficiencies so that they can provide more care for the same costs or provide the same care at a greater ''profit'' (i.e., less cost) [1,13,14].

Both the patient and the health care system (or payer) are concerned with humanistic outcomes. Humanistic outcomes are those that describe the impact of a therapy on some aspect of human quality of life, longevity, pain and suffering, or emotional satisfaction [1]. Quality of life can be defined as an individual's overall satisfaction with life and general personal well-being [15]. Health-related quality of life (HRQOL) includes those aspects of quality of life that are affected by one's health. From the patient's perspective, drug therapy of infection should preserve or improve HRQOL by maximizing positive humanistic outcomes and minimizing negative humanistic outcomes. In acute infection, the obvious payoff occurs when the infection is resolved and the patient is discharged from the hospital with no permanent sequelae. In chronic infection such as that which occurs when an individual has contracted the human immunodeficiency virus (HIV), discussion of humanistic outcomes take on more than one dimension. Current treatment regimens such as HAART (highly active antiretroviral therapy) do not eradicate the infection but instead suppress viral activity to the point where its impact on the body's T-helper cells is minimal. This comes at a price, that price being that the patient must be willing to tolerate side effects that range from annoying to uncomfortable to life-threatening. The patient and physician must attempt to find the trade-off between the HAART combination that offers the best promise for longevity with the least impact on quality of life.

Humanistic outcomes can be difficult to use in a pharmacoeconomic analysis. Although most health care providers, administrators, and researchers agree that it is important to assess humanistic aspects of care, there is no consensus on standard measurement techniques [8]. Because of the subjective nature of quality of life, it is difficult to correlate improvements in HRQOL to clinical improvements [8]. In the HAART example above, for instance, the patient's viral load may be brought to undetectable levels (clinical improvement) while the patient reports a decrease in HRQOL (from side effects). Another difficulty with applying humanistic outcomes to pharmacoeconomic analysis is that it is frequently difficult to place an economic value on them. Although everyone can agree that prolonging life is mostly desirable, it is nonetheless very difficult to answer the question: What is the dollar value of an extra year of life? The answer again depends on the perspective of the answerer. A third-party payer might value the extra year of life differently than a patient or a health care provider. Entire subdisciplines in health economics are devoted to the issue of assessing and placing value on humanistic and quality of life outcomes in health care. Although the subjects are beyond the scope of this chapter, two such areas of study are contingent valuation methodology (CVM) [16] and time trade-off (standard gamble) [17] analysis. Readers desiring to learn more on these subjects are directed to the vast body of information in the medical literature.

4 METHODOLOGICAL CONSIDERATIONS IN CONDUCTING PHARMACOECONOMIC ANALYSES

The validity of a pharmacoeconomic analysis is influenced a great deal by the methodology one chooses to employ in doing the analysis. To be valid and useful, an analysis must use methods that are most appropriate to the disease state in question in the health setting of interest. Selection of the type of analysis and securing the data inputs on which the analysis is based are critical steps in conducting a good, sound pharmacoeconomic analysis.

As stated elsewhere in this chapter, there are at least four major types of pharmacoeconomic analyses: cost minimization, cost-benefit, cost-utility, and cost effectiveness are all analysis types [1,8]. In analyzing the pharmacoeconomics of an infectious disease agent or protocol, one of the four types is usually more suitable than the others. However, in some cases two or more methods are equally valid. Some methods may in theory produce results with greater validity but may be too difficult to put into practice or may be judged unethical.

Choice of the analysis type should be based on the goals of the analyst or organization doing the analysis. A government entity concerned with formulating public policy or allocating scarce resources will have different goals and requirements than a managed care organization desiring to enhance economic efficiency in its hospitals. Researchers seeking to advance the body of knowledge in the discipline will have still different goals and requirements. Organizations seeking to formulate public policy or allocate resources are likely to find cost-benefit analysis to be more useful [1,8]. If two treatment choices are deemed to be equal in outcomes, an organization is likely to find cost minimization analysis to be useful [1,8]. In most cases, the organization is seeking to provide the most effective treatment for the least expenditure. In this case it is likely that cost-effectiveness analysis is most useful.

Regardless of which overall analysis type is chosen, there remains the question of which methodology to use in conducting the analysis. The analyst has a number of methodological techniques to choose from, each with its own optimal applications, strengths, and weaknesses. These techniques include cost comparisons, mathematical models, simulations, and decision analysis.

Cost comparison is the simplest methodological technique, and it is most applicable to cost-minimization analysis. This technique is also sometimes called cost identification. When all the costs of therapy are known or identified, they are tabulated and compared. Because all therapies are deemed to have equal outcomes, the therapy with the lowest identified cost is considered to have an economic advantage.

Mathematical models and simulations are very frequently used in cost effectiveness and cost-benefit analyses [18]. A mathematical model is a model that seeks to precisely describe in mathematical terms all of the costs and consequences of a particular therapeutic option. Simulations are quite similar to mathematical models except in one critical aspect. Generally speaking, mathematical models represent static points in time, whereas simulations attempt to show change over a time course [11]. Hence, a ''simulation clock'' (i.e., a mechanism to account for time change in regular increments) is a critical part of a simulation. Simulations, when done on a computer, allow changing events to be represented graphically, perhaps making it easier for the intended audience to ''see'' the differences among competing alternatives. Mathematical models and simulations are more alike than different in that they both require precise identification of costs and consequences in mathematical terms. Generally speaking, mathematical models are used more often in pharmacoeconomics than simulations, though a few exceptionally well done simulations can be found in the literature [19]. The reader seeking to learn more about simulations and their application to medical decision making should consult the references at the end of this chapter [18–22].

As stated above, the mathematical model expresses the costs and consequences of treatment choices in mathematical terms. When applied to cost-effectiveness analysis, this means that the analyst must develop an equation that expresses as precisely as possible the relationship between the variables (inputs) that influence the costs and outcomes of each treatment course. Variables will, of course, differ with each disease state or drug type being analyzed. Some potentially important variables to consider when developing a mathematical model include the acquisition cost of the drug, the cost of administering the drug, nursing costs, the probability of incurring additional visits, additional visit costs, the probability of hospitalization, hospitalization costs, the probability of adverse drug

TABLE 2 Advantages and Disadvantages of Modeling

Advantages	Disadvantages
Allows evaluation of multiple options and prediction of outcomes.	It may be difficult to validate findings.
Can be used to predict outcomes associated with rare events.	Decision makers unfamiliar with the technique may be skeptical.
Does not endanger or inconvenience patients or providers.	Data may be difficult to get and/or apply.
Costs are much lower than an observational study.	It usually requires assumptions.

Source: Adapted from Ref. 18.

events (ADE), the cost of ADE, the probability of treatment failure, the cost of treatment failure, the probability of additional laboratory monitoring, the costs of additional laboratory monitoring, the probability of treatment success, and biological measures of outcome.

Mathematical models can be further categorized as stochastic or deterministic [11]. If none of a model's inputs involve probabilities, the model is said to be deterministic. If one or more of the model's inputs involve probability distributions, the model is said to be stochastic. For example, in a pharmacokinetic model the mathematical relationships describing the drug's absorption, distribution, and elimination are known and can be represented by specific equations, and the model is considered deterministic. In a model such as one for the treatment of community-acquired pneumonia, several variables may involve probability distributions. The likelihood of successful resolution of infection, of seeking retreatment after treatment failure, of experiencing an ADE severe enough to require treatment, or of presenting with an infection caused by a resistant organism are all governed by probabilities of occurrence, and the model is considered stochastic. A stochastic model in which the inputs from one stage are dependent on the outputs from another stage is termed a Markov chain or Markov model [11].

Still another type of mathematical model, which can be either stochastic or deterministic, is the analytical hierarchy model. This type of model is also called a multiattribute utility theory (MAUT) model [20,21]. The key feature of this model is the fact that all categories of model inputs are weighted by relative importance to the decision maker prior to running the model. For example, a health care system choosing among new antibiotics for formulary inclusion may place a higher weight on the attribute "coverage of resistant organisms" than on the attributes of price, probability of ADE, or cost of administration. In this case the "utility," or health system's valuation, will have additional influence

TABLE 3 Types of Mathematical Models

Type	Description
Stochastic	Involves probability distributions, uncertainty in values of variables
Deterministic	No probabilities involved; all variables specifically stated and all mathematical relationships known
Analytical hierarchy	Involves valuation, weighting of specific model attributes by end users

on the model's behavior and results. The types of mathematical models and their characteristics are described in Table 3.

4.1 Decision Analytic Modeling

Another type of modeling that is very useful in pharmacoeconomics is decision analytic (DA) modeling. Decision analytic models seek to quantify the expected value of a particular course of action by examining the probabilities of events occurring after the decision and the outcomes (payoff) that result from the event [11,22]. These models involve the construction of a decision tree, with each branch representing an outcome probability. The analyst can compare competing choices and select the decision that offers the best expected value for the health system. In cost-effectiveness analysis the ''winner'' is usually the treatment path that yields the lowest expected value in dollars. In cost-benefit analysis, the ''winner'' is usually the treatment path that yields the highest expected value in dollars. A simplified example of a decision tree is shown in Fig. 1.

The case in Fig. 1 illustrates the basic principles of decision trees. In standard notation, a square box represents a decision node (e.g., treat with A or B), circles represent chance (probability) nodes, and triangles represent terminal

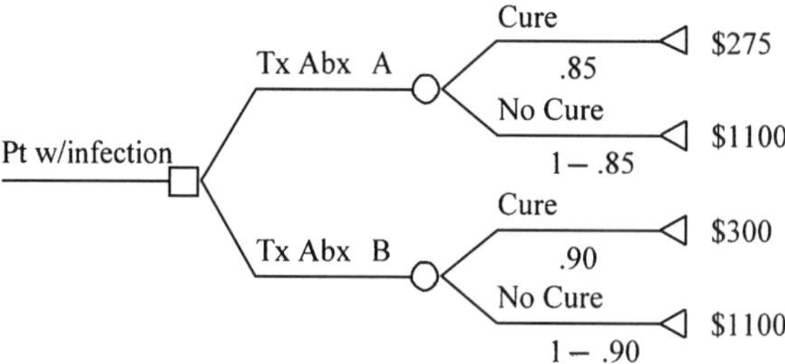

FIGURE 1 Antibiotic A vs. antibiotic B in acute infection.

(payoff) nodes. Multiplying the probabilities at each chance node by the payoffs and summing the results gives the *expected value* of each choice. In the example, antibiotic B has a 5% greater probability of cure but costs a little more for each course of therapy. Although it is not necessarily obvious, the most cost-effective choice in the above example is antibiotic B. Although it would appear that B is more expensive by $25 per course of therapy, when one factors in the greater probability of cure (assuming an equal cost of failure of $1100) the expected value of B becomes $380 [(.90 × $300) + (.10 × $1100)] versus an expected value of $399 [(.85 × $275) + (.15 × $1100)] for A. Thus, one can say that *on average* over a large number of cases B will actually work out to be less expensive than A by approximately $19 per case. In practice, decision trees are usually more complex than the example shown above. There may be many branches representing probabilities and associated payoffs for ADEs, complications, re-treatment, etc. Decision trees are nonetheless very useful when one can obtain the proper data (probabilities and the associated costs) with which to construct the model. A more detailed example of a decision analysis applied to the economic evaluation of competing antibiotic regimens can be seen in a recent study by Richerson et al. [23].

4.2 Data Sources for Pharmacoeconomic Studies

The decision on which type of model to use in a pharmacoeconomic analysis is dependent upon the data available for inputs. In turn, the data available for inputs depends, in many cases, on the pharmacoeconomic question one is trying to answer. Certain data lend themselves to answering some questions more accurately than others. Certain data are inappropriate for answering some types of questions. Thus, it is wise for the analyst not to approach the matter of data considerations too cavalierly when planning a pharmacoeconomic study.

In order to increase the scientific quality and integrity of pharmacoeconomic studies, consensus guidelines have been developed by some countries and by professional and academic organizations. Australia and Canada adopted national guidelines on health economic analysis [24,25], and the International Society for Pharmaceutical Outcomes Research has developed an international consensus statement on pharmacoeconomic methodology [26]. Each of these documents addresses in detail the issue of data validity and applicability of data to various types of analyses.

There are a number of data sources available to use in constructing a pharmacoeconomic study or model. Data can generally tell the researcher three things that may be used in a pharmacoeconomic study: the likelihood of outcomes associated with the treatment or nontreatment of disease, the treatment patterns associated with the therapy, and the costs associated with the therapy and/or disease state [27]. Some researchers have coined the term "transition probabilities" to refer to the first of these. The data must be incorporated into the analysis in a manner that is rational and appropriate to the assumptions of the analysis.

Table 4 shows the data types that may be used in conducting a pharmacoeconomic analysis or constructing a pharmacoeconomic model. The data types will vary in their applicability to different types of pharmacoeconomic analyses. Obviously, one of the best sources for data in a health care system is local research [8]. An advantage of using local research data is that a well-designed local research project can tell the analyst more about the probable costs and consequences of treatment decisions at his or her hospital than data from other facilities that may or may not have had similar patients and prescribing practices. A disadvantage to using local research data is that it takes considerable time and resources to conduct a good study [8,28]. By the time the study is designed and implemented and the findings analyzed, market conditions may have changed and rendered the results nonapplicable. Also, many hospitals are under budgetary pressures that do not allow the staffing or other resources needed to conduct a well-designed study.

4.3 Evaluating Pharmacoeconomic Studies

Often those in health care will need to evaluate other pharmacoeconomic studies, either for the purpose of making a formulary or treatment decision or for the purpose of gathering data for their own models. In those cases, it is important to make sure that the pharmacoeconomic study is valid and applicable to the health care system in question. There are several key questions that one must ask in evaluating a pharmacoeconomic analysis; these are listed in Table 5.

The first question listed in Table 5 is especially important when reviewing a study or analysis that makes conclusions about the pharmacoeconomics of a given treatment option. A clearly defined clinical question that is scientifically relevant and capable of being answered by the study design is a *must*. It simply does not make sense to attempt to ascertain the economic advantage of a therapy if the study was not properly designed to determine a relevant clinical outcome. For example, it is common to find articles in which one antibiotic is claimed to be economically superior to another but the data supporting the conclusion come from analyzing a subgroup that just happened to respond better to treatment because they had a particular variant of the infecting organism that was unanticipated at the start of the trial. Similarly, it is also important to know whether all of the interventions compared have been shown to be clinically effective. For example, it may be invalid to determine that a very low cost antibiotic is ''more cost-effective'' than another when in fact the low cost antibiotic is no longer considered clinically effective because of increasing microbial resistance.

Other important questions surround economic models. First and foremost, the model's assumptions must be rational and a realistic representation of real-

Table 4 Data for Pharmacoeconomic Studies

Data type	Examples	Comments
Transition probability (Probability of response, ADE, morbidity, mortality, etc.)	Local research	High internal validity, but may not be generalizable.
	Clinical trials	High internal validity; must be evaluated for rigor, applicability.
	Meta-analysis	Pooled data across studies; may or may not be able to generalize.
Treatment patterns (How the therapy is used in current practice, real-world and "preferred" best practices)	Databases Claims Clinical	Can be good for showing admissions, visits, LOS, prescriptions. Limitations: Shows what actually happens, not necessarily what should happen, may not be temporally related to therapy.
	DUE	Good data source for local prescribing patterns, drug usage patterns. Pharmacy database usually easily accessible.
	Delphi (expert opinion)	Sometimes the only way to get certain information. Limitations: No standard guidelines for selection of Delphi panel; data considered subjective; response bias may be a problem.
Costing information (How much the treatment or nontreatment of disease costs, direct and indirect costs, burden of illness)	Claims data	Good source of data on local (health system) patients. However, it may be difficult to associate claims dollars with real dollar cost of the illness.
	Wholesaler info; MAC rates	Good for model inputs; use for actual acquisition costs in health system.
	Epidemiological data	Use to determine burden of illness.
	Local research, DUE, expert opinion	Good for determining costs at local institution, high internal validity.

Table 5 Key Questions for Evaluating Pharmacoeconomic Studies

Is the analysis based on a study that answers a clearly defined clinical question about an economically important issue?
Does the type of analysis match the objectives of the organization or person conducting the study? Is it appropriate?
Does the analysis seek to answer questions for which it is not structured?
Is the quality of the data appropriate to the conclusions of the analysis?
Is there real or perceived bias in the way in which the analysis was structured?
If an economic model, was the model tested for sensitivity of its inputs?
Were the model's assumptions realistic in comparison to "real life"?
Whose viewpoint are costs and benefits being considered from?
Have all the interventions compared been shown to be clinically effective?
How were costs and benefits measured?

Source: Adapted from Refs. 14 and 22.

life occurrences [7,15]. Failure and retreatment rates, probability of laboratory monitoring, and likelihood of additional visits are some areas where modelers sometimes make unrealistic assumptions that may bias a model's results. Another important consideration for economic models is sensitivity testing [15,18,29]. The model's inputs should be tested around a range of values to determine how changing these values affect the model's results. If the model's results appear to be similar across the likely range of possible input values, then the model is said to be *robust*. On the other hand, if the model's results vary greatly when small but realistic changes are made in its inputs, then it is less valid. A final consideration that should be given to economic models is whether or not the model is transparent and reproducible. All of the major governmental and academic bodies that have developed guidelines have included recommendations that the model's inputs and mathematical relationships be transparent (i.e., equations and variables clearly shown). They also recommend that the model be constructed in a manner that would make it possible for other researchers or analysts to duplicate the model and its findings [16–18]. Models that have hidden ("black box") relationships may be considered of questionable validity.

The rapid development of new drug technologies combined with direct-to-consumer advertising, increased patient access to care, and finite resources will require that decision makers have the analytical tools necessary to make important health-related resource allocation decisions. This chapter has attempted to introduce the reader to some of the available pharmacoeconomic methodologies used to assess the cost and outcomes of competing drug therapy options, including effective antimicrobial therapy.

REFERENCES

1. Juergens JP, Szeinbach SL, Smith MC. Will future pharmacists understand pharmacoeconomic research? Am J Pharm Educ 1992;56:135–140.
2. Pritchard C. Trends in economic evaluation. Office of Health Economics Briefing, No. 36, April 1998.
3. Vital and Health Statistics Series 13, No. 129.
4. Drummond MF, Stoddart GL, Torrance GW. Methods for the Economic Evaluation of Health Care Programmes. New York: Oxford Univ Press, 1987.
5. Eisenberg JM. Clinical economics: A guide to the economic analysis of clinical practice. JAMA 1989;262:2879–2886.
6. Quenzer RW, Pettit KG, Arnold RJ, Kaniecki DJ. Pharmacoeconomic analysis of selected antibiotics in lower respiratory tract infection. Am J Managed Care 1997; 3:1027–1036.
7. Lee JT, Sanchez LA. Interpretation of ''cost-effective'' and soundness of economic evaluations in the pharmacy literature. Am J Hosp Pharm 1991;48:622–627.
8. Bootman L. Pharmacoeconomics (''The Green Book'').
9. Websters' New Riverside University Dictionary. Boston: Riverside, 1988.
10. Rupp MT, Kreling DH. The impact of pharmaceutical care on patient outcomes: What do we know? Drug Benefit Trends 1997;9(2):35–47.
11. Tse, CS Outcomes measurement across the continuum of care. Med Interface 1997; 10(11):103–107.
12. Kenreigh CA, Wagner LT. Medscape Pharmacists Treatment Update. Hillsboro: Medical Education Collaborative, Inc., June 1999.
13. McDonald RC, Coons SJ. An Introduction to Health Economics. Indianapolis: Eli Lilly, 1993.
14. Greenhalgh T. Papers that tell you what things cost (economic analysis). Br Med J 1997;315;596–599.
15. Jones AJ, Sanchez LA. Pharmacoeconomic evaluation: Applications in managed health care formulary decision making. Drug Benefit Trends 1995;7(9):12,15,19–22,32–34.
16. Morrison GC, Gyldmark M. Appraising the use of contingent valuation. Health Econ 1992;1(4):233–243.
17. Dolan P, Gudex C, Kind P, Williams A. The time trade-off method: Results from a general population study. Health Econ 1996;5(2):141–154.
18. Dean BS, Gallivan S, Barber ND, Van Ackere A. Mathematical modeling of pharmacy systems. Am J Health Syst Pharm 1997;54;2491–2499.
19. Lightwood JM, Glantz SA. Short-term economic and health benefits of smoking cessation: Myocardial infarction and stroke. Circulation 1997;96:1089–1096.
20. Schumacher GE. Multiattribute evaluation in formulary decision making as applied to calcium channel blockers. Am J Hosp Pharmacy 1991;48(2):301–308.

21. McCoy S, Chandramouli J, Mutnick A. Using multiple pharmacoeconomic methods to conduct a cost-effectiveness analysis of histamine H2 receptor antagonists. Am J Health Syst Pharm 1998;55(suppl 4):S8–S12.
22. Summers KH, Hylan TR, Edgell ET. The use of economic models in managed care pharmacy decisions. J Managed Care Pharm 1998;4:42–50.
23. Richerson MA, Ambrose PG, et al. Pharmacoeconomic evaluation of alternative antibiotic regimens in hospitalized patients with community acquired pneumonia. Infect Dis Clin Pract 1998;7:227–233.
24. Commonwealth of Australia Dept of Human Services & Health. Guidelines for the pharmaceutical industry on preparation of submissions to the Pharmaceutical Benefits Advisory Committee including major submissions involving economic analysis. Canberra: Australian Govt Pub Service, 1995.
25. Canadian Coordinating Office for Health Technology. Guideline for Economic Evaluation of Pharmaceuticals: Canada. Ottawa: CCOHTA, 1994.
26. International Society for Pharmaceutical Outcomes Research. Consensus Statement on Pharmacoeconomic Studies. Philadelphia: ISPOR, 2000.
27. Nuijten MJC. The selection of data sources for use in modeling studies. Pharmacoeconomics 1998;13(3):305–315.
28. Else BA, Armstrong EP, Cox ER. Data sources for pharmacoeconomic and health services research. Am J Health-Syst Pharm 1997;54:2601–2608.
29. Brennan A, Akehurst R. Modelling in health economic evaluation. What is its place? What is its value? Pharmacoeconomics 2000;17(5):445–459.

17

Utilizing Pharmacodynamics and Pharmacoeconomics in Clinical and Formulary Decision Making

Paul G. Ambrose
Cognigen Corporation, Buffalo, New York

Annette Zoe-Powers
Bristol-Myers Squibb Company, Plainsboro, New Jersey

René Russo
Rutgers University, Piscataway, New Jersey

David T. Jones
University of California at Davis, Sacramento, California

Robert C. Owens, Jr.
Maine Medical Center, Portland, Maine
and University of Vermont College of Medicine, Burlington, Vermont

1 INTRODUCTION

Managed care organizations (MCOs), community hospitals, and university teaching hospitals are challenged to control total organizational cost while maintaining high quality patient care and services. Most health care institutions have implemented processes, including pharmacy and therapeutics committees (P&Ts) and formularies, in an effort to control drug costs. In essence, a formulary is a list of products that have been reviewed and approved by the Pharmacy and Therapeutics Committee. Moreover, the goal of the P&T and formulary process is to optimize clinical outcomes while controlling or minimizing cost. Despite these efforts, drug and organizational expenditures continue to increase. Because many antibiotic regimens could be considered appropriate for the treatment of a given infectious disease, the challenge is to find the most cost-effective regimens. It should be realized, however, that a low drug cost does not necessarily correlate to a low organizational cost. For instance, although a drug with a high acquisition price compared with standard therapy may increase total drug costs, it may significantly decrease the institutional expenditures in other areas. Unfortunately, few prospective, randomized clinical data are available comparing new therapeutic modalities and standard regimens under usual care conditions.

Consequently, it is crucial to develop methods to treat infections that are both clinically sound and economically effective. The application of pharmacodynamic and pharmacoeconomic concepts to issues involving the use of antimicrobial agents provides a data-driven paradigm to achieve these goals. This approach often identifies the best agent to maximize bacterial killing, the appropriate dose, and the most cost-effective agent to select for formulary inclusion and clinical use. In order to understand the discussion contained in this chapter, a basic understanding of pharmacodynamic theory and pharmacoeconomic concepts is essential. For a complete review of these concepts the reader is encouraged to review Chapters 5, 7, 9, and 16 as they form the basis for the discussion that follows.

In this chapter, pharmacodynamic and pharmacoeconomic principles are used to guide clinical and formulary decisions. Through the use of contemporary antimicrobial agents as real-life illustrations, the reader will become cognizant on how these concepts can be applied to formulary decision making and in the clinical practice of medicine and pharmacy. Moreover, agents from a variety of antimicrobial classes (e.g., cephalosporins, fluoroquinolones, and macrolides) and modes of bacterial killing (time-dependent versus concentration-dependent) will be used as examples. Obviously, the following evaluations are not meant to be complete unto themselves but rather are intended to outline the use of pharmacodynamic and pharmacoeconomic data in the decision-making process.

2 CEFEPIME VERSUS CEFTAZIDIME

2.1 Background

Cefepime and ceftazidime are intravenously administered β-lactam antibiotics that exhibit a broad spectrum of antibacterial activity that includes aerobic gram-positive and gram-negative bacteria. Due to their spectrum of activity, these agents have emerged as standard therapy for a number of serious nosocomial infections such as hospital-acquired pneumonia and the empirical therapy of febrile neutropenia.

2.2 Pharmacokinetics

The pharmacokinetic parameters of cefepime and ceftazidime in adults are presented in Table 1 [1,2]. From these data it is apparent that the two agents are similar pharmacokinetically in terms of volume of distribution, clearance, percent urinary excretion, and protein binding. However, cefepime has an approximately 25% longer serum half-life and a slightly larger area under the serum concentration–time curve (AUC). For this reason, cefepime is dosed on a twice-daily schedule, whereas ceftazidime must be dosed three times daily in those patients with normal or moderately reduced renal function (Cl_{cr} ≥50–60 mL/min). The pharmacokinetics of both agents vary with degree of renal function. Following a 1000 mg dose of cefepime in patients with glomerular filtration rates (GFRs) of less than 60 mL/min, serum half-life and AUC increase from 2.3 to 4.9 h and from 131 to 292 μg · h/mL, respectively [3]. Similarly, following a 1000 mg dose of ceftazidime in patients with GFRs less than 50 mL/min, serum half-life and AUC increase from approximately 1.9 to 4.0 h and 130 to 270 μg · h/mL, respectively [1,4].

2.3 Microbiology

Comparative antimicrobial activities of cefepime and ceftazidime against various pathogens are presented in Table 2 [5]. From these data, it appears that cefepime has lower minimal inhibitory concentration (MIC) values than ceftazidime against most gram-positive aerobes, especially *Streptococcus pneumoniae* and *Staphylococcus aureus*. This is significant because gram-positive aerobes, primarily staphylococci, are a leading cause of serious nosocomial infection. In fact, *S. aureus* is the second most common cause of hospital-acquired pneumonia.

Against aerobic gram-negative microorganisms, including *Pseudomonas aeruginosa*, the microbiological activity of cefepime is similar to that of ceftazidime; however, notable exceptions exist. Unlike ceftazidime, cefepime has been shown to have enhanced stability in the presence of Bush-Jacoby-Mederios group 1 β-lactamases, which when induced, can render all other currently available cephalosporins inactive [6,7]. Not unexpectedly, therefore, cefepime demonstrates significantly lower MICs against isolates such as *Enterobacter* species and *Citrobacter freundii* that elaborate this enzyme. In addition, cefepime exhibits appreciably more activity against *Klebsiella pneumoniae*. These observations carry considerable clinical relevance, because *P. aeruginosa*, *K. pneumoniae*, *Enterobacter* species, and *Citrobacter* species are the first, third, fourth, and fifth most likely pathogens in hospital-acquired pneumonia, respectively. Although it

TABLE 1 Pharmacokinetic Parameters of Cefepime and Ceftazidime Following 1 g Doses[a]

Agent	C_{max} (μg/mL)	Half-life (h)	AUC (h · μg/mL)	V_{ss} (L)	Clearance (mL/min)	% Urinary excretion	% Protein binding
Cefepime	82	2.3	150	18	120	85	20
Ceftazidime	69	1.8	130	18	115	85	10–20

C_{max}, peak serum concentration; AUC, area under the serum concentration–time curve; V_{ss}, volume of distribution at steady state.

TABLE 2 Comparative In Vitro Microbiological Activity of Cefepime and Ceftazidime

Organism (no. tested)	Antimicrobial agent	MIC_{50}	MIC_{90}	Percent susceptible
Gram-positive				
Staphylococcus saprophyticus (16)	Cefepime	2	4	100.0
	Ceftazidime	16	>16	12.5
Streptococcus				
Serogroup A (23)	Cefepime	≤0.12	≤0.12	100.0
	Ceftazidime	≤0.12	≤0.12	100.0
Serogroup B (57)	Cefepime	≤0.12	≤0.12	100.0
	Ceftazidime	0.25	0.5	100.0
Enterococcus species (133)	Cefepime	>16	>16	8.3
	Ceftazidime	>16	>16	1.5
Staphylococcus aureus, Oxacillin-susceptible (632)	Cefepime	2	2	99.2
	Ceftazidime	4	8	94.8
Staphylococcus epidermidis, Oxacillin-susceptible (110)	Cefepime	1	8	91.9
	Ceftazidime	8	16	61.5
Gram-negative				
Citrobacter freundii (75)	Cefepime	≤0.12	1	97.3
	Ceftazidime	0.5	>16	77.3
Enterobacter cloacae (198)	Cefepime	≤0.12	2	100.0
	Ceftazidime	0.25	>16	75.8
Escherichia coli (1354)	Cefepime	≤0.12	≤0.12	99.9
	Ceftazidime	≤0.12	0.25	99.8
Klebsiella pneumoniae (319)	Cefepime	≤0.12	≤0.12	100.0
	Ceftazidime	≤0.12	0.5	98.4
Morganella morganii (52)	Cefepime	≤0.12	≤0.12	100.0
	Ceftazidime	≤0.12	4	100.0
Proteus mirabilis (196)	Cefepime	≤0.12	≤0.12	100.0
	Ceftazidime	≤0.12	≤0.12	100.0
Serratia marcescens (68)	Cefepime	0.25	0.5	98.5
	Ceftazidime	≤0.12	0.5	97.1
Pseudomonas aeruginosa (569)	Cefepime	2	8	90.0
	Ceftazidime	2	16	87.7
Stenotrophomonas maltophilia (51)	Cefepime	>16	>16	19.6
	Ceftazidime	8	>16	54.9

Source: Ref. 5.

is tempting to conclude from in vitro microbiological observations that cefepime is a preferential choice over ceftazidime, the significance, if any, of these observations will become apparent in the pharmacodynamic discussion below.

2.4 Pharmacodynamics

An accurate prediction of clinical outcome requires the use of pharmacodynamic concepts that integrate microbiological and pharmacokinetic data. Cefepime and ceftazidime, like all other β-lactam antimicrobial agents, kill bacteria in a time-dependent fashion. Once the drug concentration exceeds the MIC of the pathogen, killing occurs at a zero-order rate, and increasing drug concentration does not result in a proportionally increased rate of kill. Thus, the goal with β-lactam antimicrobial agents is to maintain their duration or time above the MIC for as long as possible over any one dosing interval. As mentioned in Chapter 5, a reasonable time period for β-lactam antimicrobial agents to exceed the MIC is 40–60% of any single dosing interval [8]. Earlier, comparisons of in vitro activity against several clinically relevant pathogens between cefepime and ceftazidime were made. In the following analysis, we will explore the potential clinical significance of these observations.

Time versus plasma concentration curves of cefepime and ceftazidime are presented in Figs. 1 and 2, respectively. Following a 1000 mg intravenous dose of cefepime every 12 h, serum levels remain above the MIC of most organisms over the entire dosing interval. Against *P. aeruginosa*, however, cefepime serum concentration time above the MIC ($T >$ MIC) is approximately 50% of the dosing interval. Following a 1000 mg intravenous dose of ceftazidime every 8 h, a somewhat different picture emerges. The serum concentration of ceftazidime remains above the MIC over the entire dosing interval for only *E. coli* and *K. pneumoniae*. Against *P. aeruginosa* and *S. aureus*, serum ceftazidime $T >$ MIC is approximately 50%. Moreover, against *C. freundii* and *E. cloacae*, for only 25% of the dosing interval does the ceftazidime serum concentration remain above the MIC.

Based on these observations, one would expect similar clinical outcomes when either agent is used to treat infections involving *E. coli* or *K. pneumoniae*, because both agents maintain drug concentrations over the entire dosing interval. However, against *C. freundii* and *E. cloacae*, it would be predicted that cefepime is the superior agent, because cefepime maintains levels over 100% of the dosing interval compared with 25% for ceftazidime. Indeed, the literature is replete with case reports describing failure of ceftazidime when used to treat serious infections involving these pathogens [9]. In fact, because these organisms can elaborate Bush-Jacoby-Mederios group 1 β-lactamases, third generation cephalosporins are not recommended for infections when these organisms are likely to be involved. On the other hand, cefepime's advantage against *S. aureus* would not be expected to be of clinical relevance, because ceftazidime maintains serum levels above the

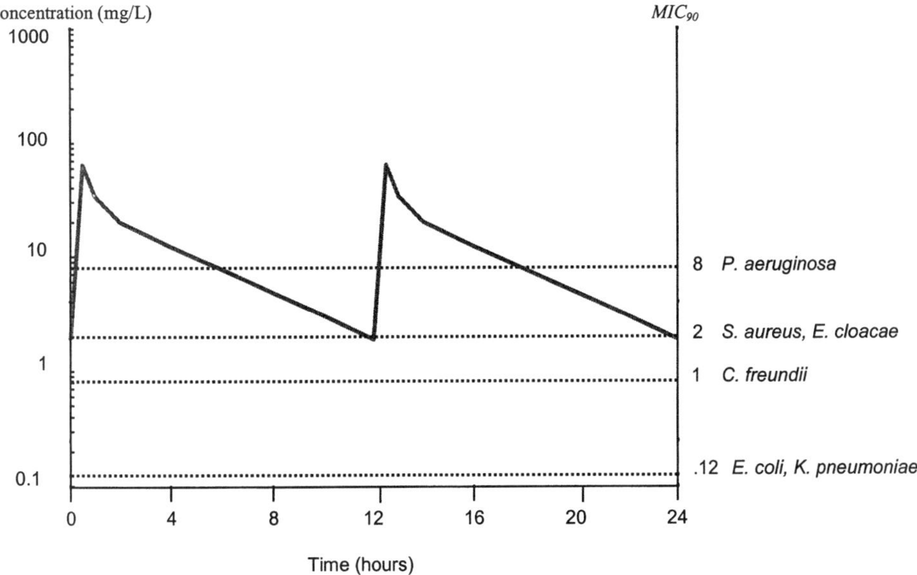

FIGURE 1 Concentration–time profile of cefepime following a 1 g dose every 12 h with MIC values of selected bacteria superimposed.

MIC for approximately 50% of the dosing interval. Moreover, one would predict similar outcomes against *P. aeruginosa* for the same reason [10].

2.5 Pharmacoeconomics

As mentioned earlier, few prospective, randomized clinical data are available comparing new therapeutic modalities and standard regimens under usual care conditions. Naturalistic trials are a study design approach that compares one drug regimen, such as a new drug, with one or more commonly used therapies under usual care conditions. In other words, naturalistic studies compare clinical and other outcome measures of competing therapeutic alternatives based upon how the drugs are actually used in clinical practice rather than in the strict confines of traditional clinical trials. This information is crucial, especially as new products are introduced to the market, because health care providers must make clinical and economic decisions concerning these agents. Two such studies have directly compared cefepime and ceftazidime and are reviewed briefly below.

Ambrose et al. [1] compared the cost effectiveness of cefepime and ceftazidime in intensive care unit patients with hospital-acquired pneumonia. The efficacy, safety, and cost effectiveness of each agent were evaluated in a prospective,

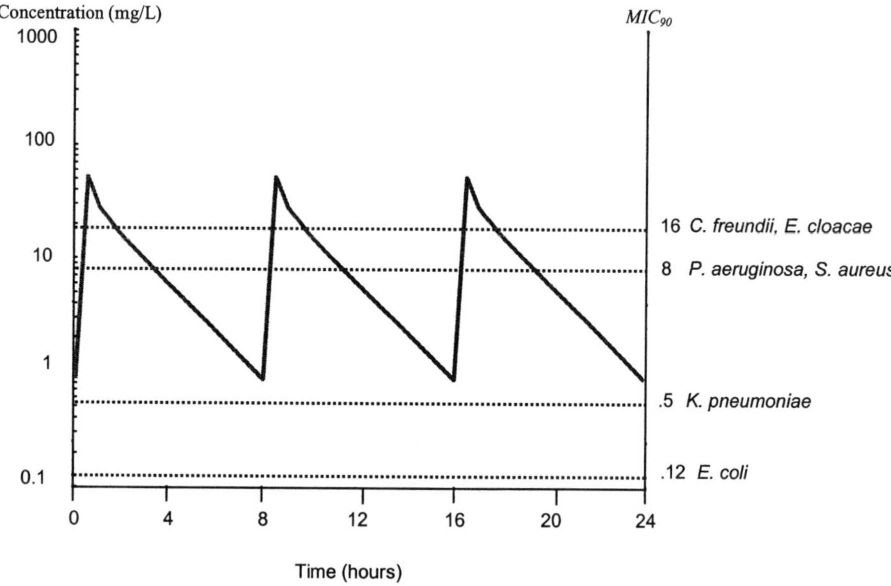

FIGURE 2 Concentration–time profile of ceftazidime following a 1 g dose every 8 h with MIC values of selected bacteria superimposed.

noninterventional, investigator-blinded study involving 100 patients. Clinical success rates were 60% and 78% for patients treated with ceftazidime and cefepime, respectively ($P = 0.05$). Microbiological eradication rates were 55% for ceftazidime and 77% for cefepime ($P = 0.04$). In those patients in whom *P. aeruginosa* were isolated, the organism was eradicated in 70% (14/20) of cefepime patients and 50% (7/14) of ceftazidime patients. Interestingly, the authors noted that the MICs of *P. aeruginosa* and *S. aureus* were higher for ceftazidime than for cefepime at the study institution and that the resultant pharmacodynamic differences may be the reason for their observations. The frequency of concomitant antibiotic use was less in the cefepime group [ceftazidime 74% (37/50), cefepime 44% (22/50); $P = 0.004$], particularly with the use of vancomycin. Cefepime was more cost effective than ceftazidime (ceftazidime $24,528.10, cefepime $19,996.21). Sensitivity analysis of efficacy rates demonstrated that ceftazidime would have to be 50% more effective than cefepime to change the economic outcome. The authors concluded that cefepime was clinically more efficacious and more cost effective than ceftazidime in similar patients with hospital-acquired pneumonia [11].

Owens et al. [12] compared the cost effectiveness of cefepime dosed 1000–2000 mg every 12 h and ceftazidime dosed 1000–2000 mg every 8 h as empirical monotherapy for febrile neutropenia. The efficacy, safety, and cost effectiveness of each agent were evaluated in a prospective, noninterventional, evaluator-blinded study involving 99 patients.

Patients were stratified by risk for infection in accordance with the IDSA, FDA, and HIS guidelines (i.e., cancer type, age, and fever). Clinical assessments were made at 72 h of therapy and at 7 days post-therapy or at discharge from the hospital. Clinical success was defined as apyrexia maintained, clinical signs and symptoms improved, and organism eradicated (when applicable), no relapse or new infection, and survival. Failure was defined as inability to eradicate the pathogen, death due to infection; and discontinuation of study agent because of nonresponse.

Clinical success rates were 80% and 96% for patients treated with ceftazidime and cefepime, respectively ($P = 0.028$). Moreover, the frequency of CDC/IDSA-unsupported vancomycin addition to therapy occurred significantly ($P = 0.001$) less often in the cefepime group (14%) than in the ceftazidime group (46%).

The authors found that cefepime was more cost effective than ceftazidime (ceftazidime $50,128; cefepime $31,407). Sensitivity analysis of efficacy rates demonstrated that cefepime efficacy would have to decrease by 50% to change the economic outcome. The authors also noted that the elimination of ceftazidime from the formulary was associated with a favorable impact on *Enterobacter cloacae* susceptibility in the study units.

2.6 Conclusion

Based upon this pharmacodynamic analysis, it would be predicted that clinical outcomes would be improved if cefepime were chosen over ceftazidime for the treatment of nosocomial infection. This prediction is supported by comparative pharmacoeconomic data obtained from studies naturalistic in design. Therefore, it may be reasonable to select cefepime over ceftazidime for formulary inclusion.

3 CLARITHROMYCIN VERSUS AZITHROMYCIN

3.1 Background

Azithromycin and clarithromycin are two of the most commonly prescribed antibiotics in the United States. Because of their convenient dosing schedule and activity against respiratory tract pathogens, azithromycin and clarithromycin are primarily used to treat infections such as community-acquired pneumonia, sinusitis, and bronchitis.

3.2 Pharmacokinetics

The pharmacokinetics parameters in adults of both macrolides are shown in Table 3. The bioavailability and volume of distribution are similar between the two drugs. However, azithromycin has a markedly longer half-life ($t_{1/2}$) than clarithromycin, 68 h and 3–4 h, respectively [13,14]. As a result, azithromycin can be dosed just once daily for 5 days. Clarithromycin undergoes metabolism through oxidative and hydrolytic pathways that produce several metabolites. Conversely, azithromycin is not highly metabolized, with 75% of the parent compound being excreted unchanged [15]. Because the macrolides rapidly distribute into tissues, resulting in high concentrations within the cells, the serum concentration of macrolides is markedly lower than that of β-lactam antibiotics.

3.3 Microbiology

The microbiological activity of macrolides against various bacteria is shown in Table 4. In vitro studies have shown that both agents are active against *S. pneumoniae* and *M. catarrhalis*. Based solely on MIC data, azithromycin appears to be more active against *H. influenzae* than clarithromycin. However, the combination of clarithromycin and its active metabolite 14-hydroxyclarithromycin has been demonstrated to have additive or even synergistic activity against *H. influenzae* [16].

3.4 Pharmacodynamics

As mentioned earlier, macrolides such as erythromycin and clarithromycin and azilides like azithromycin are generally considered concentration-independent killing agents. As with β-lactam agents, the duration of time that the drug concentration exceeds the MIC of the infecting pathogen at the site of infection is the primary determinant of efficacy for macrolides and azilides [4]. How long the levels of these agents should remain above the MIC remains controversial, as these agents have a prolonged post-antibiotic effect (PAE) with gram-positive cocci and *Haemophilus influenzae* [17,18]. Craig et al. [17] postulated that the PAE allows these drugs to yield maximal efficacy in murine thigh infections when concentrations exceed the MIC for significantly less than 50% of the dosing interval (i.e., 30–35%). Due to an extended PAE and long serum half-life, the proper pharmacodynamic correlate for azithromycin may be the AUC/MIC ratio rather than $T >$ MIC.

Other investigators suggest that the concentration of the drug at the site of infection, specifically where bacteria attach to the mammalian cell, is significantly higher than the concentration in the serum. This is due to macrolides and azilides, especially azithromycin, being highly concentrated inside mammalian cells. As the drug egresses out of the cell, a drug concentration gradient exists that is

TABLE 3 Steady-State Pharmacokinetic Parameters of Azithromycin and Clarithromycin Following 500 mg (Day 1) and 250 mg (Days 2–5) Doses and 500 mg Doses, Respectively[a]

Agent	C_{max} (µg/mL)	Half-life (h)	AUC (h · µg/mL)	V_{ss} (L)	Clearance (mL/min)	% Urinary excretion	% Protein binding
Azithromycin	0.24	68	2.1	2160	630	6.5	7–51
Clarithromycin	2.85	4.8	20.84	191	437	30	42–70

[a] C_{max}, peak serum concentration; AUC, area under the serum concentration–time curve; V_{ss}, volume of distribution at steady state.
[b] Protein binding varies at different concentrations.

TABLE 4 Comparative In Vitro Microbiological Activity of Azithromycin and Clarithromycin

Organism (no. tested)	Antimicrobial agent	MIC_{50}	MIC_{90}
Gram-positive			
Streptococcus pyogenes (105)	Azithromycin	0.03	0.03
	Clarithromycin	0.016	0.016
Staphylococcus aureus, BLA neg (54)	Azithromycin	0.13	0.13
	Clarithromycin	0.06	0.06
Streptococcus pneumoniae, penicillin-susceptible (26)	Azithromycin	0.03	4
	Clarithromycin	0.016	2
Penicillin resistant (15)	Azithromycin	0.5	>16
	Clarithromycin	0.25	>16
Gram-negative			
Haemophilus influenzae (1137)	Azithromycin	2	2
	Clarithromycin	8	16
Moraxella catarrhalis (723)	Azithromycin	0.06	0.06
	Clarithromycin	0.06	0.12

Source: Refs. 40–42.

highest at the mammalian cell surface and lowest in the serum. In this paradigm, the drug concentration in the serum is a poor correlate for that at the site of infection [19].

Azithromycin's long serum half-life (approximately 68 h), which results in low serum concentration over an extended period of time, has raised concern regarding its propensity to select for macrolide-resistant isolates [20]. Leach et al. [21] prospectively studied the impact of community-based azithromycin treatment on carriage and resistance of *Streptococcus pneumoniae*. Single-dose azithromycin (20 mg/kg) was given to children in a remote Aboriginal community in Australia with trachoma and their household contacts who were children. Carriage rates of pneumococci resistant to azithromycin immediately before treatment with azithromycin and 2–3 weeks, 2 months, and 6 months after treatment were 1.9%, 54.5%, 34.5%, and 5.9%, respectively. In this study, the authors concluded that the selective pressure of azithromycin allowed the growth and transmission of pre-existing azithromycin-resistant strains.

Similarly, azithromycin was evaluated in an open clinical, microbiological, and pharmacokinetic study in hospitalized patients with acute exacerbation of chronic bronchitis [22]. Patients received 500 mg on the first day, followed by 250 mg once daily for 4 days. Cultures of *Haemophilus influenzae* during and after treatment showed many infections persisting. Geometric mean MICs of

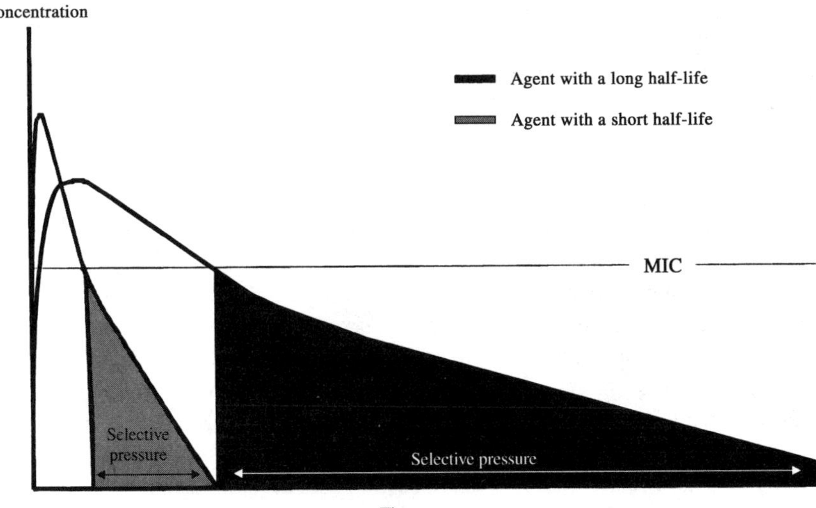

FIGURE 3 Pharmacodynamic concept: Darwin's window of natural selection. Schematic illustration of the serum pharmacokinetic profile of two oral drug regimens over one dosing interval. If the serum concentration–time curves of two drugs, one each with a short or long serum half-life, are compared with an MIC value superimposed, a period or "window" of potential Darwinian selection appears. For the agent with a short half-life, the duration of time between when the drug concentration falls below the MIC and its total elimination from the body is short relative to that of the agent with a much longer half-life.

azithromycin for these organisms rose from 1.23 mg/L pretreatment to 4.87 mg/L a week after the end of treatment.

One explanation for these observations relates to azithromycin's long serum half-life and the duration of time subinhibitory concentrations of drug exist [23]. If the serum concentration–time curves of two drugs, one each with short and long serum half-lives, are compared with an MIC value superimposed, a period or ''window'' of potential Darwinian selection appears (Fig. 3). For the agent with a short half-life, the duration of time between when the drug concentration falls below the MIC and its total elimination from the body is short relative to that of the agent with a much longer half-life. For an agent with a 68 h half-life, such as azithromycin, the drug is not totally eliminated from the body for 5–7 half-lives or 14–20 days after the end of therapy. Therefore, this period of natural selection or ''Darwin's window'' may be the pharmacodynamic explanation for the aforementioned observations.

3.5 Pharmacoeconomics

Health economic models have been used to investigate the cost consequences of different treatment options in community-acquired respiratory tract infections [11,24,25]. Two recent studies evaluated the relationship between cost of care and either first-line antibiotic clinical efficacy or microbiological eradication rate for the treatment of community-acquired pneumonia and acute exacerbation of chronic bronchitis [25,26]. These studies used a Markov model that was populated with health care resource estimates obtained from a panel of physicians (including general practitioners and pulmonology specialists). Cost was determined by multiplying utilized resource items by the price of each item and evaluated from the perspective of the third-party payer.

Use of these models has led to several significant observations. First, the least expensive antibiotic is not necessarily the most cost-effective treatment modality; second, not unexpectedly, treatment failure resulted in the increased utilization of health care resources. These resources included physician office visits, laboratory tests, antibiotics, and hospital admissions. Consequently, clinical efficacy rate was found to be a key cost driver due to the high cost of treatment failure. This was especially true of treatment failures that resulted in hospital admissions.

These observations are supported by a retrospective review of the medical literature since 1990, which investigated the relationship between clinical efficacy and microbiological eradication rates. The review found 12 comparative studies of acute exacerbation of chronic bronchitis in which both clinical and microbiological success rates were reported for 27 treatments involving 15 different antibiotics. A significant correlation ($r = 0.90$) was found between clinical failure rates and microbiological eradication failure rates. Hence, a key cost driver in the treatment of acute exacerbation of chronic bronchitis is the eradication rate of the causative bacterial pathogens by the first-line antibiotic. Failure to eradicate the causative pathogens increases the risk of treatment failure, with its associated additional treatment costs.

In a prospective, randomized comparative study, Weiss [26] evaluated the efficacy and safety of azithromycin, clarithromycin, and erythromycin in the therapy of patients with the clinical diagnosis of acute exacerbation of chronic bronchitis. Although the clinical efficacy rates were higher for azithromycin (80%) and clarithromycin (85%) compared with erythromycin (70%), 40% of the azithromycin group requested and received prescription refills. The financial impact of this observation is not limited to the mere cost of an additional prescription for azithromycin, which is minimal compared to the burden placed on the health care system in the form of additional physician office visits and potential hospitalizations.

3.6 Conclusion

Based upon the foregoing pharmacodynamic analysis, it would be predicted that the use of azithromycin as first-line antibiotic treatment might result in the more rapid selection of resistant strains of respiratory tract pathogens and treatment failure. Moreover, clinical and microbiological failure of first-line therapy remains the key cost driver in patients with community-acquired respiratory tract infections. For these reasons, it may be reasonable to select clarithromycin over azithromycin for formulary inclusion and clinical use.

4 GATIFLOXACIN VERSUS LEVOFLOXACIN

4.1 Background

Fluoroquinolones, such as gatifloxacin and levofloxacin, have become popular choices for the empirical treatment of community-acquired pneumonia, acute exacerbation of chronic bronchitis, and sinusitis. These agents are different from earlier quinolones due to their increased in vitro activity against *Streptococcus pneumoniae*, which is the most common and difficult pathogen associated with community-acquired respiratory tract infection. The increased popularity of gatifloxacin and levofloxacin has paralleled the rising resistance rates among pneumococci and *H. influenzae* to many traditional antimicrobial agents such as the cephalosporins and macrolides.

4.2 Pharmacokinetics

The pharmacokinetic profiles of gatifloxacin and levofloxacin are presented in Table 5. These two agents are similar with regard to volume of distribution, percent urinary excretion, and protein binding. Gatifloxacin demonstrates a slightly longer half-life, whereas levofloxacin has a slightly larger area under the serum concentration–time curve (AUC). Both agents are administered once daily. Both agents are primarily excreted as unchanged drug from the kidney with negligible hepatic metabolism. Both agents' pharmacokinetics vary with renal function, and doses should be decreased accordingly in those patients with renal insufficiency. As with many of the newer generation fluoroquinolones, the oral bioavailabilities of gatifloxacin and levofloxacin are near 100%, making these ideal agents for oral antimicrobial therapy.

4.3 Microbiology

Comparative antimicrobial in vitro activities of gatifloxacin and levofloxacin against various pathogens are presented in Table 6. One of the notable differences

TABLE 5 Pharmacokinetic Parameters of Gatifloxacin and Levofloxacin Following 400 mg and 500 mg Doses, Respectively[a]

Agent	C_{max} (μg/mL)	Half-life (h)	AUC (h · μg/mL)	V_{ss} (L)	Clearance (mL/min)	% Urinary excretion	% Protein binding
Gatifloxacin	4.2	8–10	51.3	140	161	83.5	20
Levofloxacin	8.7	7	72.5	111	99	72.6	30

C_{max}, peak serum concentration; AUC, area under the serum concentration–time curve; V_{ss}, volume of distribution at steady state.

TABLE 6 Comparative In Vitro Microbiological Activity of Gatifloxacin and Levofloxacin

Organism (no. tested)	Antimicrobial agent	MIC_{50}	MIC_{90}
Gram-positive			
Enterococcus faecalis (100)	Gatifloxacin	0.25	2
	Levofloxacin	1	2
Enterococcus faecium (40)	Gatifloxacin	2	4
	Levofloxacin	2	8
Staphylococcus aureus	Gatifloxacin	0.06	0.13
Meth-S (90)	Levofloxacin	0.13	0.25
Meth-R (63)	Gatifloxacin	0.13	16
	Levofloxacin	0.5	16
Staphylococcus epidermidis	Gatifloxacin	0.13	0.25
Meth-S (39)	Levofloxacin	0.5	0.5
Meth-R (26)	Gatifloxacin	0.13	0.25
	Levofloxacin	0.5	1
Streptococcus pneumoniae	Gatifloxacin	0.25	1
Pen-S (30)	Levofloxacin	1	2
Pen-R (15)	Gatifloxacin	0.25	0.5
	Levofloxacin	1	2
Streptococcus pyogenes (47)	Gatifloxacin	0.25	0.5
	Levofloxacin	1	1
Streptococcus agalactiae (38)	Gatifloxacin	0.25	0.5
	Levofloxacin	0.5	1
Gram-negative			
Citrobacter freundii (52)	Gatifloxacin	0.06	1
	Levofloxacin	0.03	0.5
Enterobacter cloacae (63)	Gatifloxacin	0.016	0.06
	Levofloxacin	0.03	0.06
Escherichia coli (30)	Gatifloxacin	0.008	0.016
	Levofloxacin	0.016	0.03
Haemophilus influenzae (46)	Gatifloxacin	0.008	0.016
	Levofloxacin	0.03	0.06
Klebsiella pneumoniae (61)	Gatifloxacin	0.03	0.13
	Levofloxacin	0.03	0.13
Moraxella catarrhalis (11)	Gatifloxacin	0.008	0.16
	Levofloxacin	0.008	0.06
Morganella morganii (41)	Gatifloxacin	0.06	0.25
	Levofloxacin	0.03	0.06
Proteus mirabilis (37)	Gatifloxacin	0.13	0.25
	Levofloxacin	0.03	0.25
Pseudomonas aeruginosa (50)	Gatifloxacin	4	32
	Levofloxacin	2	32
Serratia marcescens (55)	Gatifloxacin	0.25	4
	Levofloxacin	0.25	8
Stenotrophomonas maltophilia (50)	Gatifloxacin	0.25	4
	Levofloxacin	0.25	8

Source: Refs. 43, 44.

in these in vitro data involves the pneumococci. Gatifloxacin exhibits up to four times greater potency than levofloxacin against isolates of *S. pneumoniae*, which, as mentioned earlier, is the most common and most virulent pathogen associated with community-acquired respiratory tract infection. Although it is tempting to conclude from this in vitro microbiological observation that gatifloxacin is a preferential choice over levofloxacin, the clinical relevance, if any, of this observation will become apparent in the following pharmacodynamic discussion.

4.4 Pharmacodynamics

The pharmacodynamic properties of fluoroquinolone antibiotics have been well elucidated. Gatifloxacin and levofloxacin, like all fluoroquinolones, eliminate bacteria most rapidly when their concentrations greatly exceed the MIC of the targeted organism. This type of activity is referred to as concentration-dependent or time-independent killing [27–30]. Although peak/MIC ratios of greater than 10–12:1 correlate with optimal bactericidal activity, the AUC/MIC ratio is the important parameter determining the efficacy of fluoroquinolones.

Data obtained from animal models, in vitro pharmacodynamic studies, and clinical outcome studies indicate that the magnitude of the AUC/MIC ratio can be used to predict response. Forrest et al. [30] demonstrated that an AUC/MIC ratio of 125 was associated with the best bacterial eradication rates in the treatment of infections caused by gram-negative pathogens. For gram-positive bacteria, it appears that the AUC/MIC ratio may be lower. An in vitro model of infection demonstrated that for levofloxacin and ciprofloxacin, an AUC/MIC ratio of approximately 30 was associated with a 4 log kill, while ratios less than 30 were associated with a significantly reduced extent of bacterial killing and in some instances bacterial regrowth [31]. In like fashion, Lister and Sanders [32] reported that for levofloxacin and ciprofloxacin, an AUC/MIC ratio of 32–64 was associated with maximal eradication of *S. pneumoniae* in an in vitro model of infection. These data are supported by data from animal models of infection where survival was associated with an AUC/MIC ratio of 25–30 against pneumococcus [33]. Finally, for gatifloxacin and levofloxacin, bacteriological eradication was associated with an AUC/MIC ratio greater than 33 in patients with community-acquired pneumonia and acute exacerbation of chronic bronchitis [34].

Clinicians often make such interquinolone comparisons based upon AUC/MIC ratios. Typically, this is accomplished by using mean AUC values, usually obtained from normal healthy volunteers, and MIC_{90} values from the literature. When making comparisons in this manner, variability in pharmacokinetic (AUC) and microbiological (MIC) data is not accounted for [35]. Thus, the metrics developed applies only to a minimum number of clinical instances.

Pharmacodynamic modeling using Monte Carlo simulation is one approach that takes into account variability in microbiological and pharmacokinetic data.

Monte Carlo simulation estimates the probability of achieving a pharmacodynamic outcome. This is accomplished by selecting an AUC value from a population of actual patients (in proportion to their probability of occurrence) and pairing it with an MIC value from a clinical isolate (also in proportion to the probability of occurrence). This is done for thousands of iterations, resulting in a probability distribution that reflects the chance that a pharmacodynamic target will be achieved in a patient treated with a given drug.

Ambrose et al. performed such an analysis using gatifloxacin and levofloxacin pharmacokinetic data obtained from adult patients (18 years or older) enrolled in clinical trials conducted at multiple centers [36] and susceptibility data for *S. pneumoniae* from almost 2000 isolates [37]. The gatifloxacin data set included 64 acutely ill patients, all of whom had community-acquired infections; the pharmacokinetic data set for levofloxacin included 172 acutely ill patients, all of whom had community-acquired infections [38]. AUC and MIC probability distributions based on these data were then plotted for both agents, and a 5000-patient Monte Carlo simulation was performed.

Following standard 500 mg doses of levofloxacin, the probability of achieving an AUC/MIC ratio of greater than 30 against *S. pneumoniae* was 80% (Fig. 4). With standard 400 mg doses of gatifloxacin, the probability of achieving

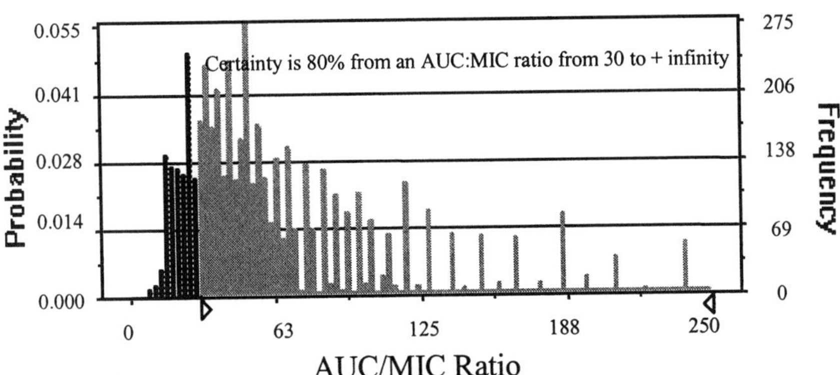

FIGURE 4 Pharmacodynamics of levofloxacin against *Streptococcus pneumoniae*. Results of a 5000 patient Monte Carlo simulation based upon the variability in the pharmacokinetics in the population of patients modeled and the MIC variability observed in a large susceptibility surveillance program. The dark-colored bars represent the number of simulated patients with AUC/MIC ratios less than 30; whereas the light-colored bars represent the number of simulated patients with AUC/MIC ratios of 30 or greater. The probability of attaining an AUC/MIC ratio of at least 30 is approximately 80%.

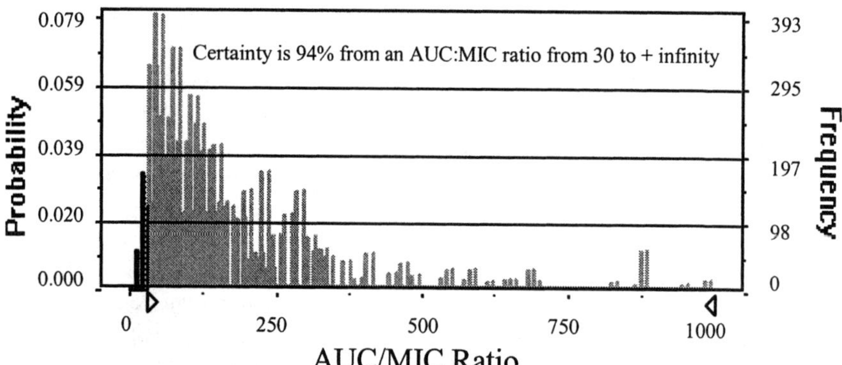

FIGURE 5 Pharmacodynamics of gatifloxacin against *Streptococcus pneumoniae*. Results of a 5000 patient Monte Carlo simulation based upon the variability in the pharmacokinetics in the population of patients modeled and the MIC variability observed in a large susceptibility surveillance program. The dark-colored bars represent the number of simulated patients with AUC/MIC ratios less than 30; whereas the light-colored bars represent the number of simulated patients with AUC/MIC ratios of 30 or greater. The probability of attaining an AUC/MIC ratio of at least 30 is approximately 94%.

an AUC/MIC ratio of greater than 30 for *S. pneumoniae* was 94% (Fig. 5). These data suggest that in treating patients with community-acquired pneumonia due to *S. pneumoniae*, the pharmacodynamic target hit rate is greater for gatifloxacin than for levofloxacin. Interestingly, these pharmacodynamic target hit rates mirrored the bacteriological eradication rates observed in randomized, double-blind, multicenter, phase III clinical trials involving these two agents [39]. Unfortunately, currently there are no comparative pharmacoeconomic data available for these two agents.

4.5 Conclusion

Based upon the foregoing pharmacodynamic analysis, it would be predicted that the use of gatifloxacin would achieve a greater pharmacodynamic target hit rate against pneumococci than levofloxacin. In the era of multidrug-resistant pneumococci, this may result in the less rapid selection of resistant strains if gatifloxacin is used preferentially over levofloxacin. However, more clinical data will be needed to confirm or refute this hypothesis. Nonetheless, due to the aforementioned pharmacodynamic differences between these two agents, it may be reasonable to select gatifloxacin over levofloxacin for the treatment of community-acquired respiratory tract infections.

5 SUMMARY

In this chapter, pharmacodynamic theory and pharmacoeconomic principles were used as a guide for rational decision making. The use of these principles can be applied to any drug or drug class and should be considered an aid in a data-driven decision-making paradigm. Our purpose was not to convince the reader to select one antimicrobial agent over the other in the examples given, but to illustrate how pharmacodynamic and other data can and have been used for decision making.

REFERENCES

1. Product information. Fortaz (Ceftazidime sodium), Glaxo Pharmaceuticals, June 1994.
2. Product information Maxipime (Cefepime hydrochloride), Bristol-Myers Squibb Company, January 1996.
3. Barbhaiya RH, Knopp CA, Forgue ST, Matzke GR, Guay DRP, Pittman KA. Pharmacokinetics of cefepime in subjects with renal insufficiency. Clin Pharmacol Ther 1990;48:268–276.
4. Ambrose PG. Ceftazidime. Antibio Clin 1997;1:44–49.
5. Marshall SA, Aldridge KE, Allen SD, Fuchs PC, Gerlach EH, Jones RN. Comparative antimicrobial activity of piperacillin-tazobactam tested against more than 5000 recent clinical isolates from five medical centers. Diagn Microbiol Infect Dis 1995; 21:153–168.
6. Hiraoka M, Inoue M, Mitsuhashi S. Hydrolytic rate at low drug concentration as a limiting factor in resistance to newer cephalosporins. Rev Infect Dis 1988;10:746–751.
7. Chong Y, Lee K, Kwon OH. In-vitro activities of cefepime against *Enterobacter cloacae, Serratia marcescens, Pseudomonas aeruginosa* and other gram-negative bacilli. J Antimicrob Chemother 1993;32(suppl 3):21–29.
8. Quintiliani R, Nicolau DP, Nightingale CH. Clinical relevance of penicillin-resistant *Streptococcus pneumoniae*. Infect Dis Clin Prac 1996;5:S37–S41.
9. Chow JW, Fine MJ, Shales DM, Quinn JP, Hooper DC, Johnson MP, et al. *Enterobacter* bacteremia: Clinical features and emergence of antibiotic resistance during therapy. Ann Intern Med 1991;115:585–590.
10. Owens RC, Ambrose PG, Quintiliani R. Ceftazidime to cefepime formulary switch: Pharmacodynamic and pharmacoeconomic rationale. Conn Med 1997;225–227.
11. Ambrose PG, Richerson MA, Stanton ME, Bui K, Nicolau DP, Nightingale CH, et al. Cost-effectiveness analysis of cefepime compared with ceftazidime in intensive care unit patients with hospital-acquired pneumonia. Infect Dis Clin Prac 1999;8: 245–251.
12. Owens RC, Owens CA, Holloway WJ. Comparative evaluation of the cefepime Q12 hour dosing interval as empirical therapy for febrile neutropenic patients. Pharmacotherapy 1999;19:496–497.

13. Product information. Zithromax (azithromycin), Pfizer Inc., June 1996.
14. Product information. Biaxin (clarithromycin), Abbott Laboratories, August 1994.
15. Shepard RM, Fouda HG, Johnson RC, et al. Disposition and metabolism of azithromycin in rats, dogs and humans. Int Congr Infect Dis, Montreal, Quebec, July 15–19, 1990, abstr 184.
16. Jorgenson JH, Maher LA, Howell AW. Activity of clarithromycin and its principal human metabolite against Haemophilus influenzae. Antimicrob Agents Chemother 1994;35:1524–1526.
17. Craig WA, Rikardsdottir S, Watanable Y. In vivo and in vitro post-antibiotic effects of azithromycin. Abstracts of the 32nd Interscience Conference on Antimicrobial Agents and Chemotherapy, Anaheim, September 1992.
18. Odenholt-Tornqvist I, Lowdin E, Cars O. Post-antibiotic effects and post-antibiotic sub-MIC effects of roxithromycin, clarithromycin, and azithromycin on respiratory tract pathogens. Antimicrob Agents Chemother 1995;39:221–226.
19. Nightingale CH. This volume, Chapter 9.
20. Jackson MA, Burry VF, Olson LC, Duthie SE. Breakthrough sepsis in macrolide-resistant pneumococcal infection. Pediatr Infect Dis 1996;15:1049–1050.
21. Leach AJ, Shelby-James TM, Mayo M, Gratten M, Laming AC, Currie BJ, Mathews JD. A prospective study of the impact of community-based azithromycin treatment of trachoma on carriage and resistance of Streptococcus pneumonia. Clin Infect Dis 1997;24:356–362.
22. Davies BI, Maesen FPV, Gubbelmans R. Azithromycin (CP-62,993) in acute exacerbations of chronic bronchitis: An open clinical, microbiological and pharmacokinetic study. J Antimicrob Chermother 1988;23:743–751.
23. Guggenbichler JP, Kastner U. Influence of antibiotics on the normal flora. Infect Med 1998;15(suppl A):15–22.
24. van Barlingen H, Volmer T, Lacey LF. The clinical failure rate of first-line antibiotic treatment is the key cost driver in the treatment of patients with severe community-acquired lower respiratory tract infections. Abstracts, 6th Intl Symp on Quinolones, Denver, CO, November 1998.
25. Lacey LF, Volmer T, Harris AM. The microbiological eradication rate of first-line antibiotic treatment is a key cost driver in the treatment of acute exacerbation of chronic bronchitis. Abstracts, 6th Intl Symp on Quinolones, Denver, CO, November 1998.
26. Weiss LR. A clinical study of macrolide therapy in a select patient population. Abstracts, 4th Intl Conf on the Macrolides, Azilides, Streptogramins and Ketolodes, Barcelona, Spain, January 1998.
27. Preston SL, Drusano GL, Berman AL, Fowler CL, Chow AT, Dornseif B, et al. Levofloxacin population pharmacokinetics and creation of a demographic model for prediction of individual drug clearance in patients with serious community-acquired infection. Antimicrob Agents Chemother 1998;42:1098–1104.
28. Drusano GL, Johnson DE, Rogan M, Standford HC. Pharmacodynamics of a fluoroquinolone antimicrobial agent in a neutropenic rat model of *Pseudomonas* sepsis. Antimicrob Agents Chemother 1993;37:483–490.
29. Dudley MN. Pharmacodynamics and pharmacokinetics of antibiotics with special reference to the fluoroquinolones. Am J Med 1991; 91(suppl. 6A):45S–50S.

30. Forrest A, Nix DE, Ballow CH, Schentag JJ. Pharmacodynamics of intravenous ciprofloxacin in seriously ill patients. Antimicrob Agents Chemother 1993;37:1073–1081.
31. Lacy ML, Lu W, Xu X, Nicolau DP, Quintiliani R, Nightingale CH. Pharmacodynamic comparisons of levofloxacin and ciprofloxacin against *Streptococcus pneumoniae* in an in vitro model of infection. Antimicrob Agents Chemother 1999;43: 672–677.
32. Lister PD, Sanders CC. Pharmacodynamics of levofloxacin and ciprofloxacin against *Streptococcus pneumoniae*. J Antimicrob Chemother 1999;43:79–86.
33. Vesga O, Craig WA. Activity of levofloxacin against penicillin-resistant Streptococcus pneumoniae in normal and neutropenic mice. Abstracts, 36th Interscience Conf on Antimicrobial Agents and Chemotherapy, New Orleans, Sept 15–18, 1996.
34. Ambrose PG, Grasela DM. Pharmacodynamics of fluoroquinolones against Streptococcus pneumoniae: Analysis of phase-III clinical trials. Abstracts, 40th Interscience Conf on Antimicrobial Agents and Chemotherapy, Toronto, Sept 17–20, 2000.
35. Ambrose PG, Quintiliani R. Limitations of single-point pharmacodynamic analysis. Pediatr Infect Dis J 2000;19:769.
36. Ambrose PG, Grasela DM. Effect of pharmacokinetic and microbiological variability on the pharmacodynamics of gatifloxacin and levofloxacin against Streptococcus pneumoniae. Abstracts, 39th Interscience Conf on Antimicrobial Agents and Chemotherapy, San Francisco, Sept 26–29, 1999.
37. Jones RN, Pfaller MA, Doern GV, Beach M. Antimicrobial activity of gatifloxacin, a newer 8-methoxy fluoroquinolone, tested against over 23,000 recent clinical isolates from the SENTRY antimicrobial surveillance program. Abstracts, 37th Interscience Conf on Antimicrobial Agents and Chemotherapy, San Diego, Sept 24–27, 1997.
38. Preston SL, Drusano GL, Berman AL, Fowler CL, Chow AT, Dornseif B, et al. Levofloxacin population pharmacokinetics and creation of a demographic model for prediction of individual drug clearance in patients with serious community-acquired infection. Antimicrob Agents Chemother 1998;42:1098–1104.
39. Mayer H, Pierce P, Ambrose PG. Bacteriologic eradication of gram-positive organisms: Gatifloxacin and levofloxacin. Abstracts, Am Thoracic Soc, Chicago, May 5–10, 2000.
40. Fung-Tomc J, Huczko E, Stickle T, Minassian B, Kolek K, Denbleyker K, Bonner D, Kessler R. Antibacterial effects of cefprozil compared with those of 13 oral caphems and 3 macrolides. Antimicrob Agents Chemother 1995;39(2):533–538.
41. Doern GV, Brueggemann AB, Pierce G, Hogan T, Holley HP, Rauch A. Prevalence of antimicrobial resistance among 723 outpatient clinical isolates of Moraxella cattarhalis in the United States in 1994 and 1995. Antimicrob Agents Chemother 1996; 40(12):2884–2886.
42. Doern GV, Brueggeman AB, Pierce G, Holley HP, Rauch A. Antibiotic resistance among clinical isolates of Haemophilus influenzae in the United Sataes in 1994 and 1995. Antimicrob Agents Chemother 1997;41(2):292–297.

43. Bauerfeind A. Comparison of the antibacterial activities of the quinolones BAY 12-8039, gatifloxacin, trovefloxacin, clinafloxacin, levofloxacin and ciprofloxacin. J Antimicrob Therapy 1997;40:639–651.
44. Goldstein EJC, Citron DM, Merriam CV, Tyrell K, Warren Y. Activity of gatifloxacin compared to those of five other quinolones versus aerobic and anaerobic isolates from skin and soft tissue samples of human and animal bite wound infections. Antimicrob Agents Chemother 1999;43(6):1475–1479.

Index

About the Editors

CHARLES H. NIGHTINGALE is Vice President for Research and Director of the Institute for International Healthcare Studies at Hartford Hospital, Connecticut, as well as Research Professor at the University of Connecticut School of Pharmacy, Storrs. The author of over 450 journal articles and 215 published abstracts, Dr. Nightingale is a Fellow of the American College of Clinical Pharmacology and the Infectious Disease Society of America, as well as a member of the American Society for Clinical Pharmacology and Therapeutics, among others. An Editorial Board Member for numerous publications, Dr. Nightingale received the B.S. degree (1961) from Fordham University, Bronx, New York, the M.S. degree (1966) from St. John's University, Jamaica, New York, and the Ph.D. degree (1970) from the State University of New York at Buffalo.

TAKEO MURAKAWA is Supervisor of the Development Division of Fujisawa Pharmaceutical Co., Ltd., Osaka, Japan, and a Lecturer at the Graduate School of Pharmaceutical Sciences at Kyoto University, Japan. The author or coauthor of numerous books and scientific papers, Dr. Murakawa is a member of the American Society for Microbiology, the Japanese Society of Microbiology, and the Japanese Society of Chemotherapy, among others. An Editorial Board Member for the *Asian Journal of Drug Metabolism and Pharmacokinetics*, Dr. Murakawa received the Ph.D. degree (1974) in medical sciences from Toho University, Tokyo, Japan.

PAUL G. AMBROSE is Director of Infectious Diseases, Cognigen Corporation, Buffalo, New York, as well as an Adjunct Faculty Member of Albany College of Pharmacy, New York, and Assistant Clinical Professor of the University of the Pacific School of Pharmacy, Stockton, California. The author or coauthor of over 50 books, book chapters, and journal articles, Dr. Ambrose serves on the Editorial Board of *Antibiotics for Clinicians* and the *Journal of Infectious Disease Pharmacotherapy*. Additionally, Dr. Ambrose is a member of the Infectious Disease Society of America and the Society of Infectious Disease Pharmacists. A member of the Subcommittee on In-Patient Medication Use for the National Committee for Clinical Laboratory Standards, Dr. Ambrose received the Pharm.D. degree from the University of the Pacific, Stockton, California.

ISBN 0-8247-0561-0

90000

9 780824 705619